Bio-Imaging
Principles, Techniques, and Applications

R. Vadivambal
University of Manitoba
Winnipeg, Canada

Digvir S. Jayas
University of Manitoba
Winnipeg, Canada

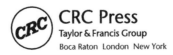

CRC Press
Taylor & Francis Group
Boca Raton London New York

CRC Press is an imprint of the
Taylor & Francis Group, an **informa** business

CRC Press
Taylor & Francis Group
6000 Broken Sound Parkway NW, Suite 300
Boca Raton, FL 33487-2742

First issued in paperback 2018

© 2016 by Taylor & Francis Group, LLC
CRC Press is an imprint of Taylor & Francis Group, an Informa business

No claim to original U.S. Government works

ISBN-13: 978-1-4665-9367-1 (hbk)
ISBN-13: 978-1-138-74963-4 (pbk)

Visit the Taylor & Francis Web site at
http://www.taylorandfrancis.com

and the CRC Press Web site at
http://www.crcpress.com

Dedicated to our spouses:
Mrs. Manju Jayas
Mr. Natarajan Thiagarajan

Contents

Preface

Human beings are blessed with senses to observe objects and make decisions about the type and quality of objects, but their decisions can be affected by fatigue, improper lighting conditions, lack of experience, or a combination of these. On the other hand they are not so blessed when they are inflicted by diseases and require diagnostic tools to detect and identify these diseases. Digital image processing with associated sensing elements operating in the broad range of the electromagnetic spectrum has emerged as a prominent technique in almost every field for making such decisions. Although the imaging technique originated more than a century ago, tremendous growth has been seen in the last two decades, especially with growth in the hardware and software industries providing a significant boost. Imaging is a broad term that encompasses a variety of techniques focused on different types of imaging. Imaging was originally developed for applications in the medical field and remote sensing. As technology grew, the technique has occupied an irreplaceable part in every walk of life.

The term *bio-imaging* refers to imaging of biological materials, which are the basis of the food and agriculture, health, aquaculture, forestry, and environmental industries. New technology originally invented for applications in other industries is gradually adopted by the food and agriculture industry.

Imaging includes various types of techniques from simple imaging in the visible spectrum to other regions of the electromagnetic spectrum such as X-ray, thermal, and hyperspectral imaging. In the food and agriculture industry, automation of various processing operations has occurred to a large extent and automation based on imaging is the latest trend. The idea for this book sprouted when we realized a need to gather together the principles and applications of various imaging techniques in the food and agriculture industry. Some of the imaging techniques are commercially available, whereas others are in the research phase. Research studies on the potential of imaging in food- and agriculture-related applications are published in international journals and many techniques are being further developed to meet the growing demands of the industry. This book provides a collection of various imaging techniques, their working principles, and their applications in the food, agriculture, and some bio-medical sectors.

The first chapter deals with introduction and the need for biological imaging. The second chapter discusses various image acquisition and processing techniques, and the third chapter elaborates on classification techniques. From the fourth chapter onward the discussion is of an imaging technique and its applications based on the food and agriculture industry. A summary of most of the imaging-based research work in the food and agriculture industry is discussed in the applications section of each chapter along with the advantages and limitations of every technique. The concluding chapter summarizes imaging-based automation techniques with the focus on the current trends and the future of imaging in the food and agricultural sector.

Acknowledgments

We sincerely thank the University of Manitoba for providing us with the lab facilities to conduct research and prepare manuscripts. We express our sincere thanks to our colleagues who were encouraging and positive throughout this time. Special thanks to our family members for being so supportive and motivating from the beginning to the end of preparation of this book. When they see the finished product, they will be able to appreciate that we were really working during odd hours and not just browsing the Internet.

Our sincere thanks to David Fausel, project coordinator, and Michael Slaughter, acquiring editor, at CRC Press/Taylor & Francis Group for agreeing to publish our work and guiding us through the process of publication.

A considerable amount of preparation of this book was done during travels by Digvir S. Jayas on Air Canada flights. He sincerely thanks Air Canada, its flight attendants and concierges, in general, but concierges in Winnipeg, namely, Don Boulet, Sarah Hardy, Conrad Hill, Janice Hudson, Glenn Rusnak, and John Ticzon, for their assistance in making his flights very comfortable with the perfect working environment during the flights and in the Maple Leaf lounges. Their pleasant personalities and willingness to accommodate his requests for changes and the best seats are gratefully acknowledged.

Authors

Dr. Digvir S. Jayas, distinguished professor, was educated at the G.B. Pant University of Agriculture and Technology, Pantnagar (India); the University of Manitoba (Canada); and the University of Saskatchewan (Canada). Before assuming the position of vice president (research and international), he held the position of vice president (research) for two years and associate vice president (research) for eight years. Prior to his appointment as associate vice president (research), he was associate dean (research) in the Faculty of Agricultural and Food Sciences, department head of Biosystems Engineering, and interim director of the Richardson Centre for Functional Foods and Nutraceuticals. He is a registered professional engineer and a registered professional agrologist.

Dr. Jayas is the vice president (research and international) at the University of Manitoba, Winnipeg, Canada. He held a Canada Research Chair in stored-grain ecosystems and conducts research related to drying, handling, and storing grains and oilseeds, and digital image processing for grading and processing operations in the agri-food industry. He has authored or coauthored more than 800 technical articles in scientific journals, conference proceedings, book chapters, and conference papers dealing with the issues of storing, drying, handling, and quality monitoring of grains. He has collaborated with researchers in several countries but has had significant impact on development of efficient grain storage, handling, and drying systems in Canada, China, India, Ukraine, and the United States.

Dr. Jayas has received awards from several organizations in recognition of his research and professional contributions. He is the recipient of the 2008 Dr. John M. Bowman Memorial Winnipeg Rh Institute Foundation Award, as well as the 2008 Natural Sciences and Engineering Research Council (NSERC) Brockhouse Canada Prize. In 2009, he was inducted as a Fellow of the Royal Society of Canada. He has received professional awards from the Agriculture Institute of Canada, Applied Zoologists Research Association (India), American Society of Agricultural and Biological Engineers, Association of Professional Engineers and Geoscientists of Manitoba, Canadian Institute of Food Science and Technology, Canadian Academy of Engineering, Canadian Society for Bioengineering, Engineers Canada, Engineering Institute of Canada, Indian Society of Agricultural Engineers, Manitoba Institute of Agrologists, National Academy of Agricultural Sciences (India), National Academy of Sciences (India), Partners-in-Research Sigma Xi, the University of Manitoba, and the University of Saskatchewan.

Dr. Jayas serves on the boards of many organizations including, NSERC, ArcticNet, Composite Innovation Centre, Engineers Canada, ISIS Resource Centre, Genome Prairie, International Centre for Infectious Diseases (ICID), MabNet, Manitoba Institute of Agrologists (MIA), Research Manitoba, Cancer Care Manitoba Projects Grants and Awards Committee, TRIUMF, and TRTech. He is also chair of the board of directors of RESOLVE, a prairie research network on family violence and of the advisory board of the Richardson Centre for Functional Foods and Nutraceuticals, a research center dedicated to the discussion, discovery and development of functional foods. He has served as president of the Agriculture Institute of Canada, Association of Professional Engineers and Geoscientists of Manitoba, Canadian Institute of Food Science and Technology, Canadian Society for Bioengineering, and Manitoba Institute of Agrologists. He is currently the president of Engineers Canada.

Dr. Rajagopal Vadivambal is a post-doctoral fellow at the University of Manitoba, Canada. She holds a doctoral degree in biosystems engineering from the University of Manitoba, Canada, and a bachelor's in agricultural engineering from Tamil Nadu Agriculture University, Coimbatore, India. In her research career, she has published more than fifteen research papers in national and international journals related to grain quality, grain storage issues, microwave drying and disinfestation, and thermal imaging. She has presented research articles at many national and international conferences and has authored chapters in books related to the food and agriculture industry. She has won several awards including the W.E. Muir Award, the Academic Award, and the University of Manitoba Graduate Fellowship for her outstanding performance during her doctoral education. She has also won the Tamil Nadu Agriculture University Merit Scholarship and Tamil Nadu State Council for Science and Technology Award. She is a registered professional engineer and has worked on collaborative projects with researchers from India, Canada, China, and Nigeria.

chapter one

Introduction to bio-imaging

1.1   Introduction

Digital image processing began in the 1960s for space applications and in the early 1970s for medical applications, remote sensing, and astronomy. The growth of image processing technology from the 1960s to the current era was enormous and the application of image processing technology can be seen today in almost every field. Research interest in image processing for the food and agriculture industry began in the late 1970s and a few real-time applications were developed in later years of the 1980s and early 1990s. Researchers understood the potential for image processing in the biological industry and began to focus on conducting research for the possibilities of using image processing in agriculture and food industry. There are various techniques in imaging involving different principles and equipment, including optical, X-ray, thermal imaging, X-ray computed tomography (CT), hyperspectral imaging, and magnetic resonance imaging (MRI). This book describes in detail the present applications of imaging in bio-industries; extensive research that has been conducted using optical, X-ray, X-ray CT, MRI, and thermal imaging for various operations and processes in the food and agriculture industry; and the future potential for imaging applications in the bio-industries.

Food safety has become one of the top priorities around the world and the importance of food safety is well understood by everyone involved in the food supply chain including producers, processors, transporters, retailers, and consumers. Food safety standards are periodically reviewed worldwide with the intention of increasing the standard of food safety and maintaining the quality of agricultural products and processed food materials supplied to the consumers. As safety standards are raised, conservative technologies cannot sustain the needs and hence pave the way for new technologies. Also, incidence of foodborne illness due to deadly bacterial contamination has demanded more strict and advanced technologies. Food safety measures are adopted for all types of food including fresh fruits and vegetables, dairy, processed food, frozen food, bakery and confectionery, and meat products.

Fresh fruits and vegetables are an important part of a healthy diet and there is an increased awareness among consumers on the need for higher consumption of fresh produce. Globally, 1.575 billion tonnes of fruits and vegetables were produced in 2011 (Fruit Logistica, 2012). Global meat production has tripled in the last four decades and increased by 20% in the last decade alone (Worldwatch Institute, 2011). Food production is increasing every year to meet the demands of the growing population and food safety standards are becoming more stringent. The meat industry has strict regulations on quality due to several outbreaks of foodborne illness. *Quality* is a well-rounded term that encompasses nutritional quality, appearance and texture, microbial safety, and noncontamination. In order to meet food safety standards, every product on the supermarket aisle should have undergone vigorous monitoring and testing throughout the supply chain from farm to consumer. Hence, more sophisticated and rapid testing methods are necessary.

Agriculture is the most important industry necessary to feed the world. The agriculture sector has seen tremendous growth and requires constant technology improvements to increase the food production for the growing population. Global grain production reached a record high 2.4 billion tonnes in 2012, an increase of 1% from the previous year. Global grain production has nearly tripled since 1961 and the per capita consumption has increased from 285 kg in 1961 to 350 kg in the last decade (Worldwatch Institute, 2012). To increase production and to meet the ever-increasing demands, conventional technologies are constantly being replaced by emerging technologies. Soil preparation and testing, irrigation, water management, fertilizer/herbicide application, weed management, maturity detection, harvesting, and storage are the major areas in agriculture that require careful monitoring. Applications of biological imaging have been able to provide useful input to improve and develop most of these operations.

Aquaculture is one of the fastest growing industries and the world's fish food supply has grown tremendously. About 148 million tonnes of fish was supplied in 2010 (total value of US \$217.5 billion) through fisheries and aquaculture (FAO, 2012). With an increase in production, increased concern about safety arises and the potential of physical, chemical, and biological hazards needs careful monitoring and testing before the product reaches consumers. On the nutritional perspective, it is also necessary to study and analyze composition such as fat protein content and other nutritional constituents required for labeling.

Increase in the world population has resulted in an increase in demand for food production and supply. With limited resources, such as availability of land and natural resources, only technology can fill the gap between the growing demand and limited supply. Hence, there is a great dependency on technology, which has resulted in adoption of newer technologies in every field. One of the important technologies adopted by the food and agriculture industry in the last couple of decades is imaging technology.

1.1.1   What is bio-imaging?

Biological imaging is a computer vision technology that uses artificial vision rather than human vision to observe, capture, process, and present an object of interest. Biological imaging is the technique of acquiring images of biological materials using a variety of imaging equipment and processing the images using various techniques to acquire information and knowledge that can help achieve the objective. Imaging is a modern technique used in most major industries, including medicine, space, construction, manufacturing, agriculture, food, and animal science. Conventional techniques used in many industries are being replaced by imaging techniques. Imaging techniques and applications have seen rapid growth and tremendous improvement in the past two decades. Although originally developed for medical applications, researchers in the food and agriculture industry have explored the possibilities of using optical, X-ray, X-ray CT, MRI, and infrared thermal imaging. Computer vision technology has been adopted by many industries and the food industry ranks among the top ten users (Gunasekaran, 1996).

Biological imaging is a sophisticated technology and needs a setup of equipment to carry out the imaging. Each kind of imaging requires different equipment, but the basic components in any imaging system are essentially the same. Biological imaging systems are comprised of the following basic components: a camera, illumination, frame grabber, and image processing hardware and software.

A camera is the primary component that captures the image of the biological material or the area of interest. There are a wide variety of sensors used including a charge-coupled device (CCD) camera, X-ray, X-ray CT, ultrasound, and MRI. Of these sensors, a CCD camera is the most commonly used sensor for evaluating external characteristics, such as color, shape, size, and surface texture. For evaluating internal quality characteristics, advanced image acquisition sensors, such as X-ray, X-ray CT, MRI, and ultrasound, are used (Du and Sun, 2004a). Illumination is the lighting source and proper illumination is very important in capturing good quality images. Good lighting increases the clarity of the captured image, which produces better results. A good quality image requires a low level of image processing algorithms and improves the accuracy of the image by enhancing the contrast between the area of interest and the background. When the illumination is poor, even the highest level of image processing techniques will not provide good results. The frame grabber (or digitizer) is a device that aids in the conversion of the analog video signal from the camera into a digital signal that can be stored for further processing. This process of conversion of pictorial images into digital form is called digitization. Image processing hardware performs arithmetic and logical operations, and software enables users to write codes to analyze the captured images. There is a wide variety of each of these components available based on the requirement of the particular imaging application.

Image processing consists of a series of steps that need to be performed to obtain the necessary output. Biological image processing consists of the following basic steps: image acquisition, image preprocessing, enhancement, segmentation, representation and description, and recognition. Image acquisition is the process of acquiring the raw binary data from the image of the area of interest. Preprocessing is the process of reducing the unwanted features in the images. Image enhancement is the technique of making the image clearer and highlighting the area of interest. Image segmentation is the process of dividing or segmenting the image into many parts. Segmentation is followed by representation in which data are represented as a boundary or whole region depending on whether the objective is to focus on the external shape characteristics or the internal features. Image description is the process of obtaining useful quantitative information from the image features. Image recognition is the process of identifying an object based on its description. These are the primary steps involved in image processing and there are a lot of techniques involved in every stage of image processing.

1.1.2   Need for bio-imaging

Quality is the most important word in any industry, particularly in the food and agriculture industry since the output product is directly related to the health and well-being of the population. With increased awareness on quality, the need for accurate and objective quality determination technology has increased. The need for biological imaging became significant as awareness and expectation among consumers increased regarding the safety aspects of food and agricultural products. In the food and agriculture industry, contamination of the product is a major concern and there are various sources of contamination that can happen at different stages of the supply chain.

The various stages involved in food material production from raw material to final product for consumption are shown in Figure 1.1. The figure shows the minimum stages involved in the processing of most of the raw materials; and many more complicated processing stages are involved in many other products. At every stage of the supply chain, there are chances of physical, chemical, or biological contamination that could occur to the product. Physical contamination includes dirt, metal, glass, pins, plastic, bones, or anything other than the desired product. The chemical sources of contamination include pesticides, insecticides, cleaning supplies, or any other chemical product that is not supposed to be present in the product. Biological contamination includes insects, pests, or other mold or fungal infection. Other than these contaminants, the product itself may become spoiled due to undesirable atmospheric conditions such as high or low temperature, moisture, and

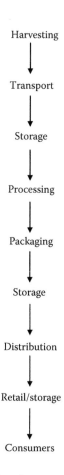

Harvesting

Transport

Storage

Processing

Packaging

Storage

Distribution

Retail/storage

Consumers

Figure 1.1 Stages involved in food production from raw material to final product.

humidity. Hence, raw material, whether grain, fruits, vegetables, meat, nuts, dairy, or any other food material, needs continuous monitoring throughout the supply chain starting from harvesting until it is delivered to consumers for consumption. Incorporating imaging techniques in each of these steps increases the efficiency of the process, ensures quality, and helps to attain higher quality standards, thereby maintaining food safety.

Many of the quality monitoring operations in the food and agricultural industry are performed by human inspection, which is very labor intensive, tedious, inconsistent, and subjective, and sometimes produces less accurate results. For instance, grading of fruits and vegetables based on color, size, maturity, and firmness is performed by manual labor, which is very time consuming and subjective. Other examples of operations dependent on human inspection include: pistachios (Keagy et al., 1996), pecans (Kotwaliwale, 2007), and onions (Tollner et al., 2005) that are damaged, deformed, or off color are manually removed; mangoes receive a physical examination before being fed into the processing line (P. Thomas et al., 1995; Yacob et al., 2005); the manual deboning of poultry (Graves, 2002); and the manual detection and control of physical hazards including metals and bones in the majority of meat and poultry processing plants (Morales, 2002).

There are many disadvantages in manual inspection of quality analysis of agricultural and food materials. Manual inspection may result in fatigue and boredom for employees, which may affect the accuracy of the results. It is labor intensive and may result in low rate of performance compared to automated systems. Manual inspection may raise hygiene issues, especially in meat and poultry processing plants, because there is more possibility of contamination spreading from one person to another or from one piece of meat to another (Chen, 2003). Automated imaging technologies have started to replace some human-dependent quality assessments. Computer vision and image processing techniques are rapid, consistent, and nondestructive, for the internal quality assessment of agricultural commodities and various food products. Due to the high speed of the computer vision system, whole product lines can be tested rather than random sampling of lots as done during manual inspection. Over the last two decades, numerous studies have been conducted on the viability of imaging technology for quality assessment in the food and agricultural industry. The major challenge in using imaging technologies for industry is the heterogeneous nature of the product and the diversity in the shape, size, and color of the food products as compared to other industrial products.

1.1.3   Ease of use and cost effectiveness of bio-imaging

Biological imaging is very quick and objective, and produces consistent results compared to conventional techniques. The most important advantage of imaging in the food and agriculture industry is the noncontact and nondestructive nature of the technology, which results in unaltered samples. Another important application is the detection of internal defects in agricultural and food materials, which is not possible in conventional human-dependent testing. Imaging technology provides repeatability and relatively high plant throughput without affecting the accuracy of the results (Gunasekaran, 1996). Numerous agricultural and food products require vigorous internal quality evaluation before being labeled for consumer consumption. The applications of various imaging techniques, such as X-ray, X-ray CT, MRI, optical, and thermal imaging, in the food and agricultural industry are numerous and provide quality monitoring for various operations.

The most important advantage of X-ray imaging is the nondestructive nature of the technique to capture internal features of the sample, which enables detection of defects. X-ray is more convenient and less costly than MRI in postharvest nondestructive detection methods (Yacob et al., 2005). An X-ray imaging system is unaffected by the temperature of the products and it is safe to be used in the product temperature range of –20°C to 90°C.

Metal detectors are more commonly used in detection of undesired foreign objects in food and are installed in many industries. But of late, the X-ray imaging system has replaced metal detectors due to the ability of X-ray imaging to detect metal or thin products in the range of 0.5 to 0.7 mm and the ability to detect glass contaminants in the range of 1.5 to 3 mm (Labs, 2012). Since X-ray detection is based on the density of the products, it is possible to detect many contaminants in food. Metal detectors cannot be used for products packaged in metalized films, foils, or aluminum trays, whereas X-ray systems can be used for all types of product packaging (Labs, 2012). Not only is X-ray imaging used to detect product contamination, but it can also find missing or broken products, monitor fill levels, estimate product mass, and detect improperly sealed packages. The cost of X-ray imaging is two to three times higher than metal detectors, but in terms of food safety it serves the purpose much better (Astley, 2012; Labs, 2012). When product contamination occurs, food and beverage manufacturers face huge profit loss due to product recalls and related settlement issues. Food and beverage manufacturers save millions of dollars annually by using X-ray inspection units (Scott, 2013). Fat analysis is also critical for food manufacturers in order to inform health-conscious customers, and dual energy X-ray absorptiometry (DEXA) is the most accurate method to analyze fat (Woolford, 2011a).

MRI is a noninvasive technique and requires minimal or no sample preparation. This technique can be used to study both homogeneous and heterogeneous food samples (S. Wang et al., 2011). MRI permits capturing image in any plane through an object (Clark et al., 1997). Water is the major component of most food materials and MRI can be used to study the moisture migration in food materials, which makes it the most valuable technique to study food samples. Cost of MRI is high and requires sophisticated data analysis. There is a lack of MRI equipment designed specifically for the food industry (S. Wang et al., 2011).

Infrared imaging is a noncontact, nondestructive technique that allows on-line testing during production and gives valuable information without impeding productivity and consuming time. Infrared imaging does not need an external source of illumination as required by other imaging techniques. Hence, thermal imaging provides a means for seeing at nighttime or under conditions of poor illumination. Thermography lowers operating costs through periodical inspection of equipment with a thermal camera, thereby preventing costly failure and subsequent shutdown of process lines.

In computer vision, by installing imaging equipment at intermediate points in the production process, defective product could be detected and eliminated or sent back for fixing rather than eliminating it at the end of the process. Imaging technologies could replace human inspectors, which could save in the long term the costs of providing workers with salaries and benefits.

1.2   Current applications

In the food industry, imaging applications are primarily used in internal quality evaluation of fresh fruits and vegetables; detection of insect infestation in grain, vegetables, fruits, and nuts; detection of fungal infestation in grain; and temperature mapping of various food products. In packaged food, imaging is useful for detection of foreign bodies such as wood, nail, glass, metal, or other unwanted substances in the food material. Imaging is also useful for on-line monitoring of sealed food containers for cracks or other contamination. In the meat industry, imaging is used for detection of bone, determination of body composition of animals, and estimation of meat yield.

X-ray imaging systems have replaced many metal detector units in the food processing industry due to their advantages over metal detectors. X-ray imaging systems are installed in many processing plants, including bottling mushroom plants, pie and sausage production plants, and bakery and confectionery units, to inspect and eliminate contaminants such as glass, stone, metal, plastic, and rubber that are as little as 1 mm. In meat processing plants and the fish industry, X-ray imaging is used to detect bones in fish fillets, chicken fillets, and chicken nuggets. X-ray units are also used for identifying contaminants in food products packed in rigid containers such as cans, bottles, and jars.

The integration of X-ray systems and robots have revolutionized the food industry. The X-ray system monitors the internal quality of the product and passes on the information to the robot assigned to the system, which passes on the product for packaging or for further processing depending on the assessment of the X-ray system (Li, 2006). Another application is inspecting the quality of lettuce and removal of the core. Fresh lettuce is monitored for stone and insect damage, and the images provide core position and orientation so that lettuce can be aligned in such a way to enable automatic core removal (Li, 2006).

MRI imaging has found many applications in the food industry. MRI imaging could provide useful information on internal processes such as oil and moisture distribution, crystallization of frozen food, fermentation monitoring in beer and dairy products, and monitoring of the extrusion process. Most of these analyses were previously done using lab testing that required more time and manual testing. But MRI imaging could immediately provide much useful information on product and process control in the production line, which could save lots of time and labor. MRI imaging is useful in postharvest agricultural operations to monitor and provide internal characteristics of fruits and vegetables such as bruising, cracks, and split pits in apples, tomatoes and potatoes.

Thermal imaging is used in the food industry for noncontact temperature measurement of food products. Temperature is a very important parameter and higher or lower temperature of the product decreases the shelf life or spoils the product or sometimes may even result in compromising on the safety of the product due to survival of microorganisms, which makes the product totally unsafe for consumption. Thermal imaging has various applications such as monitoring temperature of various products, monitoring temperatures of ovens, proper filling of frozen meals, and ensuring the proper sealing of multicompartment and microwavable meals (FLIR, 2012).

1.3   Research studies and potential future applications

1.3.1   Agriculture

X-ray imaging could be used for detection of glass contamination in horticultural peat (Ayalew et al., 2004). The application of X-ray CT in agriculture is being explored by researchers to determine airflow resistance of wheat, barley, and flax (Neethirajan et al., 2006a); and for nondestructive measurements of tree rings (Okochi et al., 2007). X-ray CT study of internal structures of hard and soft wheat has revealed that discontinuity of protein in soft wheat resulted in different image patterns for soft and hard wheat (Dogan, 2007).

The potential application of MRI in agriculture was investigated by Posadas et al. (1996) to determine 3D flow within soil samples. Nuclear magnetic resonance (NMR) studies on wood and wood products, such as methods to characterize structure of wood lignin, structural changes that occur during pulping and bleaching process, and the kinetics of the pulping process, are described by Maunu (2002).

Hull thickness is an important quality characteristic of seeds, which affects the dehulling ability, nutritional characteristics, and cooking times. Clements et al. (2004) studied the optical coherence tomography (OCT) technique to measure hull thickness and identify thin-hulled lupin seeds.

1.3.2   Grain

Many research studies are conducted with various imaging techniques on different types of grain to monitor grain quality. Application of X-ray for detection of insect infestation in wheat has been studied by many researchers (Schatzki and Fine, 1988; Keagy and Schatzki, 1991; Karunakaran et al., 2003a,b, 2004a, 2005; Haff and Slaughter, 2004; Fornal et al., 2007). Other studies include classification of vitreousness in wheat (Neethirajan et al., 2006b, 2007a), detection of fungal infection in wheat (Narvankar et al., 2009), and detection of sprout damage in wheat (Neethirajan et al., 2007b).

MRI could be used for measurement of stress cracking in maize (Song and Litchfield, 1990), moisture distribution in maize kernels (Ruan and Litchfield, 1992) and wheat (Song et al., 1998), measurement of change of moisture profile in rice (Takeuchi et al., 1997), and mapping the water distribution in wheat after boiling and steaming for a certain period of time (Stapley et al., 1997). MRI was used to study the structural changes in rice during cooking by monitoring the water distribution (Horigane et al., 1999).

Thermal imaging was used for detection of insect infestation in grain (Manickavasagan et al., 2008a), surface temperature distribution in grain after microwave heating (Manickavasagan et al., 2006), and detection of sprout damage in wheat (Vadivambal et al., 2010a).

Optical coherence tomography, a noninvasive imaging technique, was used to acquire images of internal structures of rice grain to identify waxy and nonwaxy grain (Jiang et al., 2010).

1.3.3   Fruits and vegetables

Research studies are widely conducted for quality monitoring of fresh fruits and vegetables using different imaging techniques. Applications of X-ray imaging for classification of split-pit and normal peaches (Han et al., 1992); detection of bruises and watercore in apples (Schatzki et al., 1997; Kim and Schatzki, 2000); quality determination of pecans (Kotwaliwale et al., 2007), apples, pears, and peaches (Ogawa et al., 2003); detection of defects in onions (Tollner et al., 2005); and detection of insect damage in mangoes (P. Thomas et al., 1995) have been reported.

The potential application of X-ray CT has been studied to detect watercore in apples (Herremans et al., 2012); ripening assessment in mangoes (Barcelon et al., 2000); internal quality evaluation of peaches (Barcelon et al., 1999), apples, breads, and cereals (Herremans et al., 2011); and maturity of green tomatoes (Brecht, 1991). X-ray CT imaging to study ice crystals formed during freezing in food was explored by Mousavi et al. (2007).

For quality determination of fruits and vegetables, MRI could be used for detection of bruises (Zion et al., 1995) and watercore loss in apples (Clark et al., 1998), characterization of pulp of apples and pears (Werz et al., 2010), water mobility during osmotic dehydration of strawberries (Evans et al., 2002), core breakdown in pears (Lammertyn et al., 2003), internal structure and effect of freezing courgettes (Duce et al., 1992), sensory analysis of potatoes (Martens et al., 2002), and measurement of tomato maturity (Zhang and McCarthy, 2012a). Thermal imaging was used in a potato storage facility to optimize the temperature of the facility (Geyer et al., 2004). Thermal imaging can also be used to monitor and assess the surface drying time of citrus fruits (Fito et al., 2004).

Optical imaging using digital or video cameras is possible for grading various fruits such as apples (Nakano, 1997), peaches (Nimesh et al., 1993), strawberries (Liming and Yanchao, 2010), raisins (Omid et al., 2010), mandarins (Blasco et al., 2009); and vegetables such as potatoes (Heinemann et al., 1996), tomatoes (Edan et al., 1997; Jahns et al., 2001), onions (Shahin et al., 2002). Imaging using color cameras to detect defects in apples were studied by Xiao-bo et al. (2010) and Puchalski et al. (2008). In supermarkets, cashiers must identify the correct species and variety of fruit to determine its price, which is a tough task. Rocha et al. (2010) introduced a system for automatic classification of fruits and vegetables in supermarkets based on color, texture, and appearance.

OCT, a nondestructive, high-resolution imaging technique, could be used to determine internal defects such as watery scale, neck rot, or bruises in onions (Meglinski et al., 2010). OCT was used to control and monitor the thickness and homogeneity of the wax layer in apples, which is an essential feature for long-term storage of apples (Leitner et al., 2011).

1.3.4   Other foods

Research studies were conducted on the application of X-ray imaging for internal defect detection in chestnuts (Lü et al., 2010), detection of pinholes in almonds (Kim and Schatzki, 2001), and detection of insect damage in pistachio nuts (Keagy et al., 1996).

The detection of foreign bodies in hazel nuts and quality analysis of individual nuts using thermal imaging was studied by Warmann and Märgner (2005). Presence of unwanted foreign materials such as wooden sticks, stones, metal chips, and cardboard in almonds and raisins were detected using thermal imaging by Ginesu et al. (2004). Application of thermal imaging to detect cherries in chocolate chunks, and leaves, stalks, pedicels, and thorns in a variety of fruits was studied by Meinlschmidt and Märgner (2002). Liu and Dias (2002) explored the potential of thermal imaging as a nondestructive means of identify packaging defects such as cracking, delamination, and voids.

The three-dimensional cellular microstructure of food products such as aerated chocolate, mousse, marshmallows, and muffins was analyzed by Lim and Barigou (2004) using X-ray tomography, which could help the modern food processing industry to understand the microstructure of various food products. X-ray CT could be used for characterizing the microstructural properties of chicken nuggets (Adedeji and Ngadi, 2009), cereal food products (Dalen et al., 2007), French fries (Miri et al., 2006), extruded starches (Babin et al., 2007), corn flakes (Chaunier et al., 2007), bread and biscuits (Falcone et al., 2005; Frisullo et al., 2010a), and chocolate (Frisullo et al., 2010b).

MRI could be used to observe moisture migration in confectionaries (Troutman et al., 2001) and to study rehydration properties of extruded pasta (Hills et al., 1996). In the food industry, determination of various food components is very essential for raw material acceptance, quality assurance, pricing, and labeling of various nutritional contents. The MRI technique is used for determination of various food components such as water and fat content in ground beef, high-fat deboned chicken, and fresh pork (Keeton et al., 2003); fatty acid composition in palm, olive, safflower, and corn oils (Miyake et al., 1998); quantification of glycerol in red wines (Hatzakis et al., 2007); and the deuterium/hydrogen value in maple syrup (Martin, 2001). Laghi et al. (2005) studied the potential of MRI to determine the internal quality of eggs.

Shahin and Symons (2001) developed an on-line classification system for grading of lentils based on color features. Patel et al. (1998) developed a computer vision method using video camera (Sony chip CCD) to detect defects such as blood spots, dirt stains, and cracks in eggs.

1.3.5 Meat

The meat industry requires stringent quality testing and continuous monitoring of the product. X-ray CT was used as an imaging technique to determine: meat yield and carcass composition in live cattle (Nade et al., 2005), genetic improvements in carcass composition in sheep (Karamichou et al., 2007), and the microstructure of processed meat (Frisullo et al., 2009).

The various potential applications of MRI in the meat industry are estimation of poultry breast meat yield (Davenel et al., 2000), measurement of interdiffusion of sodium ions in pork (Guiheneuf et al., 1997), *in vivo* determination of body composition in animals (Baulain, 1997), measurement of the lean meat percentage of pig carcass (Collewet et al., 2005), meat quality determination by muscle characterization (Laurent et al., 2000), fat and muscle distribution in meat (Tingle et al., 1995), and water interaction in meat (Renou et al., 2003).

Costa et al. (2007) explored the potential of thermal imaging to determine the fat content of pork and ham. The pelleting process used in the poultry feed industry was studied and the temperature of the pelleting process was monitored by noncontact thermal imaging methods (Salas-Bringas et al., 2007).

1.3.6   Aquaculture

Fish and fish products are an important source of protein and micronutrients, and play an important role in maintaining good health and a balanced diet for the population. Imaging applications have found a place in aquaculture industry to a great extent. A new method for prediction of fat and pigment concentration in live and slaughtered Atlantic salmon using digital photography, visible and near infrared (NIR) spectroscopy, and X-ray CT has been developed by Folkestad et al. (2008). X-ray CT was used to determine the fat and protein content, and fillet yield of live and anesthetized common carp (species of oily freshwater fish) (Hancz et al., 2003), determination of carcass composition of Atlantic salmon (Rye, 1991), carcass composition of rainbow trout (Gjerde, 1987), and fillet composition (Romvári et al., 2002). In muscle-based food such as fish fillets, interaction between water and macromolecules influence quality characteristics like texture and juiciness. Jørgensen and Jensen (2006) studied the water distribution in fish products in relation to various quality attributes.

MRI was used to study the anatomy and reproductive condition of live Sydney rock oyster (Smith and Reddy, 2012), and the effect of freeze-thawing on cod and mackerel (Nott et al., 1999a). Chanet et al. (2009) studied the anatomy of fresh and alcohol-preserved common carp using MRI techniques and concluded that MRI could be used to examine species even if they are preserved for a very long time (38 years for their specimen). The possibility of using MRI to determine the body growth and gonad development of oysters (*Crassostrea gigas*) and European flat oysters (*Ostrea edulis*) was studied by Hatt et al. (2009) and Davenel et al. (2010), respectively. Pouvreau et al. (2006) investigated the internal morphology and anatomy of pacific oysters using MRI. Davenel et al. (2006) used MRI techniques to determine the sex and characterize gonad development of pacific oysters. The soft tissues of freshwater mussels have been examined by MRI and noteworthy observations were made on the structure, function, and integrity of mussels by Holliman et al. (2008). MRI was used to visualize and study the major organs and muscular-skeletal framework of fresh and frozen-thawed rainbow trout (Nott et al., 1999a).

Production of feed pellets for fish is more complex than any other animal feed. X-ray CT and MRI technologies are used to determine how the various feed ingredients and production parameters, such as grinding, affect the structure and composition of fish feed (Jonkers, 2012). Length measurement of fish is important to grade the fish and also to direct the fish for the proper size filleting and head cutting machines. Strachan (1993) developed a computer vision system for length measurement of fish using a video camera (Sony DXC 325PK) and an image processing algorithm.

1.3.7   Packaged food

A major challenge in development of multicomponent food is the lack of understanding in the moisture migration phenomena. MRI could be used to monitor the moisture distribution in multicomponent food (Ramos-Cabrer et al., 2006), which could help control moisture migration and maintain the textural quality of the multicomponent food system. Moisture migration in cereal-based food using MRI was studied by Weglarz et al. (2008). Altan et al. (2011) monitored the salt uptake and moisture loss in feta cheese during brining using MRI and NMR relaxometry. MRI has been used to measure the internal spatial distribution of temperature during on-line immersion in hot water or after microwave heating, and the results suggested that temperature distribution during microwave heating of baby food is heterogeneous and proper care should be taken when heating baby food in microwaves (Amin et al., 2007). Melado et al. (2011) have studied the texture analysis of cereals to describe the rehydration and milk diffusion processes.

Detecting spoilage in packaged food is a major challenge for the food packaging industry because packaged foods require destructive testing of the sample and time-consuming procedures. MRI could be used to inspect food quality because the main indicator of food spoilage is a lowered pH value. In MRI, changes in pH value directly relate to the changes in free induction decay (FID) and hence the spoiled food could be detected (Haystead, 1999). Pascall et al. (2006) examined the use of MRI for detecting bacterial contamination in soy milk and cheese sauce.

Rehydration properties and crispiness are important parameters of breakfast cereals and OCT was used as a noninvasive technique to monitor the thickness and homogeneity of sugar coatings as well as the pore size distribution of the cereals (Leitner et al., 2011). Foils are used as a major food packaging material and the foils have special properties to avoid light and gases penetrating into the package, thereby protecting the food material inside the foil. Generally foil thickness is measured by a radiographic method that uses hazardous materials and it is not possible to determine thickness of individual layers. Optical coherence tomography, a noncontact and nondestructive method, could be used for on-line analysis and quality control of multilayered foils used in food packaging industry (Hanneschläger et al., 2011).

1.4 Conclusions

Biological imaging has found numerous applications in the agriculture, food, and related bio-industries. In the food industry, X-ray imaging has replaced metal detectors for determination of physical contaminations in a wide variety of products such as fresh vegetables and fruits, processed and packaged food, grain, meat, fish, and dairy products. Thermal imaging has found application in temperature mapping of food and related products to detect spoilage and contamination. There is a lot of research and potential for MRI for determination of moisture migration and water distribution in the food materials and related quality monitoring applications. X-ray CT has the great potential to determine the fat and protein content of aquaculture products and meat, and for assessment of the meat yield of various live and slaughtered poultry and other animals. X-ray CT has provided great visualization into the microstructure of various cellular food products. Although imaging technology has proved to have applications in bio-industries, there is still huge potential to be explored. Many applications are still in the research phase showing prominent results and have few stumbling blocks for commercialization purposes. It is quite evident that in the near future biological imaging will be the most irreplaceable technique in the agriculture and food-related industries.

chapter two

Image acquisition and processing

2.1 Introduction

A black-and-white image is a spatial representation of any scene or an object that can be stated as a 2D function: $f(x, y)$, where x and y represent the spatial coordinates. The gray level denotes the image intensity, which is defined as the amplitude of f at any pair of coordinates (x, y). The gray level interval from minimum to maximum value is called the gray scale, which is represented numerically as 0 and L, where 0 denotes the pure black and L denotes the white color with the intermediate values as shades of gray. A digital image is comprised of a finite number of elements that has a particular value and location, and these elements are named as picture elements or pixels. In an image, the number of pixels is based on the size of the 2D sensor array present in the camera for acquisition of the image.

The history of digital imaging dates to the 1920s with applications in the newspaper industry when pictures were sent through submarine cable. However, the basis for the modern computer dates to the 1940s with the introduction of two concepts: memory to hold a stored program and conditional branching, which are the basic foundations of the central processing unit. The first computers capable of image processing originated in the 1960s and the image processing field began to grow steadily. The application of X-ray imaging in medicine started in the 1950s, and invention of computerized axial tomography (CAT) or computerized tomography (CT) in the 1970s is the most crucial event in medical applications of digital image processing (Gonzalez and Woods, 2002). The original applications of image processing were in space programs and medicine, but later the applications of image processing began to grow widely. In the last couple of decades, many research and development works have been conducted related to image processing applications in the food and agriculture industry. A wide variety of imaging applications have replaced traditional methods for food quality monitoring, classification and grading of food materials, and evaluating the processing methodologies in the agri-food sector. Image processing is a wide subject area and many techniques that depend on the subject material and the requirement of the application are involved. This chapter deals with image acquisition and processing techniques adopted in the food and agriculture industry, and examples of imaging techniques adopted with various food materials will be presented.

The most common image processing applications consist of six major steps: image acquisition, preprocessing, segmentation, image representation and description, object recognition, and classification. Image processing can be classified into three levels of processing: low, intermediate, and high. Low-level processing involves the initial steps in image processing, that is, image acquisition and preprocessing. Intermediate-level processing includes the next level of processing, that is, segmentation of the image and image representation and description. The high level of image processing is the latter stage in processing, that is, image recognition and interpretation of images with the help of statistical classifiers or artificial neural networks (ANNs) (Brosnan and Sun, 2004).

2.2   *Image acquisition*

Image acquisition is the preliminary step of any image processing application. Image acquisition consists of acquiring the image of an object or scene of interest using different types of sensors. Image acquisition can be performed by a single sensor, sensor strips, and sensor arrays. The most common single sensor is the photodiode, which is made of silicon materials, and its output voltage waveform is directly proportional to the light. The sensor strip, which consists of an in-line arrangement of sensors, provides imaging element in one direction and motion perpendicular to sensor strip results in imaging in the other direction. Sensor arrays are arranged in the form of 2D arrays and the typical sensor of a 2D array is the charge-coupled device (CCD) array found in digital cameras (Gonzalez and Woods, 2002). Image acquisitions using other systems such as X-ray, thermal camera, and hyperspectral camera, are performed based on the requirements of the application.

With the numerous ways to acquire images, digital images need to be generated from the sensed data. The continuous sensed data can be converted into a digital image by two processes, namely, sampling and quantization. Sampling is the process of digitizing the coordinate values of an image, whereas quantization is the process of digitizing the amplitude values of an image. The process of sampling and quantization results in a matrix consisting of real numbers. If an image $f(x, y)$ is sampled and the resulting image has A rows and B columns, then coordinate value (x, y) becomes discrete. At the origin, the coordinate value of (x, y) is $(0, 0)$, and along the first row the next coordinate value is represented as $(0, 1)$. The digital image A × B could be written as follows. The equation represents a digital image. Every element in the matrix is called the picture element or pixel (Gonzalez and Woods, 2002).

$$F(x,y) = \begin{bmatrix} f(0,0) & f(0,1) & f(0,2)... & f(0,\text{B-1}) \\ f(1,0) & f(1,1) & f(1,2)... & f(1,\text{B-1}) \\ ... & ... & ... & ... \\ f(\text{A-1},0) & f(\text{A-1},1) & f(\text{A-1},2)... & f(\text{A-1},\text{B-1}) \end{bmatrix}$$

2.2.1   *Illumination*

Illumination is a crucial component of any image acquisition process and the quality of an acquired image can be significantly influenced by the illumination source and conditions. It is less expensive to identify and propose the best possible light source than to apply complex image processing algorithms to improve low-quality images. The performance of an image processing system is directly affected by illumination and to obtain the best possible results, the objects should be illuminated such that object surfaces are very clear (Yi et al., 1995). The various lighting techniques for machine vision and the common issues associated with machine vision lighting are elaborated by Mersch (1987). Using computer-aided design (CAD), Cowan (1991) developed a procedure to determine the location of the camera and sensor to acquire high-quality images. Yi et al. (1995) developed an optimal positioning for the sensor and light source using optimization approach. Kopparapu (2006) proposed a procedure to achieve uniform illumination of an object or scene being imaged with different light sources and stated that an external light source is essential to maintain uniform illumination. The simulation results showed that the suggested methodology was suitable for uniform illumination of the scene or an object.

Proper lighting is very important and fundamental for acquiring good quality images in machine vision applications. Although illumination is a critical factor, there are not well-established rules for selecting proper illumination. To acquire an image of an object, light must originate from a source, and reflect from the object what needs to be collected by the lens to form an image. In any application involving image processing, controlled illumination should be provided to minimize distractions in the image.

The various factors affecting illumination are the angle of illumination, quality of light, wavelength of light, lighting control, and surface conditions of the object (Global Innovative Technology Company Ltd., 2011). The lighting techniques can be categorized into three types: front lighting, back lighting, and structured lighting. In front lighting, the light originates from the same side the camera is located, whereas in backlighting the light originates from behind the object (Figure 2.1). In bright field illumination, most of the directly reflected light is captured by the sensor and hence the lighting direction is perpendicular to the surface of the object and the surface appears bright. In dark field illumination, the light is reflected away from the camera and the angle of incident light rays to the surface of the object is large. Hence, in dark field illumination, the surface appears dark, but the features such as scratches on the surface of the object appear bright in the image (Pernkopf and O'Leary, 2003). The major uses of backlighting are for viewing translucent objects or for silhouetting opaque objects. The structured lighting is the technique of projecting a light pattern on the surface of object at a known angle to acquire the dimensional information (Figure 2.2). The structured lighting is advantageous in assembly lines for the implementation of process control and helps in decreasing process variation, increasing precision and thereby reducing the overall cost (Coherent, 2011).

The major light sources for machine vision applications are fluorescent, light-emitting diodes (LEDs), quartz halogen lamps (fiber optics), metal halide, strobe light (Xenon), and high presssure sodium lights (Martin, 2007). Of these, fluorescent, LEDs, and quartz halogen lamps are used in small- to medium-scale applications, whereas others are used in typically large-scale areas, which require a very bright source of illumination. The major advantages of LEDs are higher life expectancy, ability to form many configurations within the same array, higher stability, and the ability to strobe at high power and speed. The main disadvantage is that large arrays are required to light larger areas and some features are difficult to see with a single color source. Quartz halogen (fiber optic) lamps have greater intensity and are available in

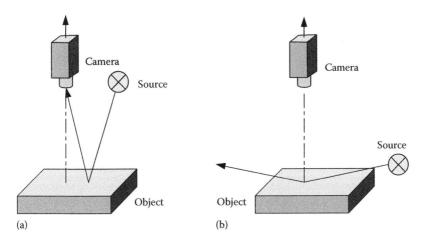

Figure 2.1 Lighting techniques for image acquisition. (a) Bright field, illumination; (b) dark field, illumination. (From Pernkopf, F., and P. O'Leary, *NDT&E International*, 36, 609, 2003. With permission.)

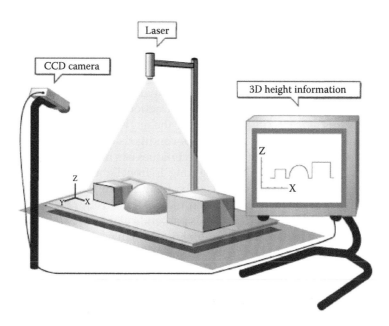

Figure 2.2 Structured lighting. (From Coherent, 2011, What is Structured Light, http://www.coherent
.com/products/?1826/What-is-Structured-Light#; accessed October 1, 2013. With permission.)

many configurations, but the drawback is that they have low efficiency especially for blue light.
Fluorescent lights function at various spectral ranges, have long life, and are efficient, however
the disadvantages are that intensity control is not available in some lamps and there is availability of the limited range of configurations (Martin, 2007; Melles Griot, 2013).

2.2.2   Image acquisition using different types of sensors

There are basically three types of sensor arrangement to capture digital images: single
sensor, sensor strips, and sensor array. The most common single sensor is the photodiode,
which is made of silicon materials and the voltage output is proportional to the light.

To bring down the cost and lower the complexity, digital cameras are manufactured
with single sensors incorporated with a color filter array (CFA) to acquire the three primary colors (red, green, blue) at the same time instead of three separate sensors (Figure 2.3)
(Lukac et al., 2006). With a single sensor, two-dimensional images can be generated by relative motion in the x and y direction between the sensor and the area to be imaged.

A linear arrangement of sensors forms a sensor strip, which has imaging elements in
one direction and perpendicular motion to the strip results in imaging in the other direction. This type of sensor arrangement could be seen in flatbed scanners. Sensor strips
mounted in circular or ring configurations are used in medical imaging such as X-ray CT.
Sensors arranged in two-dimensional arrays are most commonly used in digital cameras
and light sensing instruments. The sensor arrays may be either a CCD or complementary
metal-oxide semiconductor (CMOS) (Gonzalez and Woods, 2002).

2.2.2.1   Image acquisition using X-ray

X-ray image acquisition is performed by positioning the object between the X-ray source
and detector, which provides a two-dimensional projection of a three-dimensional object.

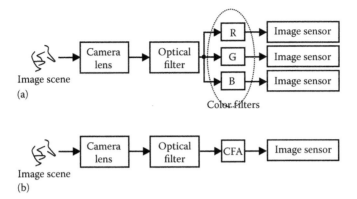

Figure 2.3 Image acquisition using (a) three sensors and (b) a single sensor. (From Lukac, R. et al., *Signal Processing*, 86, 1559, 2006. With permission.)

Conventional X-ray imaging is based on film radiographs, whereas modern imaging consists of digital detectors that capture the X-ray intensity through direct electronic means and produce high-quality digital images. The speed of image acquisition is higher in digital radiography compared with traditional methods and also provides much greater flexibility in storing and processing digital images. A schematic representation of image acquisition of X-ray radiography is shown in Figure 2.4.

Detectors or sensors for X-ray imaging include many types: imaging plates (IP), single crystal detectors, and compound detectors. Of the single crystal detectors, there are many types such as silicon (Si) photodiodes, silicon avalanche photodiodes (APD), CCD, CMOS, and flat panel image sensors (Hamamatus, 2013). The important properties of X-ray detectors are field coverage, sensitivity, quantum efficiency, geometrical characteristics, noise characteristics, uniformity, acquisition speed, dynamic range, frame rate, and cost (Yaffe and Rowlands, 1997). Izumi et al. (2001) developed and tested a flat panel X-ray sensor, which is a combination of X-ray detection material and thin film transistor (TFT) array. These flat panel X-ray image sensors are of two types: indirect and direct conversion. In the sensors based on indirect conversion, X-ray information is first converted to visible light using scintillators and then photodiodes convert the visible light into electric signal.

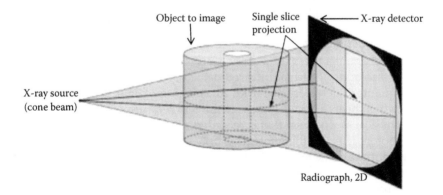

Figure 2.4 Schematic of image acquisition of X-ray radiography. (From Heindel, T.J. et al., *Flow Measurement and Instrumentation*, 19, 67, 2008. With permission.)

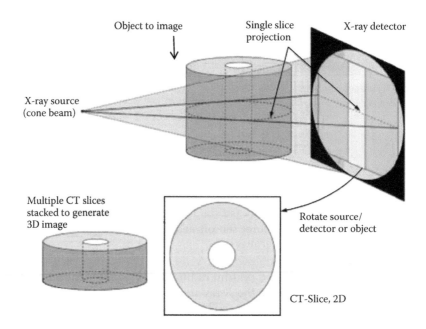

Figure 2.5 Schematic of image acquisition of X-ray computed tomography radiography. (From Heindel, T.J. et al., *Flow Measurement and Instrumentation*, 19, 67, 2008. With permission.)

In direct conversion sensors, X-ray information is directly converted to electrical signals. The advantages of flat panel X-ray sensors over conventional sensors are improved image quality, electronic filing, and networking.

In X-ray CT image acquisition, the object is illuminated by the X-ray source, and the X-ray intensity that is transmitted is projected to an imaging device. Projections are collected from hundreds of orientations and are then reconstructed to produce cross-sectional images of the object (Figure 2.5). A two-dimensional detector array is used to receive multiple slices and every slice represents one horizontal row of pixels (Heindel et al., 2008). The image acquisition and formation in X-ray CT consist of three stages: the scanning phase, which produces data but not an image; the reconstruction stage, which processes the data acquired and forms a digital image; and the third stage, which is the formation of a visible image produced by the digital-to-analog conversion process (Sprawls, 1995).

2.2.2.2 Thermal imaging detectors

The critical component of a thermal imaging unit is the detector that determines the thermal and spatial resolution. Thermal infrared detectors are of two types: thermal detector, and photon or quantum detector (Rogalski, 2012). Thermal detectors depend on the infrared radiation, which heats up and increases the temperature of the detector, which triggers a certain physical mechanism that is recorded as a measure of radiation falling on the element. In a photon detector, the interaction between the incident radiation and detector material occurs at the atomic level to produce a voltage across the detector or a change in the electrical resistance. This mechanism involves a photon absorption by an electron and hence shifting from one quantum energy level to the next level. Cadmium mercury telluride (CMT), platinum silicide (PtSi), indium antimonide (InSb), and quantum well devices are the various types of photon detectors. Other materials, which are used as detectors with limited applications, are indium arsenide, lead sulfide, and lead tin telluride. The most commonly used thermal detectors are pyrovidicon, resistive bolometer arrays, ferroelectric/pyroelectric arrays, and bimetallic cantilever arrays (Thomas, 2009).

Thermal imaging cameras can be classified into cameras with cooled detectors and uncooled detectors. A cooled infrared detector is placed in a vacuum-sealed cryogenic container and is very sensitive to small temperature differences. Cooled thermal detectors have very low thermal noise, that is, the infrared radiation comes from sources other than the object of interest, and are effective in detecting small temperature differences even from a long distance. Since the cryogenic cooling contains mechanical devices with moving parts, they require maintenance periodically. Also, the cooling detector owing to its cryogenic cooling has increased size, and is complex and expensive. Mercury cadmium telluride (HgCdTe) and indium antimonide (InSb) are commonly used cooled detectors. The uncooled detectors are commercially used in many applications because of their compact size, reduction in complexity, and are economic compared to other detectors. The microbolometer is the most common form of uncooled detector and is based on the principle of microelectromechanical (MEMS) technology. When a detector material absorbs infrared radiation ranging from 7 to 13 μm, the detector temperature increases, and a change in the electrical resistance is observed. The change in electrical resistance is processed to create a thermal image. Amorphous silicon (a-Si) and vanadium oxide (Vox) are commonly used microbolometer detector materials (Sofradir EC Inc., 2013). Piotrowski and Rogalski (2004) suggested ways to increase the performance of detectors without cooling by decreasing the volume of the semiconductor thereby reducing the amount of thermal generation without reducing the quantum efficiency, field of view, and optical area of the detector. The new detector materials that show the capability to provide uncooled detection are indium arsenide antimonide (InAsSb), indium thallium antimonide (InTlSb), and indium antimonide bismuth (InSbBi).

2.2.2.3   MRI

In image acquisition using MRI, the person or object to be imaged is placed on a gantry inside a scanner, which forms a large magnetic field around the person or object (Figure 2.6). Radio frequency waves are then used to excite the nuclei of water molecules using an external coil, which are re-emitted by the patient/object. The re-emitted radio frequency waves are detected using an external coil, which are then digitized and processed using a computer (Sprawls, 2000a). The MRI system basically comprises of a scanner; a superconducting coil, which generates a static magnetic field; and a RF (radio frequency) coil, which transmits the radio-frequency excitation to the object to be imaged, and a radio frequency reception coil. MRI scanners can generate images with very high resolution. The magnetic field of commercial MRI scanners ranges from 0.2 to 0.5 T, whereas for the MRI scanners used for medical imaging range is from 1.5 to 3 T.

2.3   Image preprocessing

Image preprocessing is a preparatory step that involves the enhancement of the quality of the image. The acquired image often contains noise and distortion, which degrades

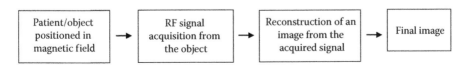

Figure 2.6 Basic flow chart of magnetic resonance imaging process.

the quality of the image. Preprocessing typically consists of enhancing the contrast, noise removal, and isolating the regions of interest. Image preprocessing techniques could be categorized into three types: image compression, which reduces the extent of computer memory required; image enhancement, which modifies the contrast and brightness of an image; and image restoration to suppress and undo defects that reduce an image quality and reconstruct an image from a noisy background (Nasir et al., 2012). Preprocessing involves either one or more of the following steps: noise reduction, gray level correction, geometrical correction, and defocussing correction (Gunasekaran, 1996). Vidal and Amigo (2012) developed a set of preprocessing techniques especially for hyperspectral images, although these techniques could be used for different types of images. There is no correct logical order to perform preprocessing techniques because it highly depends on the quality of the acquired image, the difficulty of the acquired data, availability of methods, and priority in the acquisition of data (Vidal and Amigo, 2012).

According to the size of the pixel neighborhood, image preprocessing can be classified into four groups: pixel brightness transformation, geometric transformation, local preprocessing, and image restoration. In pixel brightness transformation, the brightness of pixels is modified depending on the properties of the pixels. There are two ways of brightness correction: position dependent and gray-scale transformation. The position dependent brightness correction is based on the original brightness and the position of pixels in the image, whereas gray-scale transformation alters the brightness without considering the position of the pixels in the image. The brightness transformation could be denoted by

$$B' = T(B)$$

where B' and B represents the brightness transform from a scale of B to B'.

Geometric transformation aids in the removal of geometric distortion that occurs during the image acquisition process. A geometric transform could be defined as a vector function that maps the pixel (x, y) to a new position (x^I, y^I) (Kumar et al., 2005) (Figure 2.7).

A geometric transformation is an image preprocessing operation that defines the spatial relationship between the various points in an image and helps in the manipulation of spatial layout, that is, the size and shape of an image. Geometric transformation comprises three components: spatial transformation, resampling, and anti-aliasing. Geometric transformation is based on the idea of mapping one coordinate system into another that could be defined by spatial transformation and is a mapping function establishing a spatial correspondence on all points between the output and input images. It is essential to perform spatial transformation to

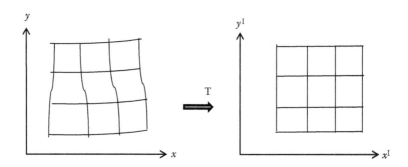

Figure 2.7 Geometric transformation.

align images that were acquired with different sensors at different times, to correct the images for lens distortion, and to correct the camera orientation effects (Wolberg, 1988).

When an image is subjected to geometric transformation, some or most of the pixels in the source image are relocated from the actual spatial coordinates to a different position in the output image. When the relocated pixels fall in between the center of the pixel location instead of directly mapping onto a pixel location, the pixel value is estimated by sampling the neighboring pixels' values, which is termed *resampling*. This resampling is also termed *interpolation*, and it affects the output image quality (Research Computing, 2005).

Anti-aliasing. Point sampling is an ideal sampling method in which the value of every sampling point is acquired independently of its neighbors, which means each input point could influence only one output point. But in point sampling, the intervals between the samples are disposed and the information is lost. The data lost could be recovered by interpolation or reconstruction, only if the input signal varies smoothly, but if the intervals are complex, the lost data could not be recovered by interpolation and the input signal is referred as undersampled and an attempt to reconstruct results in a condition called aliasing. Aliasing is most evident when spatial mapping produces large-scale changes such as magnification or minimization. In magnification, the output contains at least as much information as the input. But in minimization, clear loss of data occurs, which requires appropriate filtering to integrate properly all the information mapping to the pixel. The filtering used to counter the aliasing is referred as anti-aliasing (Wolberg, 1988).

2.3.1 Local preprocessing

Preprocessing techniques result in a new brightness value for the output image by employing a neighborhood of pixels from an input image. This operation is termed *filtration*. Based on the goal of processing, preprocessing operations can be classified into two groups: smoothing and gradient operators. Smoothing is the process of suppressing the noise and any other fluctuations present in the image. The disadvantage of smoothing is that it blurs the sharp edges, which contain valuable information about the image. The objective of gradient operators is to identify locations in the image where the image functions are subjected to rapid changes. Gradient operators act as high pass filters and suppress the low frequency in frequency domain.

2.3.2 Image restoration

The basic purpose of image restoration is to suppress or undo the defect that decreases the image quality and reconstruct an uncorrupted image from a noisy or blurred image. The quality of the image may be degraded due to defects in the optical lens, motion between the camera and object, nonlinearity in optical sensors, improper focus, or atmospheric factors, which may affect the images obtained from remote sensing. Image restoration is the process to reconstruct or recover a degraded image with the use of prior knowledge of the degradation process. A simple version of image restoration process is (Humbe et al., 2011)

$$y(i, j) = D[f(i, j)] + n(i, j)$$

where $y(i, j)$ is the degraded image, $f(i, j)$ is the original image, D denotes the degradation process, and $n(i, j)$ is the external noise.

Image restoration techniques perform an operation that is inverse of the imperfections that appear on the image. Blur identification is performed to estimate the attributes of the imperfect imaging system from the blurred image. The blur identification and image restoration together is often termed as blind image deconvolution (Khare and Nagwanshi, 2011).

Image restoration techniques can be classified into two types based on the knowledge of point spread function (PSF) that explains the response of imaging system to point input and analogous to impulse response. The two techniques are blind image restoration and non-blind image restoration. Blind image restoration is a technique in which reconstruction of the original image from the degraded image is performed even with very little or no knowledge of point spread function. Blind image deconvolution (BID) algorithm is an example for blind image restoration. Non-blind restoration is a technique where original images are reconstructed from degraded images with the knowledge of how the image was degraded. Deconvolution using a Wiener filter (DWF), deconvolution using a regularized filter (DRF), and deconvolution using the Lucy–Richardson algorithm (DLR) are examples of non-blind restoration algorithms (Kaur and Chopra, 2012).

In the blind image deconvolution technique, an estimate of PSF is made and using that estimate the image is deblurred. This technique could be performed either iteratively or non-iteratively. By using the iterative approach, each iteration improves the PSF estimation, and by using the calculated PSF the resultant image can be improved. Wiener filtering performs the deconvolution using inverse filtering (high pass filter) and a compression operation (low pass filter) to remove the noise. When limited information is available about the additive noise and constraints like smoothness are applied on image, regularized filtering is applied. It is an approximation of Wiener filter and provides results close to that of Wiener filtering. The Lucy–Richardson algorithm is an iterative technique and requires a good understanding of the degradation process. PSF is known but with little or no information on noise. Kaur and Chopra (2012) performed an analysis of various image restoration techniques on different image formats and compared the various techniques based on metrics like peak signal-to-noise ratio (PSNR), root mean square error (RMSE), and mean square error (MSE). Figure 2.8 shows a portable network graphics (.png) input image of an onion and the images obtained by various restoration techniques.

2.3.3   Noise

The major sources of noise that occur in an image arise during the process of image acquisition or transmission. There are various factors that affect the performance of sensors. For instance, environmental conditions such as lighting, temperature, and other external factors during image acquisition, and the quality and suitability of the sensor element also affect the quality of the image and result in the presence of noise in an image. The various types of noise that occur are Gaussian noise, Rayleigh noise, uniform noise, exponential noise, and salt and pepper noise. There are various filters such as mean filters (arithmetic, geometric, and harmonic mean filter), order-statistics filters (median, maximum and minimum, and midpoint filter), and adaptive filters (Gonzalez and Woods, 2002). Humbe et al. (2011) applied the various image restoration techniques for images acquired through remote sensing of an agricultural field. Various types of filters such as median filters, spatial filters, Wiener filters, and wavelet filters were applied for the images of agricultural field data. They provided a comparison between restoration techniques and provided guidelines for choosing restoration techniques for agricultural applications. Spatial filtering techniques detect and sharpen boundary discontinuities by exploring the distribution of pixels of varying brightness.

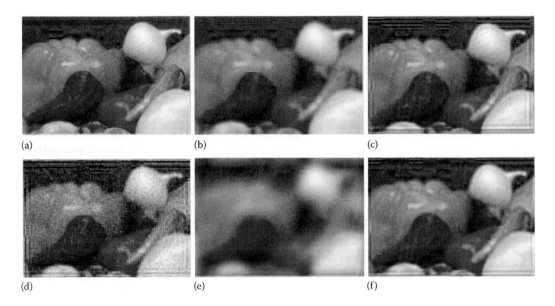

(a)   (b)   (c)

(d)   (e)   (f)

Figure 2.8 Restoration techniques. (a) Original image, (b) blurred image, (c) image restored using BID, (d) image restored using DWF, (e) image restored using DRF, and (f) image restored using DLR. (From Kaur, A., and V. Chopra, *International Journal for Science and Emerging Technologies with Latest Trends*, 2, 7, 2012. Open access.)

The algorithm is referred to as spatial filter because it suppresses or deemphasizes certain frequencies and emphasizes (or pass) other frequencies. Figure 2.9 shows the spatial filter applied on an agriculture field with low pass and high pass filters. Median filtering under certain conditions removes noise while preserving edges and hence is widely used in image processing. Figure 2.10 shows the median filtered image of an agricultural field.

2.4 Image segmentation

Image segmentation is basically the segmenting of an image into regions that correspond to various objects or various parts of an object. Each pixel in an image is assigned to any one of the regions or categories. A segmentation of an image is good if all the pixels in the

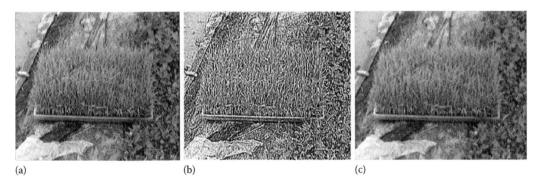

(a)   (b)   (c)

Figure 2.9 Spatial filters applied on agricultural field image. (a) Original image, (b) low pass spatial filter, and (c) high pass spatial filter. (From Humbe, V.T. et al., *International Journal of Machine Intelligence*, 3, 138, 2011. With permission.)

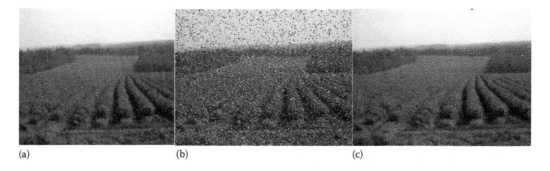

(a)   (b)   (c)

Figure 2.10 Median filters applied on agricultural field image. (a) Median filtered image, (b) salt and pepper noisy image, and (c) salt and pepper median filtered image. (From Humbe, V.T. et al., *International Journal of Machine Intelligence*, 3, 138, 2011. With permission.)

same category have similar gray scale value and the neighboring pixels that belong to different categories have different gray scale values.

Segmentation is generally performed based on three approaches: thresholding, edge based, and region based. Du and Sun (2004b) stated that the image segmentation technique for monitoring the quality of food can be classified into four categories: thresholding, region based, gradient based, and classification based. There is no standard segmentation technique, but choice of technique is dependent on the application and the type of image to be processed. For medical image processing, segmentation techniques have been classified into two major categories: based on gray-level features or texture features (Sharma and Aggarwal, 2010).

The segmentation technique has been applied in many studies involving various types of food product analyses. The segmentation technique has been used to evaluate pork color (Lu et al., 2000), marbling in pork (Faucitano et al., 2005) and ham (Cernadas et al., 2002), defect detection in fresh ham (Marty-Mahe et al., 2003), to measure fat and lean tissues in dry cured hams (Carnier et al., 2004; Sánchez et al., 2008), to conduct quality analysis of tuna (Mateo et al., 2006), and to determine pores and porosity in cooked ham (Du and Sun, 2006a). Table 2.1 shows the types of segmentation techniques applied in various food and agricultural applications.

2.4.1 Thresholding

The input in thresholding is either a gray scale or color image, and the output is a binary image with black pixels corresponding to background and white pixels corresponding to foreground (or vice versa). Segmentation is performed by intensity threshold, and every image pixel is compared with the threshold and classified based on whether the intensity is higher or lower than the threshold value. Thresholding is a technique that partitions the pixels in the image into background and object based on the relationship between the value of the gray level and threshold value. Thresholding is a gray value determination operation, which is denoted by

$$G(x) = 0, \text{ if } x < T$$

$$G(x) = 1, \text{ if } x \geq T$$

where T is the threshold value and x represents the gray value (Pronost, 2013).

Table 2.1 Segmentation Techniques Adopted in Food and Agricultural Applications

Type of segmentation	Application	Reference
Otsu and SVM	Image segmentation for apple sorting and grading	Mizushima and Lu, 2013
k-means clustering	Detection of infected fruit (apple)	Dubey et al., 2013
Thresholding	Image segmentation of fried chip and dried apple slices for quality measurement	Kang and Sabarez, 2009
Region based	Segmentation for food classification	Somatilake and Chalmers, 2007
Thresholding	Image thresholding by histogram segmentation for rice and fish	Arifin and Asano, 2006
Thresholding	Segmentation of color food image	Chang and Chen, 2006
Thresholding	Automatic method for pore structure characterization of pork ham	Du and Sun, 2006
Thresholding	To investigate the shrinkage of cooked beef affected by cooling	Zheng et al., 2006
Histogram	Quality analysis of tuna meat	Mateo et al., 2006
Thresholding	Segmentation of color food images (pear, mandarin, plum)	Mery and Pedreschi, 2005
Region-based segmentation	To segment complex food images such as pizza	Sun and Du, 2004
Region based	To recognize marbling in Iberian ham for design of an expert computer system	Cernadas et al., 2002
Thresholding	Defect segmentation on Golden Delicious apples	Leemans et al., 1998

Thresholding could be further classified into simple or adaptive and global or local based on how the threshold value is calculated. Simple thresholding is performed by a fixed value based on previous observations, whereas in adaptive thresholding, the original image is divided into subimages and a different threshold value is calculated for each subimage. Global thresholding determines one threshold value for the image and the segmentation is performed by scanning every pixel and labeling them as object or background based on whether the pixel gray level is higher or lower than the threshold value. With local thresholding, a different threshold value is calculated for every pixel within a neighborhood (Unay and Gosselin, 2006).

If the background of the image is relatively uniform, global thresholding could be used to binarize the image using pixel intensity, whereas adaptive or local thresholding could be used if there is a large variation in background intensity. A major problem with global thresholding is that changes in illumination may cause some brighter regions and some darker regions in the image, which has actually nothing to do with the image. In such cases of uneven illumination, local thresholding could be performed instead of having a single global threshold.

In food quality analysis, histogram-based segmentation or adaptive thresholding is recommended because these are robust and have higher accuracy compared to global thresholding. Adaptive thresholding can perform better during changes in lighting and is suitable for real-time applications and various techniques such as region growing, clustering, and region merging could be used (Gunasekaran, 2010).

Mery and Pedreschi (2005) performed segmentation of color images of various food materials. The segmentation was performed in three steps. The first step was the computation of a contrast gray image from RGB color components. The next step was the estimation of global threshold based on the statistical method. The third step was the performance of morphological operations to cover the holes present in the segmented binary image. The segmented images are shown in Figure 2.11. In segmentation of food materials, there exist two regions: the background and the foreground. The input is a color image of a pear, and the output of a segmented image is only with two colors where white represents the pear (object) and black represents the background. In the histogram shown in Figure 2.12b, the left peak denotes the background and the right peak refers to the object (pear).

Kang and Sabarez (2009) presented an algorithm for segmentation of bicolored food materials. They developed an algorithm based on CIE L*a*b* for French fries and dried apple slices. The algorithm detected multiple products in images if the product was made from the same material (either potato or apple) and same cooking method. They developed a polynomial equation from CIE L*a*b* color space using the least square fitting method. Using the developed equation, the pixels were analyzed and the pixels with values closer to the equation were considered as food material and vice versa. The Figure 2.13 shows the

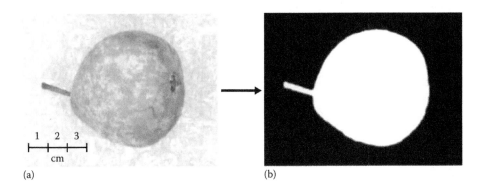

(a)   (b)

Figure 2.11 Color and segmented image of a pear. (a) Color image and (b) segmented image. (From Mery, D., and F. Pedreschi, *Journal of Food Engineering*, 66, 353, 2005. With permission.)

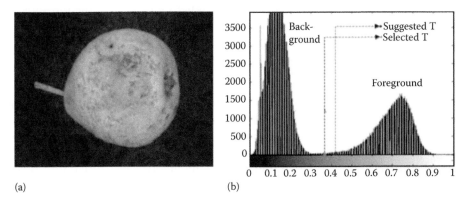

(a)   (b)

Figure 2.12 (a) High contrast monochrome image of a pear and (b) corresponding histogram. (From Mery, D., and F. Pedreschi, *Journal of Food Engineering*, 66, 353, 2005. With permission.)

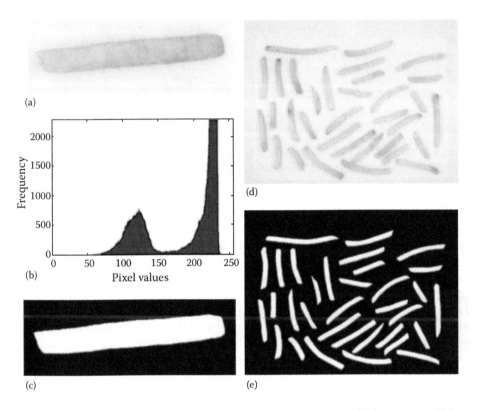

Figure 2.13 Results of segmentation. (a) Actual French fry chip image, (b) histogram of blue component of RGB, (c) segmented image using blue color threshold, (d) actual multiple French fry image, and (e) segmented image for multiple fries. (From Kang, S.P., and H.T. Sabarez, *Journal of Food Engineering*, 94, 21, 2009. With permission.)

French fry image, a histogram of blue component, and the segmented image. Their result showed that image segmentation algorithm for bicolored food materials could be used for quality measurements.

2.4.1.1 Otsu's thresholding

Otsu's thresholding is one of the best image segmentation methods available (Sahoo et al., 1988). Otsu's thresholding method provides accurate results for image thresholding for the image with bimodal distribution or multimodal distribution, but the method is not suitable if the image histogram is unimodal. Otsu's method selects the threshold values that maximize the histograms between class variance (Mizushima and Lu, 2013). A variance is a measure of region homogeneity (regions with high homogeneity correspond to low variance). In Otsu's method, the threshold is selected by minimizing the within-class variance of two groups of pixels that are separated by a thresholding operator (Sandhu, 2013).

Mizushima and Lu (2013) developed a segmentation algorithm based on Otsu's method and a support vector machine (SVM) for grading and sorting apples. The error due to segmentation was lower than 2% with the adjustable SVM. A support vector machine is basically meant to solve classification problems of two groups by creating an optimum separation hyperplane in a multidimensional space. The fundamental idea of an SVM is to determine an optimum hyperplane that could separate a data set (Vapnik, 1995). The hyperplane selection should be in a way that the margin between the hyperplane and the closest data points, called support vectors, are maximized.

2.4.2   Region-based segmentation

The main concept in region-based segmentation is to classify an image into different regions. In region-based segmentation, pixels that are neighbors and have similar values are grouped together and pixels having dissimilar values are grouped separately. Region-based segmentation can be classified into two categories: region growing and merging (GM), and region splitting and merging (SM). Region growing is the method of grouping together pixels in the neighboring region having similar properties into larger regions and the process is continued until every pixel in an image belongs to a region. When the images are segmented into regions, merging adjacent regions with similar properties is performed, which is the region growing and merging segmentation (Ikonomakis et al., 1997). Region growing and merging is a bottom-up method, whereas region splitting and merging is a top-down method that splits an image into smaller areas until specific criteria are fulfilled (Du and Sun, 2004b).

The region growing and merging method has four factors to be considered: starting seeds, the operation pattern of growing and merging, essential criteria for the tasks, and rules for ending the operations. The first starting seed factor is application specific and the maximum intensity point or the points that are homogeneous with their neighbors are selected as starting seeds. The efficiency of the algorithm is determined by the growing and merging pattern. The common growing patterns expands pixels in every direction by selecting a seed and growing its neighbors as the initial boundary and by utilizing the points on the boundary as new seeds for growing more until no seeds are found. The quality of segmentation is most affected by the third factor and is hard to select optimal region criteria and at times either too many or too few regions may be produced. When it becomes difficult to detect the edges, the region-based segmentation is better than edge-based segmentation. But region-based segmentation may result in false boundaries in the absence of edge-based methods (Sun and Du, 2004). The region-based methods are very slow in certain time-limited operations as in high-speed industrial inspection processes (Vernon, 1991). In the region splitting and merging technique, the full image is considered as one region and is iteratively split into smaller regions that have uniform color, texture, or gradient characteristics. The process of segmentation is automatically stopped when there are no more regions to be split.

Sun and Du (2004) developed a new stick growing and merging algorithm for complex food material such as pizza, which includes ham, cheese shreds, green and red peppers, and tomato sauce. The algorithm consists of constructing a number of horizontal lines with homogeneous pixels and the horizontal lines are termed *sticks*. The algorithm has four main stages: stick initialization, merging of stick, subregion merging, and modification of boundaries. Based on the algorithm, good segmentation results were obtained for pizza and other food images. The growing and merging algorithm was efficient and had reasonable speed.

Somatilake and Chalmers (2007) developed a region-based segmentation method to separate the food from the background. The algorithm automatically segments the color by applying mask on the sample image. The mask is selected at two locations on the image, such as segment A representing the background of the image and segment B representing the portion of food (banana) surface. These two segments are compared with the image and based on the color differences in a*, b* space, the image could be segmented into

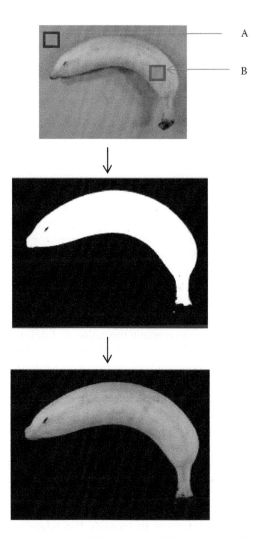

Figure 2.14 Region-based segmentation. (From Somatilake, S., and A.N. Chalmers, *Proceedings of Image and Vision Computing*, 260, 2007. With permission.)

background and sample. The selected mask when applied to the original image, would distinguish the sample from the background and the background is blacked out and the isolated food sample could be used for further analysis (Figure 2.14).

Region-based segmentation methods are mostly used for complex images with large numbers of unknown classes and are time consuming. In most of the applications related to segmentation of food image, there exists only two classes, which are food and the background or normal region, and region with defects. Hence, region-based methods are not largely used in applications related to food imaging (Zheng and Sun, 2008).

2.4.3 Edge-based (gradient-based) segmentation

Edge-based segmentation is based on idea that each object is surrounded by a border that is closed, visible, and detected based on the intensity value of the image. The basic approach is finding and following an edge. An edge can be described as the boundary between an object of interest and its background. The edges correspond to the large changes in the intensity of neighboring pixels. In edge-based segmentation, an edge filter is applied to the image to be analyzed and the pixels are grouped as edge or non-edge based on the output of the filter.

In an image processing application, if the edges of objects are determined with precision, the objects can be identified and the properties of objects, such as area, shape, and perimeter, can be accurately determined (Bolhouse, 1997). There are basically two categories of edge detection methods: gradient and Laplacian. In the gradient method, the edges are detected by locating the maximum and minimum n of the first derivative of an image. The most commonly used gradient edge detectors are Sobel, Roberts, Prewitt, and Kirsch (Russ, 1999). The Laplacian method looks for zero crossing in the second derivatives of the image to determine edges. The Canny edge detector is commonly used in food-related applications for edge detection of various food products (Du and Sun, 2004b). The Canny's edge detection algorithm also termed as optimal edge detector was enhanced by following criteria (Canny, 1986). The first criterion is low rate of error and it is critical that edges in images should not be missed and non-edges should have no response. The second feature is that the edges should be properly localized, that is, the distance between actual edge and edge pixels determined by the detector must be minimum. The next important criterion is that one edge should have only single response. By following these factors, the Canny edge detector first smoothens the image to remove the noise and determines the image gradient to focus areas with high spatial derivatives. The advantage of classical edge detectors such as Sobel Prewitt, and Kirsch is the simplicity of the detector to detect edges and their orientation, whereas the major advantages of Canny edge detectors are better edge detection especially in high noise conditions and improved signal-to-noise ratio. The disadvantages of Sobel, Prewitt, and Kirsch detectors are inaccuracy and sensitive to noise, and of Canny edge detectors are the complexity of the computation and more time consuming compared to others (Maini and Agarwal, 2009).

Du and Sun (2004b) performed a pizza base classification using thresholding-based segmentation, and the edges of the pizza base were identified by a Canny edge detector. Gujjar and Siddappa (2013) developed an algorithm for identification of basmati rice variety using image analysis. They used an edge-detection based segmentation method and applied Canny and Sobel detectors to identify the edges of rice grain. Ohali (2011) designed a date fruit grading system based on computer vision and classified the dates into three grade categories. The RGB image captured by him using a digital camera is shown in Figure 2.15a. From the image intensity histogram, a binarization threshold was estimated, which was used to convert the RGB image into the binary image shown in Figure 2.15b. By applying a Sobel edge operator, the edges that surround the binarized regions were extracted and are shown in Figure 2.15c.

Liming and Yanchao (2010) developed an automated strawberry grading system using image processing techniques. They extracted the size, shape, and color features, and developed a grading algorithm. Figure 2.16 shows the original color image, gray scale image, segmented, and edge detection images.

Du and Sun (2006b) estimated ham surface area and volume using various image processing techniques. The algorithm was based on three steps: (1) shape extraction, (2) deletion of protrusion, and (3) computation of surface area and volume using various techniques such as segmentation, edge detection, and noise reduction. The digital images were first segmented to separate the ham from the background, and median filtering was used to lower the noises in the segmented image. The edge detection was performed by the Canny edge detector method (Figure 2.17).

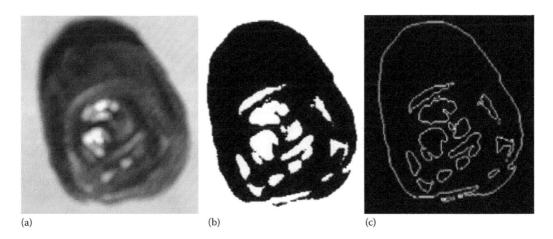

(a)   (b)   (c)

Figure 2.15 RGB, segmented, and edge-detected images of dates. (a) RGB dates image, (b) segmented image, and (c) edge detection by Sobel operator. (From Ohali, Y.A., *Journal of King Saud University—Computer and Information Sciences*, 23, 29–36, 2011. With permission.)

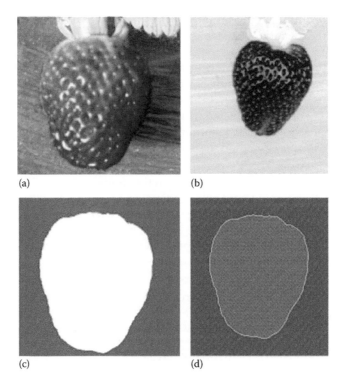

Figure 2.16 Color, gray scale, segmented, and edge detected images of strawberry. (a) Original color image, (b) gray scale image, (c) segmented image, and (d) edge detection. (From Liming, X., and Z. Yanchao, *Computers and Electronics in Agriculture*, 71S, S32, 2010. With permission.)

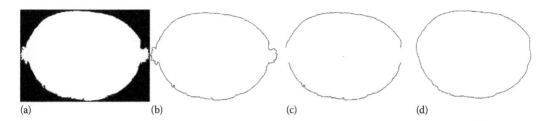

(a)   (b)   (c)   (d)

Figure 2.17 Image processing techniques applied to ham. (a) Segmented image, (b) extracted shape image, (c) protrusion deleted image, and (d) interpolated image. (From Du, C., and D.W. Sun, *Journal of Food Engineering*, 73, 260, 2006b. With permission.)

The major disadvantage of edge-based segmentation is that the method does not work efficiently when the image contains many edges because in such a case, the technique results in an oversegmented output and one is not able to determine a boundary or closed curve. To be effective, edge-based segmentation should be able to detect the global edges and the edges need to be continuous. There are other segmentation techniques such as neural-network-based segmentation, the physical-model-based approach, and clustering (*k*-means and fuzzy C-means) (Dubey et al., 2013).

Clustering partitions the data set into clusters or subsets in such a way that some common trait is shared by the data in each cluster and hence classifies the objects into different groups. There are many approaches for clustering and *k*-means clustering is a commonly used clustering algorithm and is the simplest unsupervised learning algorithm. *K*-means clustering divides the data into *k* clusters and every cluster is denoted by a changing center that originates from initial value termed *seed points*. *K*-means clustering determines the distance between the input data points and center, and allocates the input to the nearest center. The fuzzy C-means algorithm permits one data point to belong to two or more clusters.

Dubey et al. (2013) detected infected fruit parts using *k*-means clustering. The approach was to perform color segmentation automatically with *k*-means clustering and L*a*b* color space. The steps in defect segmentation using the *k*-means algorithm are:

1. Fruit image
2. Transform RGB image to L*a*b* color space
3. Classify colors into a*'b*' space using *k*-means clustering
4. Label each pixel based on *k*-means
5. Generate images that segment the input image by color
6. Determine the defected cluster

The results of the study showed that the proposed algorithm was able to detect the defective regions of apples and could also segment the defects in the stem and calyx.

2.5   *Image representation and description*

After segmentation of an image using various techniques, the resulting segmented pixels need to be represented in a suitable form for further processing. Basically image representation can be performed by one of the two ways: (1) the image can be represented with respect to its external characteristics (boundary), and (2) the image can be represented based on its internal characteristics (region comprised by pixels). When the major focus is on the shape features, external representation is chosen, whereas when the major focus is on regional characteristics such as texture and color, internal representation is chosen. After representation of the image, the description of the region based on the representation needs to be performed. For instance, when a region is represented by boundary characteristics, the boundary may be described by various features such as its length and the orientation of line joining the extreme points. The main purpose of description is to quantify the objects representation (Gonzalez and Woods, 2002).

There are various approaches for representation of segmented images: chain codes, polynomial approximation, signatures, boundary segments, and skeletons.

Chain codes—Chain codes are algorithms used to denote the shape of different objects. Chain codes represent an object's boundary, which is connected by a sequence of straight lines of specific length in the specified direction. The major drawbacks in chain codes are that the resultant chain codes are generally very long and even a small noise or imperfect segmentation along the boundary causes changes in the code, which affects the shape of the boundary.

Polynomial approximation—The objective of polynomial approximation is to represent the essence of the shape of the boundary with minimum possible polygonal segments. There are several polynomial approximation techniques such as minimum perimeter polygons, merging techniques, and splitting techniques. The major drawback is that the technique can become a time-consuming iterative process.

Signatures—The signature technique is the representation of a boundary by a one-dimensional functional representation, which could be generated in many ways. The easiest method is to represent the distance from the centroid point to the boundary as a function of an angle. The main objective of signatures is to reduce the boundary representation from actual two dimensional to one dimensional.

Boundary segments—Boundary segment is a technique where the boundary is decomposed into segments, which reduces the complexity and simplifies the process of description. This technique is useful when the boundary is comprised of one or more significant concavities that contain the shape information.

Skeletons—In the skeleton approach, the structural shape of a plane surface is reduced to a graph and this reduction could be achieved by using a thinning (or skeletonizing) algorithm to obtain the skeleton of the region (Gonzalez and Woods, 2002).

2.5.1 Methods of shape representation

Shape representation and description can be grouped in to two classes: contour based and region based. When the shape features are obtained only from the contour, the classification is termed *contour based*, whereas the classification is termed *region based* when the features are extracted from the whole region of the object rather than just the boundary information. The contour- and region-based methods are further grouped into structural (discrete) and global (continuous) methods. The global or continuous approach is a feature vector that is derived from the integral boundary of the object and do not divide the shape into segments or subparts. The structural or discrete approach usually splits the boundary of the object into segments referred to as primitives based on certain criteria. The classification of shape representation techniques is shown in Figure 2.18 (Zhang and Lu, 2004).

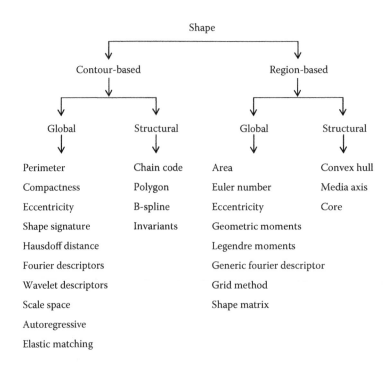

Figure 2.18 Classification of shape-based representation. (From Zhang, D., and G. Lu, *Pattern Recognition*, 37, 1, 2004. With permission.)

2.5.1.1 Contour-based global shape representation

Contour-based global shape representation technique consists of many techniques: (1) simple shape descriptors, such as area, eccentricity, major axis orientation, circularity, and bending energy; (2) correspondence-based shape matching determines the resemblance between shapes based on point-to-point matching; (3) a shape signature denotes a shape by a one-dimensional function obtained from the boundary points, and (4) boundary moments are used for reduction in dimensions of the boundary representation. There are also other methods such as elastic matching, stochastic, scale space, and spectrum transform. There is a trade-off between efficiency and accuracy in shape description. Global shape descriptors are compact but also inaccurate and hence should be combined with other shape descriptors (Zhang and Lu, 2004).

The contour-based structural shape representation technique consists of splitting the boundary into segments and consists of many methods: polygon decomposition, chain code representation, smooth curve decomposition, scale space, syntactic analysis, and shape invariants. The advantage of the structural approach is its ability to handle the occlusion problem and allow partial matching; however, there are disadvantages. The major drawback is the generation of segments or primitives because for each shape, the number of primitives needed is unknown and the success of the technique depends on the prior understanding of shape boundary features. Other drawbacks are computational complexity and the inability to record global shape features that are critical for shape representation and sensitivity to noise (Zhang and Lu, 2004).

2.5.1.2 Region-based shape representation

Region-based techniques use moment descriptors to explain shapes and includes various methods such as shape matrix, grid, media axis, and convex hull. Global region-based representation methods utilize all pixel information provided within the region and are less likely to be affected by noise and variations. Hence, they perform better with shapes containing significant defects that pose a major problem for contour-based methods (Zhang and Lu, 2004).

2.5.2 Feature extraction

2.5.2.1 Morphological features

The major types of features extracted are morphological features (which includes shape and size features), color, and textural features. The shape features of objects are the physical dimensions that are measured to characterize the appearance of the object or the surface configuration of an object. With regard to food and agricultural products, shape is an important indicator, and shape features are easier to measure using image processing techniques compared to color and textual features. The most commonly used shape features are area, perimeter, area to perimeter ratio, minor axis length, major axis length, ratio of minor to major axis length, eccentricity, Euler number, and spatial moments.

Area—The area of an object is the total number of pixels of an object boundary and its inner surface.

Perimeter—The perimeter is the total pixel distance measuring the circumference of an object or a measure of total boundary length of an object.

Major axis length—It is the distance measured between the two end points of the longest possible line through an object. The end points (x_1, y_1) and (x_2, y_2) of a major axis are determined by calculating the pixel distance between all the combinations of border pixels in the object boundary and choosing the pair with the greatest length, where length and width could be determined by measuring the sides of the rectangle bounding the kernel.

Minor axis length—While being perpendicular with the major axis, the distance measured between the end points of the longest line through the object is the minor axis length, which is a measure of object width.

Aspect ratio or elongation (or eccentricity)—Aspect ratio is the ratio between the length of major axis to the length of minor axis.

Thinness ratio or compactness ratio—The ratio of the square of perimeter (pixel distance of boundary length) and the area.

Maximum radius—The maximum distance between a pixel on the boundary and the centroid of the object.

Minimum radius—The minimum distance between a pixel on the boundary and the centroid of the object.

Radius ratio—The ratio of the maximum radius to minimum radius.

Standard deviation of all radii—Defined as the standard deviation of distances of all pixels on the boundary from the centroid of the object denoted as σ_r.

Haralick ratio—The ratio of the mean of all the radii (μ_r) to the standard deviation of all the radii (μ_r/σ_r) (Majumdar and Jayas, 2000a).

2.5.2.1.1 Fourier descriptors.   Although there are many methods for shape representation, these methods do not capture the shape features very well and are difficult to perform normalization. Among the various methods, Fourier descriptors (FD) are better in the process, that is, they achieve good shape representation and easy normalization (Zhang and Lu, 2002). The concept of the Fourier descriptor is an extension of the Fourier transform, which uses the Fourier coefficients in the frequency domain for the shape representation. The most important advantage of Fourier representation is the detailed level of interpretation in the frequency domain (Jun et al., 2011). Fourier descriptors are those that represent the boundary of an area and shape data is obtained as a periodic function that can be expressed in a Fourier series. A Fourier transform is an estimation of an arbitrary function by trigonometric functions such as cosine and sine functions. If the function is periodical, it is expressed as a Fourier series or else it is expressed as a Fourier integral (Majumdar, 1997; Gonzalez and Woods, 2002).

2.5.2.2 Color features

Color features of an object can be extracted from the pixels within the boundary of the object and the histogram provides the brightness distribution of the object. The statistics of the brightness, such as mean, standard deviation and mode, provide useful features. The mean brightness value shows the average of brightness values of an object. The standard deviation value shows how much variation occurs in the objects brightness compared to the mean. The mode value provides the most common brightness of an object. The sum of all pixel brightness of an object corresponds to the energy or aggregate brightness of the object, which is called the object's zero-order spatial moment. The R (red), G (green), B (blue) pixel component values of an image, can be converted to H (hue), S (saturation), and I (intensity) (Majumdar, 1997).

2.5.2.2.1 Color imaging.   Color is an important feature of an image and a color space could be expressed as a model that represents color in terms of intensity values. Color model (or color space) represents a color coordinate system in which each point specifies one color. There are many color models, including RGB, HSI, HSV (hue, saturation, value), L*a*b*, and CMY (cyan, magenta, yellow). The various color models are standardized for different purposes. For instance, the RGB model is used in color monitors and video cameras, CMYK (cyan, magenta, yellow, key) color space is employed in color printers, and L*a*b* is used for uniform color space. The images acquired are all in RGB color space but due to the nonuniformity of RGB color model, it needs to be converted to other color models based on the application. The basic spectral components, red, green, and blue appear in the RGB color model (Figure 2.19). In this model, RGB values are located at three corners, and cyan, magenta, and yellow are at the other three corners with black at the origin point and white at the corner farthest away from black.

*2.5.2.2.1.1 L*a*b* model.*   L*a*b* is an international standard for measurement of color and was adopted in 1976 by the Commission International d'Eclairage (CIE, Vienna, Austria). L is the luminance component or lightness, and the value ranges from 0 to 100, a (green to red) and b (blue to yellow) are chromatic components and range from –120 to 120. The equations for conversion from RGB to L*a*b* color models are provided in Patil et al. (2011).

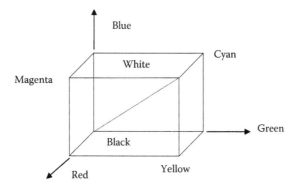

Figure 2.19 Schematic of RGB color model.

$$\begin{pmatrix} X \\ Y \\ Z \end{pmatrix} = \begin{pmatrix} 0.412453 & 0.357580 & 0.180423 \\ 0.212671 & 0.715160 & 0.072169 \\ 0.019334 & 0.119193 & 0.950227 \end{pmatrix} = \begin{pmatrix} R \\ G \\ B \end{pmatrix}$$

$$L = 116[g[y/y_n]] - 16;$$

$$a = 500[g(x/x_n) - g(y/y_n)]$$

$$b = 200[g(y/y_n) - g(z/z_n))]$$

$$g(t) = t^{1/3}, t > 0.008856; 7.787 + 16/116, \text{ if } t \le 0.008856.$$

2.5.2.2.1.2   HSI color model.   The HSI represents the hue, saturation, and intensity, and it is an important color model in image processing. Hue denotes the dominant color seen by an observer and is related to the dominant wavelength. Saturation is the relative purity of color and refers to the quantity of white light mixed with hue and intensity is the total amount of light passing through an object. Given an RGB color model, HSI components can be calculated by the following equations (Gonzalez and Woods, 2002)

$$H = \theta, \text{ if } B \le G$$

$$H = 360 - \theta, \text{ if } B > G$$

where

$$\theta = COS^{-1} \left[\frac{1/2\left[(R-G)+(R-B)\right]}{\left[(R-G)^2 + (R-B)(G-B)\right]^{\frac{1}{2}}} \right]$$

$$S = 1 - \frac{3}{R+G+B}[\min(R,G,B)]$$

$$I = \frac{1}{3}(R+G+B)$$

2.5.2.2.1.3 CMY color model.   Cyan, magenta, and yellow are the secondary colors of light, which are produced by adding primary colors of light. For instance, red and blue make magenta, green and blue results in cyan, and red plus green makes yellow. The conversion of CMY to RGB is performed using the following equation (Gonzalez and Woods, 2002):

$$\begin{pmatrix} C \\ M \\ Y \end{pmatrix} = \begin{pmatrix} 1 \\ 1 \\ 1 \end{pmatrix} - \begin{pmatrix} R \\ G \\ B \end{pmatrix}$$

Equal amounts of cyan, magenta, and yellow produce black, and a fourth color black is added to produce a CMYK color model.

2.5.2.3   *Textural features*

Texture is the surface property that describes the visual patterns and possesses critical information on the structural arrangement of the surface. Texture is an important feature that defines the characteristics of an image. In an image, texture is quantified as gray level differences or contrast that occurs in a defined area where the change occurs (Babu et al., 2010). The texture of an image measures the properties of coarseness, smoothness, and regularity. In image processing, texture is described using three approaches: statistical, structural, and spectral. The statistical approach provides textural characterization such as smooth, grainy, or coarse. Description of texture based on the structural approach deals with the arrangement of image primitives, which describes texture based on methodologically spaced parallel lines. The basic idea in the structural approach is that a complex pattern could be formed from a basic texture primitive with the help of some rules that limit the possible arrangements of the primitives to a certain extent. Spectral approaches for describing texture are based on Fourier spectrum properties and are used to identify global periodicity in an image by determining high energy and narrow peaks in the spectrum. For texture description, three features of Fourier spectrum are considered useful. They are (1) the principal direction of the textural pattern is provided by prominent peaks in the spectrum, (2) the location of the peaks in the frequency plane provides the basic spatial period of the pattern, and (3) elimination of periodic components through filtering results in nonperiodic image elements that can be described by statistical techniques (Gonzalez and Woods, 2002). The most widely used methods for applications in food processing are the statistical method, which includes pixel value, the run-length method, and the co-occurrence run length method (Anami and Burkapalli, 2009b; Narendra and Hareesh, 2011).

2.5.2.3.1 Gray level co-occurrence matrix.   The gray level co-occurrence matrix (GLCM) was first demonstrated by Haralick in the 1970s and has become an important part of image texture analysis. Texture of an image is quantified by gray level differences or contrast, and texture also quantifies the defined area in image where the change occurs. GLCM is basically a tabulation that shows how frequently various combinations of pixel brightness values or gray level values occur in an image. GLCM is a 2D matrix in which two pixels separated by a certain vector occurs in an image. The different texture characteristics could be determined by varying the vector used. When the GLCM is created, it needs to be normalized after which various texture features can be computed (Narendra and Hareesh, 2011).

The first-order texture measures do not consider the pixel neighbor relationship and are basically statistics like variance that are measured from the original image values. The second-order texture considers the relationship between groups of two pixels, normally the neighboring pixels in the original image (Hall-Beyer, 2007). A GLCM provides the probability of a particular gray value pixel that occurs at a specified direction and distance from the neighboring pixels. Six textural parameters—contrast, energy, variance, correlation, entropy, and inverse difference moment—are regarded as the most important among the fourteen parameters originally proposed (Haralick et al., 1988).

The co-occurrence matrix (i, j) calculates the co-occurrence of the pixels with gray value i, j at a distance of d. The GLCM matrix is extracted in the $0°, 45°, 90°$, and $135°$ and the matric below is generated using $0°$ and the distance between the pixels is 1.

Consider a 4×4 matrix of a simple test image and the values are image gray levels.

1	4	3	1
2	4	2	2
1	3	1	4
4	1	1	2

The following matrix shows the pixel composition matrix.

1, 1	1, 2	1, 3	1, 4
2, 1	2, 2	2, 3	2, 4
3, 1	3, 2	3, 3	3, 4
4, 1	4, 2	4, 3	4, 4

The GLCM will be constructed by first filling the top left cell by the number of times (1, 1) occurs in the whole matrix starting from top left and counting forward to the right. The first row, second column will be filled by the number of times (1, 2) occurs in the same way. The resulting matrix is shown next.

	1	2	3	4
1	1	1	1	2
2	0	1	0	1
3	2	0	0	0
4	1	1	1	0

The GLCM is then normalized by dividing every element of the matrix by a normalizing constant called C, hence

$$P(i, j) = p(i, j)/C$$

where $p(i, j)$ is the (i, j)th entry in the un-normalized GLCM, $P(i, j)$ is the (i, j)th entry in the normalized GLCM, and C is normalizing constant (Hall-Beyer, 2007).

The various textural features could be derived using the normalized GLCM as follows:

Contrast—The measure of contrast of intensity between a pixel and its neighborhood.
Correlation—The measure of how much correlation exists between a pixel and its neighbors over the whole image (Suresh and Shunmuganathan, 2012).
Energy—Also termed *uniformity*. When an image is more homogeneous, the value of energy is larger and when energy equals 1, it is a constant image, also termed *angular second moment* (ASM).
Entropy—Represents the randomness of the intensity image and images with frequent occurrences of specific color configurations result in higher values for entropy (Narendra and Hareesh, 2011).
Homogeneity—Determines the similarity of pixels or the local homogeneity of the pixel pair.
Variance—A measure of how spread out the gray level distribution is in an image. Maximum probability results in a pixel pair that is most predominant in the image. Inverse difference moments (IDMs) provide information about the smoothness of the image like homogeneity and have higher values if the gray levels of the pixel pairs are similar (Dettori and Semler, 2007).

Cluster shade and cluster prominence are skewness measures of a matrix, that is, there is a lack of symmetry (Anami and Burkpalli, 2009b).

2.5.2.3.2 Gray level run length matrix.   Gray level run length matrix (GRLM) is a method to extract higher-order statistical texture information described by Galloway (1975). GLRM is a two-dimensional matrix containing element $p(i, j/\theta)$ in which j denotes the number of occurrences of run length, and i is the gray level in a given direction θ. Five textural features that could be extracted from GLRM are (Galloway, 1975; Albregtsen et al., 2000) short run emphasis (SRE), long run emphasis (LRE), run length nonuniformity (RLN), gray level nonuniformity (GLN), and run percentage (RP). Chu et al. (1990) added two more textural features: low gray level runs emphasis (LGRE) and high gray level runs emphasis (HGRE). Short run emphasis measures the distribution of short runs and is usually large for fine textures. Long run emphasis calculates the long run distribution and is usually large for coarse structural textures. Gray level nonuniformity measures the similarity of gray level values in the image and the GLN value is small if the values of gray level are similar throughout the image. Run length nonuniformity expresses the similarity of run lengths throughout the image and has lower values if the run lengths are the same throughout the image. Run percentage determines the distribution and homogeneity of runs of an image in a particular direction. Low gray level run emphasis calculates the distribution of low gray level values and high gray level run emphasis calculates the distribution of high gray level values (Xu et al., 2004).

2.5.3 Classification of food based on shape and size features

In the quality evaluation of food, shape and size are the most commonly used object measurements and easy to determine features. The size measurement of an object is based on the measurement of width, length, area, and perimeter. Other shape and size features that are used in the quality evaluation of various foods are area ratio, aspect ratio, compactness, roundness, and eccentricity. Table 2.2 shows the classification of foods based on shape, size, color, and textural features.

Firatligil-Durmus et al. (2008) analyzed the shape characterization and geometrical properties of red and green lentils, *Lens culinaris* (Medikus). Images were acquired and seven geometrical features were determined: projected area, equivalent diameter, perimeter, MinFeret and MaxFeret (minimum or maximum diameter), circularity, and elongation. The volume and surface area of lentils were measured based on the oblate spheroid and two-sphere segment approximation. The results showed that compared with pycnometric volume measurement, the percentage difference in volume of red and green lentils were 4.4% and 4.2%, respectively and image processing provided an easy and noninvasive technique to characterize the lentils based on geometrical properties.

Sayinci et al. (2012) determined the shape and size of two orange cultivars using image processing methods. The color images were acquired through digital cameras and the various parameters calculated were equivalent diameter, projected area, length, perimeter, major width, minor width, shape factor, sphericity, surface area, geometric mean diameter, density, and elongation. PCA (principal component analysis) was applied to average values of the various properties to determine the important factors of variability. The results showed that the projected surface area, equivalent diameter, length, mass, perimeter, volume, density, geometric mean diameter, and surface area are important to distinguish the orange cultivars, and these properties can be used for sorting and various other postharvest monitoring operations.

Volume measurement of agricultural products is performed using gas displacement and water displacement methods. The gas displacement measurement technique is time consuming, whereas the water displacement method may result in harmful effects on the produce. Hence volume measurement of agricultural products was performed using imaging techniques. Koc (2007) determined the volume of watermelon using the water displacement method, ellipsoid approximation, and imaging technique. The volume of watermelon calculated by ellipsoid approximation was significantly different from the water displacement method but there was no significant variation between the volume estimated by imaging and the water displacement method.

2.5.4 Classification of food based on texture and color features

Karimi et al. (2012) determined the textural features of bread made with different processing parameters. Bread samples were prepared with different emulsifiers, in three concentrations, and at three proofing times. The sensory characteristics, specific volume, $L^*a^*b^*$ color components, porosity, hardness, and image textural features were determined. Textural features were extracted using GLCM and four image texture features, correlation, contrast, energy, and homogeneity were calculated. The contrast, correlation, energy, and homogeneity determined from GLCM showed high correlation of 0.958, 0.973, 0.966, and 0.91, respectively, with bread hardness and they concluded that image texture analysis could be used as a nondestructive method for estimation of hardness of bread.

Singh and Kaur (2012) performed inspection of bakery products using texture analysis and analyzed the texture of bread crumbs using a 2D Haar transform along with canonical

Table 2.2 Classification of Food Based on Shape, Size, Color, Texture

Feature extraction	Application	Accuracy	Reference
Color, morphology, and texture	Identification of rice variety and quality	74%–95%	Gujjar and Siddappa, 2013
Texture	Investigate the effect of processing parameters on bread quality using image textural analysis	Good correlation coefficient of 0.994 obtained between hardness of bread and image textural features	Karimi et al., 2012
Shape and size	Determination of shape and size of oranges	Size and shape could be used to successfully differentiate cultivars of oranges	Sayinci et al., 2012
Texture	Inspection of bakery products using textural analysis of images	82%	Singh and Kaur, 2012
Volume	Determination of volume of oranges	No significant difference between imaging and water displacement method	Fellegari and Navid, 2011
Texture	Classification of cashew kernels using textural features	90%	Narendra and Hareesh, 2011
Color and texture	Identification of various food grains, maize, wheat, corn, cowpeas, peas, millet; green, horse, Bengal and red gram	90.5%–95.9%	Patil et al., 2011
Color and texture	Recognition of 15 types of fruits	79%–99%	Arivazhagan et al., 2010
Color	Classification of boiled food grain using color	76%–96%	Anami and Burkpalli, 2009a
Texture	Classification of grapefruit peel disease using textural feature analysis	81.7%–96.7%	Kim et al., 2009
Shape and geometrical properties	Characterization of shape and geometrical properties of lentils	Geometric features of lentils measured using imaging	Firatligil-Durmus et al., 2008
Volume	Determination of volume of watermelon	No significant difference between imaging and water displacement method	Koc, 2007
Shape	Determination of surface area and volume of ham	Mean error compared to manual method was −1.79% and −4.96%	Du and Sun, 2006
Color	Classification of cake and biscuits	92%	De Silva et al., 2005
Shape	Classification of pizza base	86.7%–98.3%	Du and Sun, 2004b
Size	Determination of size of apples	Obtained consistent results	Rao and Renganathan, 2002
Shape	Shape analysis of Indian wheat varieties	Fifteen different wheat varieties could be identified	Shouche et al., 2001

discriminant analysis and stated that textural properties can be used for inspection of bakery products.

Patil et al. (2011) used textural and color features for classification of food grains (wheat, corn, jowar, cow peas, red gram, green gram, Bengal gram, horse gram, peas, and pearl millet) based on various color models, including L*a*b*, HSI, and YCbCr (brightness or luminance, blue minus luma, and red minus luma). The color features were extracted from color models. The three global features, namely, mean, standard deviation, and slope of regression line, were extracted from a cumulative histogram. Five local features—homogeneity, correlation, contrast, local homogeneity and entropy—were derived from the co-occurrence matrix. The extracted textural features were then used for classification using K-nearest neighbor (KNN) and minimum distance classifiers, and the highest classification accuracy was obtained in the L*a*b* color model.

Arivazhagan et al. (2010) proposed a method to classify fruits based on color and textural features. The supermarket produce data set was comprised of 15 different categories of fruits and 1633 images were used for classification. The HSV color space was selected due to its invariant properties. The five co-occurrence textural features energy, contrast, local homogeneity, cluster prominence, and cluster shade were determined from the co-occurrence matrix. The statistical features standard deviation, skewness, mean, and kurtosis were derived from the H and S components and hence one fruit image was characterized by a total of 13 features. The proposed method for fruit recognition is shown in a block diagram in Figure 2.20.

Kim et al. (2009) developed a color texture feature analysis for classification of grapefruit peel disease. Grapefruits with five disease-affected peel conditions (i.e., copper burn, canker, melanose, greasy spot, and wind scar) and healthy fruits were used for the study. The data analysis based on color co-occurrence method (CCM) involved selection of region of interest, color transformation from eight bit RGB to a six bit HSI, generation of spatial gray level dependent matrices (SGDM), texture feature calculation, selection of most useful textural features, and finally disease classification by discriminant analysis. The 13 textural features selected to construct the model were uniformity, variance, mean intensity, correlation 1, correlation 2, inverse difference, product moment, entropy, sum entropy, difference entropy, information correlation, modus, and contrast. The results of the study provided a classification accuracy of 96% and it was concluded that texture feature analysis could be used for identification and classification of diseases in citrus peel.

Narendra and Hareesh (2011) analyzed the textural features for cashew kernel classification. The textural features were extracted using GLCM and the features were used to develop a multilayer feed forward neural network model. The model was developed initially with only six textural features: energy, entropy, correlation, contrast, homogeneity,

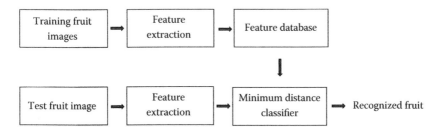

Figure 2.20 Block diagram showing method for fruit recognition. (From Arivazhagan, S. et al., *Journal of Emerging Trends in Computing and Information Sciences*, 1, 90, 2010. With permission.)

and dissimilarity. The classification accuracy of cashew kernels was only 74%. Since 6 features were inadequate for classification with higher accuracy, 15 textural features (those added were angular second moment, cluster performance, cluster shade, smoothness, mean, variance, standard deviation, third moment, and maximum probability) were extracted using GLCM. The classification accuracy of cashew kernels was around 90% and textural features could be used for classification of cashew kernels.

Savakar and Anami (2009) used color and texture features for classification of fruits, food grains, and flowers. Some food materials are easily identified by color, whereas some food materials have overlapping colors, such as ground nut and wheat, where texture becomes an ideal feature for classification. So, the authors evaluated the color and texture features for classification of various produce. The HSI color components were extracted from RGB components and the co-occurrence matrix method was adopted to obtain textural features. Nine features were considered initially but later only five textural features, namely, contrast, energy, maximum probability inverse, difference moment, and correlation, were considered because other features did not contribute effectively for classification. The average classification accuracy using color features were 87.5%, 78.4%, and 75.7%, for food grain, mango, and jasmine, respectively; the classification accuracy increased to 90.8%, 80.2%, and 85.8%, respectively for texture features. The average classification accuracies for food grain, mango, and jasmine increased to 94.1%, 84.0% and 90.1%, respectively, with combined color and texture features.

chapter three

Classification
Statistical and neural network

3.1 Introduction

Classification is a general term used in everyday life for many activities. In general, *classification* means organizing or deciding where an object fits among the groups based on its characteristics. A classification process is then made for making such judgments in a variety of other circumstances. The building of a classification procedure for a given set of data based on its characteristics and forming into groups or patterns is termed *pattern recognition*. Classification plays a major role in all aspects of life, for instance, for classifying the population into male or female. Other examples are classification of people based on income, socioeconomic status, literacy, health status, access to health, and quality of life. In every industry such as agriculture, food, veterinary, medicine, pharmacy, engineering to classify various types of products, the classification procedure is very significant. The primary purpose of classification is to provide a simplified and useful framework for analyzing data for decision-making purposes. In the food and agriculture industry, classification is vital from identification of raw materials to the completion and quality checking of finished products.

Classification could be broadly divided into unsupervised learning (also known as clustering) and supervised learning. When a set of data or observations is provided with the objective of establishing clusters or classes in the data, it is termed *unsupervised learning*. Whereas when we know that there are certain numbers of groups and the objective is to build a rule to classify new data into one of the existing groups, it is termed *supervised learning*. The various characteristics expected in a classifier are accuracy, speed of classification, comprehensibility, and time to learn (Henery, 1994).

In image processing, classification is the final stage and it involves identification of an object and classifying it into any one of the classes by comparing the characteristics of the object of interest with a known object or a known set of criteria. In supervised classification, prior knowledge of the images to be classified is known and hence, classification is simple by testing whether the computed classification agrees with the prior knowledge. In unsupervised learning, no prior knowledge of the image is available and hence the classification is tedious.

Many approaches could be used for classification and we will discuss the two major forms: statistical classification and neural network classification. A third form of classification called fuzzy logic will also be discussed in a later part of the chapter. Statistical classification is performed by grouping a set of related categories in a meaningful and standard format. The statistical approach is based on Fisher's early work on linear discrimination. Statistical classification is performed by statisticians and hence involves human contribution such as selection of variable and entire structuring of the problem.

Although neural network classification appears to be a recent development, 1890 was the beginning for neural computing when the activity of the brain was first published by William James (Nelson and Illingworth, 1990). But the actual neural network began in 1943 when McCulloch and Pitts (1943) constructed neural network models based on several assumptions as to how neurons worked. From then on, several researchers and scientists contributed to the development of the neural network field. A neural network (NN) or artificial neural network (ANN) is defined by Dr. Robert Hecht-Nielsen as "a computing system made up of a number of simple, highly interconnected processing elements which process information by their dynamic state response to external inputs" (Caudill, 1987). The human brain is made up of billions of interconnected neurons that process and transmit information through electrical and chemical signals. A neural network is primarily based on the concept of neurons in the human brain and are typically organized in layers. In the human brain, signals are collected by neurons through fine structures called dendrites. In the development of the neural network, 1986 is regarded as an important year in recent history because the back propagation learning algorithm was rediscovered by Rumelhart et al. (1986) after the initial development by Werbos (1974). From then on, ANN started to develop as an important computing technique in various fields.

3.1.1 Classifiers for pattern recognition

To categorize objects into two or more groups (called *classes*), use of a decision rule known as *classification criterion* is established based on the features extracted from the object of interest. The classification criterion is obtained from observation of known classes referred to as the *training set*. The classification criterion is then applied to a set of new data called the *test set* for the purpose of classification. Different types of classifiers are explained in many research papers and books related to pattern recognition (Jayas et al., 2000).

Different types of classifiers discussed in this chapter are statistical, neural networks, and fuzzy logic. The statistical classifiers are based on Bayes minimum error rule, which explains that to reduce the average probability of error, an object needs to be classified to a class such as to maximize the posterior probability. In many applications, the class conditional probability density function or posterior probabilities are not known and need to be calculated, which can be performed using two approaches: parametric and nonparametric. The parametric approach makes an assumption that the probability density function has a form of multivariate normal distribution, whereas the nonparametric approach does not make any assumption and determines the posterior probability from the training data set (Jayas et al., 2000). In the parametric method, the classification rules are formed based on the models of probability density function of the data. The parametric methods are restricted by the assumption of Gaussian distribution. When a density function is not Gaussian and not similar to other quantified distributions, the density function of each class can still be estimated, which is the basis for the nonparametric method. In nonparametric methods, the training examples are explicitly used as parameters and are a lazy learning method. The linear and quadratic discriminant classifiers are parametric methods, and K-nearest neighbor (KNN) is the most commonly used nonparametric method (Davies and Silverstein, 1995). Neural network classifiers are based on the structure of the human brain, which contains neurons that process the information and send out the output. There are many different forms of ANNs and architectures, and those mainly used in agriculture- and food-related applications will be discussed.

3.2   Artificial neural networks

3.2.1   Basic concept of ANNs

The concept of neural networks is to simulate the human brain, which contains a fundamental unit called a neuron. An artificial neuron is similar to a biological neuron and obtains a set of input information (x_i) that is connected via a weight factor (w_i) (Figure 3.1). The neurons add up the weighted inputs and send the results to a transfer function to produce an output. The output is either used as the network result or passed on to another neuron as input, which further processes the information. The weights are the connection strengths and are adjustable during training of the network, and there are many algorithms to regulate the weights during the training of the network (Huang et al., 2007).

A neural network is organized in layers that consist of many interconnected nodes. When patterns are presented via input layers, the input layers communicate with the hidden layers where the actual processing is performed. The one or more hidden layers then communicate with the output layer and the solutions are presented in the output layer (Figure 3.2). An artificial neural network could be used for specific applications, such as

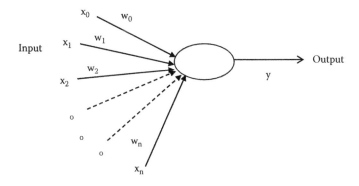

Figure 3.1 Schematic representation of an artificial neuron.

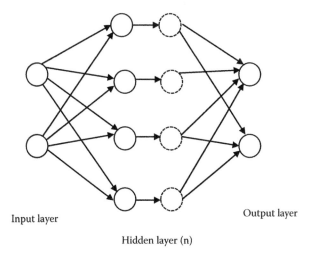

Figure 3.2 Neural network architecture.

data classification or pattern recognition through a self-learning process. A neural network has the ability to extract patterns and detect trends from a complicated or imprecise set of data (Bolo, 2007). An artificial neural network is a robust method to solve various types of problems, such as pattern classification, clustering, function approximation, forecasting, association, optimization, and control.

3.2.2 *Categorization of ANNs*

ANNs can be categorized in many ways based on their features and generally the categorization is dependent on (1) functional activity the ANN is supposed to perform such as pattern recognition or clustering, (2) the neurons' level of connectivity in the network, (3) type of learning algorithm, (4) the direction of information flow within the network, (5) the learning rule, and (6) the amount of supervision required for the ANN training phase (Basheer and Hajmeer, 2000). ANNs have been categorized in many ways. For instance, Lippmann (1987) categorized based on learning method (supervised or unsupervised) and data (continuous or binary). Simpson (1990) classified based on learning (supervised or unsupervised) and direction of data flow in the network (feedforward or feedback). Jain et al. (1996) used a four-level categorization for ANN depending on the degree of learning supervision, flow of data, learning rule, and the learning algorithm (Basheer and Hajmeer, 2000).

The architecture explains the structure of an ANN including number of nodes, hidden layers, output function, and activation function. Although there are many architectures, the most commonly used ones are feedforward, which allows information to travel only one way, and feedback networks, which have signals traveling in both the directions by introduction of loops in the network (Hua et al., 2011).

3.2.2.1 *Multilayer neural network*

A multilayer neural network (MLNN) consists of a set of neurons placed in several layers. There are usually three different layers: input, hidden (one or more), and output. The information is received by the input layer, which passes the information to the next layer (first hidden layer). The output of the first hidden layer is the input for the second hidden layer and the process proceeds to the output layer. The multilayer neural network with this type of information flow in the same direction is called a *feedforward network*. The number of neurons present in the input layer is the same as the dimensions or features of the input layer. The incoming signal is processed by amplifying, inhibiting, or attenuating through weighting factors by the hidden and output layers. For the output layer, the number of neurons is based on the number of classes being examined. Based on application requirements, the number of hidden layers and nodes present in hidden layers are determined (Jayas et al., 2000).

The MLNN is considered one of the most powerful and robust networks for pattern classification. The MLNN is trained to provide a desired output for a particular input with a predetermined error. The selection of proper network size for a particular application is an important factor. The selection of number of layers has been studied by many researchers. Chester (1990) showed that a small, three-layered network performs better than a large, two-layered network. Lippmann (1987) indicated that for any type of classification problem, no more than three layers (i.e., two hidden layers) would be required for the network. The performance of a network with three hidden layers versus two hidden layers was compared by Villiers and Barnard (1992) and the networks performed similar in most aspects. The MLNN with one hidden layer performed most of the classification and is better to use than two hidden layers, but more than two hidden layers does not increase the efficiency and may also result in lower accuracy (Ghazanfari-Moghaddam, 1996).

3.2.2.1.1 Back propagation neural network. The back propagation neural network (BPNN) is the most widely used multilayer feedforward network. It consists of an input layer, the nodes that represent the input variables, one or more hidden layers, and an output layer with nodes that represent the dependent variables. In a BPNN, the data are fed forward without any feedback, that is, all connections are unidirectional and there exists no connections between the neurons in the same layer. The neurons may be either completely or partially connected. The output errors are back propagated from the output to the input layer through the hidden layers. The BPNN is a supervised learning method, that is, the algorithms are provided with examples of input and output and the error is determined. The major focus is to minimize the error until the network learns the training data. The BPNN is versatile and used for classification, forecasting, data modeling, pattern recognition, and data and image compression (Hassoun, 1995). In a BPNN algorithm, a number of control parameters need to be set, such as learning rate and momentum rate. The learning rate is responsible for the step size, as the algorithm adjusts the weight because the algorithm converges slowly with too small steps and the algorithm becomes unstable with too large steps. The momentum rate can be determined only by experiment and it prevents the algorithm from becoming stuck in specific flat spots. An epoch is the time period when network training is performed by providing each pattern in the training set one time. The algorithm iterates through many epochs, and on each epoch the training data are presented to the network and outputs are compared and error is calculated. Based on the error, the weight is adjusted and the process is repeated (Debska and Suzowska-Świder, 2011).

3.2.2.2 Kohonen network or self-organizing map

Kohonen networks, also referred to as self-organizing maps (SOMs), are trained in an unsupervised mode. They are two-layer networks that transform high-dimensionality input data into a lower dimensional data (Kohonen, 1989). The SOM is a feedforward network with two layers: an input and an active layer. The active layer refers to two-dimensional arrays of output neuron and the nodes present in the active layer are connected to all the input nodes. The objective of the SOM is to provide training to the network so that the same type of input patterns results in physically close output neurons. Unsupervised training provides more effective solutions for biological systems than supervised learning due to the unexpected aspects of biological materials, and Kohonen's self-organizing map is the one of the most important unsupervised network systems (Huang et al., 2007).

3.2.2.3 Radial basis function neural network

Radial basis function (RBF) is a multilayer feedforward back propagation network that has three layers: input, hidden, and output (Figure 3.3). In the input layer, there is one neuron for each predictor variable and it feeds the value to each neuron in the hidden layer. The hidden layer has many neurons and the optimum number is identified based on training. The value from the output of the hidden layer is multiplied by the weights associated with the neurons and passed to the output, which adds up the weighted values and provides this sum as the output of the network. RBF networks are not as versatile as BPNNs and are relatively slower, but RBF networks train faster than BPNNs and the choice of selection between the two networks depends on the problem to be solved (Attoh-Okine et al., 1999; Basheer and Hajmeer, 2000). For instance, a clustering problem may be solved with a Kohonen network, whereas modeling of mapping problems may be performed either by RBF or BP.

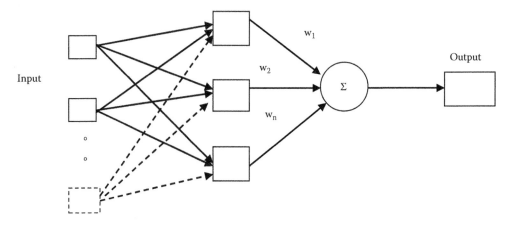

Figure 3.3 Architecture of radial basis function network.

The RBF network is similar to *K*-means clustering or a general regression neural network (GRNN) but the main difference is that a RBF usually has a variable number of neurons, normally fewer than the training points, whereas GRNNs have one neuron for each point in the training data. For classification problems with small or medium size training data, GRNNs provide more accurate results, whereas GRNNs cannot handle large training data and RBF networks are useful for such problems (Sherrod, 2003).

3.2.2.4 General regression neural network

GRNN is basically a feedforward network presented by Specht (1991) based on the nonlinear regression theory. The GRNN has an extremely parallel structure and even with minimum data in multidimensional space, the smooth transition from one observed data to another is provided by the algorithm. If sufficient data are provided, a GRNN could solve any function approximation problem. The architecture of a GRNN is shown in Figure 3.4, which has four layers: input, hidden or pattern, summation, and output. The GRNN estimates the linear or nonlinear regression on independent variables, that is, the main

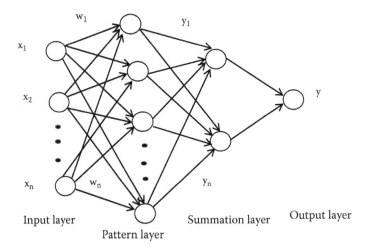

Figure 3.4 Architecture of general regression neural network.

function of the GRNN is to calculate the most possible value of output *y* when provided with the training vectors *x* (Specht, 1991; Sun et al., 2008). The GRNN does not have a training parameter but has a smoothing factor that is used when new data are provided for the network. The smoothing factor determines how closely the predictions of the network are matched with the training data (Ward Systems Group, 1998). The major advantages of the GRNN are that is has a strong nonlinear mapping capacity, flexible network structure, fault tolerance, robustness, can get better prediction even with smaller data size, and the network has the ability to deal with unstable data (J. Liu et al., 2012).

3.2.2.5 *Multilayer perceptron*

The perceptron rule derived by Rosenblatt (1962) can perform precisely only with linearly separable classes. A linearly separable class is one in which a linear hyperplane can separate one set of objects on one side of the plane and the second set on the other side of the plane. Figure 3.5 shows the two-object classification in linearly separable and nonlinearly separable classes. To handle the nonlinearly separable problem of classification, additional neuron layers need to be placed between the input and output layers, thus resulting in the multilayer perceptron architecture (Hecht-Nielsen, 1990). Since no interaction occurs between the intermediate layer and the external environment, they are referred to as hidden layers.

The multilayer perceptron (MLP) is a feedforward multilayer neural network in which the number of output and input neurons is determined based on the number of data features and classes. Unlike the input or output layer, the size of the middle (hidden) layer is not fixed. The hidden layer generally forces the network to create a simple model of the system with the potential to generalize the previously unseen patterns (Michie et al., 1994).

3.2.2.6 *Probabilistic neural network*

A probabilistic neural network (PNN) is made of four different layers: input, pattern, summation, and output. The input layer is a distribution unit that provides the same input values to all pattern units. The pattern layer forms the product of the input vector with a weight vector and performs a nonlinear operation before sending the output to the summation layer. The summation layer sums up the input from the pattern layer and the output layer provides the output of the architecture (Specht, 1990). The PNN algorithm uses a smoothing factor δ to generate the output value. The smoothing factor δ is selected based on experimentation to obtain best results, and once the network is trained different values of δ can be fed to the network (Paliwal et al., 2001).

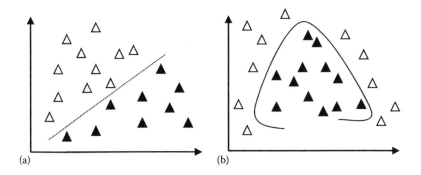

(a)   (b)

Figure 3.5 (a) Linearly separable classes and (b) nonlinearly separable classes.

The most important advantage of a PNN is that the architecture performs rapidly compared to the back propagation algorithm (Rumelhart et al., 1986). The training is easy and instantaneous in a PNN. They are suitable for real-time applications because as one pattern from each category is observed, the network starts to generalize new patterns. The generalization will improve as more patterns are observed and stored in the network. Other advantages are that by selecting an appropriate value for the smoothing factor δ, the shape of the decision surface can be made either simple or complex as required. Unlike other networks, the PNN operates entirely in parallel without a need for feedback from the individual neurons to the inputs (Specht, 1990).

3.2.2.7   Deep learning

Deep learning, also referred to as deep structured learning or hierarchical learning, has recently developed into a new research area in machine learning since 2006. Deep learning is an artificial intelligence machine learning technique in which various layers of processing information in stages in hierarchical architecture are explored for classification of patterns. A deep neural network (DNN) is a model that consists of multiple interconnected layers of hidden variables. The reasons for the increased popularity of deep learning are the significant improvement in chip processing capabilities, reduced cost of computational hardware, and recent advances in machine learning and signal processing. Researchers have found success with deep learning in various applications, including speech recognition, voice search, phonetic identification, handwriting recognition, information retrieval, and object recognition. Deep neural network models are very flexible and have the ability to learn complex nonlinear data (Deng, 2011).

3.2.3   Potential of neural network classifiers for image classification related to food and agriculture applications

The artificial neural network has been extensively used in food and related applications for classification purposes in imaging applications. Many research studies involving imaging has used different types of ANN architecture for classification of images. Table 3.1 provides the applications of ANN for image classification in various research studies.

Silva and Sonnadara (2013) studied an artificial neural network for classification of nine varieties of rice grain. Images were acquired from rice samples, and 13 morphological, 15 textural, and 6 color features were extracted from the color images of every seed sample. The MLP network consisted of four layers (one input, two hidden, and one output) and the number of nodes in the input layer was the same as the number of features. The classification accuracy of morphological model was 44% and color model was 51%. For the textural features, three models were developed for features extracted from red, green, and blue channels, and the corresponding accuracies were 61%, 59%, and 55%, respectively. The overall average classification accuracy of all three features combined was 92%. The combined feature model resulted in better classification accuracy of rice varieties rather than individual feature models.

Mukane and Kendule (2013) proposed an ANN method for classification of flowers. From a set of images for five classes of flowers, textural features were extracted. MLP architecture, a back propagation method, was used for classification of flowers and a classification accuracy of more than 85% was achieved for classification of flowers.

Savakar (2012) performed the classification of five types of bulk fruits using artificial neural networks. One thousand images were acquired for each type of fruit and color (red,

Table 3.1 Applications of Artificial Neural Networks for Classification of Images
in Food- and Agriculture-Related Research

Type of ANN architecture	Application	Accuracy	Reference
MLP	Classification of rice grain	92%	Silva and Sonnadara, 2013
MLP, GFF, RBF	Classification of pollen grains	85%	Dhawale et al., 2013
BPNN	Classification of fruits using apple, chikoo, mango, orange, and sweet lemon	92%–94%	Savakar, 2012
BPNN	Identification of Indian leafy vegetables	92%–100%	Danti et al., 2012
GRNN	Grading of tobacco leaves	93.5%	J. Liu et al., 2012
PNN	Neural network for foliage plant identification	93.08%	Kadir et al., 2011
BPNN	Classification of sprout-damaged wheat and barley	99.4% and 91.7% for healthy and sprout damaged	Vadivambal et al., 2010a,b
BPNN	Grading of *Jatropha curcas* fruit based on maturity	95%	Effendi et al., 2010
BPNN	Classification of rice varieties	93.65%	OuYang et al., 2010
MLP	Classification of cereal grains	98%	Douik and Abdellaoui, 2010
BPNN	Classification of Canadian wheat classes	80%–100%	Mahesh et al., 2008
MLNN	Classification of beans	90.56%	Kiliç et al., 2007
BPNN	Classification of barley, oats, rye, wheat, and durum wheat	98%	Visen et al., 2004a
BPNN	Classification of hard vitreous and not hard vitreous durum wheat	85%–90%	Wang et al., 2003
BPNN	Classification of barley, wheat, oats, and rye	90.9%–99.0%	Paliwal et al., 2003
MLNN	Classification of apples	96.6%	Yang, 1993
BPNN, PNN, GRNN, KNN	Classification of cereal grains	97% for wheat and oats, 88% for barley and rye	Paliwal et al., 2001
BPNN	Recognition and classification of weeds and crops	80%–100% for corn; 60%–80% for weeds	Yang et al., 2000a
MLP	Watercore sorting system for apple	92%	Kim and Schatzki, 2000
BPNN	Identification of wholesome and unwholesome poultry carcasses	91.1%–97.5% for whole carcasses; 83.3%–93.5% for carcass parts	Park and Chen, 2000
MLNN	Grading of pistachio nuts	95.9%	Ghazanfari et al., 1998

(*Continued*)

Table 3.1 (Continued) Applications of Artificial Neural Networks for Classification of Images in Food- and Agriculture-Related Research

Type of ANN architecture	Application	Accuracy	Reference
NN	Color grading of apples	95%	Nakano, 1997
Multilayer feedforward	Classification of defects in hardwood species	95%	Schmoldt et al., 1997
BPNN	Quality inspection of potatoes	74%, 73.3%, and 56% for greening, shape detection, and bruise detection, respectively	Deck et al., 1995

green, blue, hue, saturation, and intensity), and texture features (mean, range, variance, entropy, energy, contrast, correlation, inverse difference moment, and homogeneity) were extracted from the images. A multilayer feedforward model with back propagation algorithm was used for the study. In the input layer, the number of neurons was the same as the number of input features and the number of neurons in the output layer was the same as the number of fruit categories (five) that need to be classified. The classification results using color features was 89%, 90%, 87%, 88%, and 87% for apple, chikoo, mango, orange, and sweet lemon, and using textural features, the classification accuracies were higher as 90%, 93%, 90%, 91%, and 91%, respectively. The classification accuracies increased slightly with combined color and texture features to 93%, 94%, 92%, 92%, and 93%, respectively.

Narendra and Hareesh (2011) developed a multilayer feedforward with back propagation neural network model for classification of cashew kernels. In the input layer, the number of neurons was 15 (same as the number of input features) and the number of neurons in the output layer was 6 (number of categories of cashew kernels to be classified) and the number of neurons in the hidden layer was 10. A classification accuracy of 90% was obtained using an ANN model for six categories of cashew.

Effendi et al. (2010) evaluated the potential of an artificial neural network for identification of *Jatropha curcas* fruit maturity and grading the fruits based on maturity. A feedforward neural network with back propagation algorithm was used for the study. The database contained 27 images, of which 15 were used for training and 12 were used for testing. The color and shape features were extracted from the fruit for classification as raw, fruit aged, ripe, and overripe. The accuracy of classification was 95% and when assessed with different sets of images other than that used for training, the BPNN was able to classify them accordingly. As the neural network provided good accuracy of classification, the next objective was to train from live data directly from the tool.

OuYang et al. (2010) developed a BPNN algorithm for identifying five varieties of rice. Every image contained 100 kernels and after acquisition, images were segmented and features extracted. The back propagation algorithm was used to perform network training and a data set of 500 samples was used for training purposes and 250 samples were used for validation. A third data set of 250 samples was used for testing the neural network. The classification accuracies of five varieties of rice were 99.99%, 99.93%, 98.89%, 82.82%, and 86.65% for No. 5 Xiannong, Jinyougui, You166, No. 3 Xiannong, and MediumYou varieties, respectively.

Kiliç et al. (2007) developed an artificial neural network system for classification of beans based on size, color, and damage of the beans. After segmentation of the image, morphological operations were performed to determine the length, width, center, pixel coordinates, and area of each sample, because length and width are important features for classification based on size. Based on color, the samples were classified as A (white), B (yellow-green), and C (black). The beans were further classified as AA, BB, BC, CB, or CC, where the second characters A, B, and C stands for undamaged, <50% damaged, and >50% damaged, respectively. The ANN was trained using 69 samples and validated with 71 samples. Another set of 371 bean samples was used for testing and the classification accuracy was compared with the results of human inspectors. Overall classification accuracy of the system was 90.6%. The system has high reproducibility and the performance of the system was also measured based on time consumption and it performed better than human inspectors. They concluded that classification of bean images using an ANN had higher accuracy, lower misclassification, higher reproducibility, and lower time compared to human inspectors.

Visen et al. (2004a) developed neural network algorithms for classification of various types of grain such as wheat, durum wheat, rye, barley, and oats. Classification models were developed with five types of features sets: the first set consisted of 123 color features, the second of 56 textural features, the third set consisted of all color and textural features, and the fourth and fifth were the subsets of the third with the top 10 and 20 color and textural features combined. A four-layer back propagation neural network classifier was developed and trained with color and textural features. The trained network was then used to classify the various grain types. The overall classification accuracies for all types of grain were around 98% and the best classification accuracies were obtained for combined color and textural features.

Paliwal et al. (2003) compared the performance of neural network and statistical classifier for identification of various grains. Color, morphological, and textural features were extracted from the images and the classification was carried out by a four-layer BPNN and a nonparametric statistical classifier. The classification accuracies for all feature models using BPNN were 98.2%, 90.9%, 98.6%, 98.4%, and 99.0% for barley, CWAD wheat, CWRS wheat, oats, and rye, respectively, whereas the accuracies using a statistical classifier were 85.1%, 88.9%, 96.9%, 95.0%, and 96.4%, respectively. Paliwal et al. recommended the BPNN for classification of cereal grains as it provides higher classification accuracies compared to a statistical classifier.

Wang et al. (2003) developed a neural network model to evaluate the vitreousness of durum wheat. BPNN architecture was used to classify the samples as hard vitreous and amber color (HVAC), and not hard vitreous and amber color (NHVAC). The number of input was the same as the number of features used for the classification of kernels, whereas the output was equal to the number of classes that need to be separated. Samples were used from three subclasses of HVAC and six subclasses of NHVAC for the study. Several models were developed based on various combinations of classes, number of nodes in the hidden layers, and number of training epochs. Classification accuracies of 85% to 90% were obtained for HVAC and NHVAC.

Paliwal et al. (2001) evaluated the performance of various neural network architectures, including BPNN, PNN, GRNN, and Kohonen neural network (KNN). Network training was provided with morphological features as inputs and network training was provided on 70% of data and cross-validation on 20% of data. To reduce the mean square error between the observed and predicted outputs, the weights and threshold of each neuron was adjusted. To obtain the best results, the number of hidden nodes was varied and training was ended after 1000 epochs. The performance of the network was assessed based on classification accuracy, complexity of the network, and the time needed to train the network. Of the various networks evaluated, the performance of BPNN was superior to other networks and an advantage of BPNN is that it could interpret unknown patterns. The PNN displayed an acceptable performance but it required a long time for training. Since all the patterns are retained in PNN, the size of the network is large. The advantage of PNN is that when the network is trained once, more patterns for training can be included without the necessity to provide training to the network again. The performance of the GRNN was not satisfactory because it performs better in sparse data rather than a large database. The KNN showed an acceptable performance but it was not advisable for agricultural products because it lacks the ability to learn nonuniformly distributed probability density function and does not perform well in interpolation of unknown patterns (Mehrotra et al., 1996). They concluded that BPNN was the most suitable neural network classifier and GRNN was the least suitable for classification of agricultural products.

Yang et al. (2000a) explored the possibility of differentiating between weeds and crops using an ANN. The images were acquired from two experimental fields of corn, *Zea mays* (L.) and seven weed species, which occur commonly in the field. The BPNN was used for the study and the objective was just to differentiate weeds from the corn plant and it was not trained to differentiate between the species of weed. The training was conducted until completion of 2000 epochs (cycle) or a maximum acceptable sum-squared error was obtained. The ANN classified corn plants from images of weeds with an accuracy of 80% to 100%, whereas the identification of weeds from images of corn was between 70% and 80%. The accuracy of recognition was higher for corn than for weeds. The results of the study indicate the potential of an ANN for classification of plants and weeds, which can be useful for site-specific herbicide and weed control applications.

Schmoldt et al. (1997) proposed an ANN-based method for identification of bark, knots, splits, decay, and sound wood in several species of hardwoods. Computed tomography images were acquired and initial thresholding was performed to separate wood from background. A multilayer feedforward neural network was used to conduct a pixel-by-pixel defect classification. The ANN classifier has the potential to classify with an accuracy of 95% for the various defects in wood species such as oak and yellow poplar.

Nakano (1997) studied the potential of grading apples using neural networks. Based on external appearance, apples were classified into five grades: superior (AA, greater than 89% of surface is deep red), excellent (A, 70%–89% of area is red with yellowish-orange background), good (B, 50%–69% of surface area is red and yellowish-green background), poor (C, less than 50% of surface is red), and injured (D, surface of apple is injured). Two neural network models were developed, one to determine whether the surface color was normal or abnormal red, and the second model was to grade the apple into either one of five categories. The first model classified the apples almost correctly with an accuracy of 95% for normal red, poor red, and injured red color while few misclassifications happened; injured apple surfaces were classified as vines. The second model had a good classification of 92.5%, 65.8%, 87.2%, and 75.0% for superior (AA), good (B), poor color (C), and injured (D), respectively, whereas grade A (excellent) had a very low classification of 33.3%.

Egelberg et al. (1995) assessed the quality of cereal grain with the help of an instrument, GrainCheck 310™, using ANN. The classification was performed using MLP and the samples were classified as wheat, rye, oat, barley, triticale, green kernels, burned kernels, damaged kernels, wild oat, and impurities (such as dockage, stones, or weed seeds). The classification results compared well with the manual results. They concluded that the GrainCheck instrument developed for cereal grain quality assessment provided robust and consistent results, and meets the requirements of the industry.

3.3   Statistical classifiers

The statistical classification is characterized by using a probability model that provides the probability of classifying an image to a specific class rather than a simple classification. Statistical classifiers can be divided into two groups, namely, parametric and nonparametric.

3.3.1   Different types of statistical classifiers

3.3.1.1   Linear and quadratic discriminant analysis

Discriminant analysis methods determine an optical classification rule by minimizing an estimated error quantity, which is obtained by replacing a probability function with an estimated probability function. The linear discriminant analysis (LDA) is used where the two classes have normal distribution with different mean vectors but equal covariance matrices, and quadratic discriminant analysis (QDA) fits better with different covariance matrices (Schumann, 1997). The basis of discriminant analysis is to determine the relationship between a single dependent variable and a set of quantitative independent variables.

In LDA classification, grouping of data is achieved by minimizing the variance within group and maximizing the variance between groups. The LDA method focusses on determining optimal linear boundaries between the classes, a feature reduction method, and achieves maximum separation among different classes and tends to classify the unknown object based on Euclidean distance (Sharaf et al., 1986; Vasighi and Kompany-Zareh, 2012).

The LDA is a statistical method to determine the linear combination of features that provides best separation of two or more classes or objects. Linear discriminants are most commonly used to discriminate when there are two classes, although they can discriminate any number of classes. Fisher's discriminant acts as the benchmark for linear discriminant analysis between two classes (Cooke, 2002). Fisher's linear discriminant is an empirical method that is entirely based on attribute vectors. A hyperplane is selected to separate the known classes, and the points are categorized based on which side of the hyperplane they fall. LDA has the same covariance matrix, and the approach is ideal as long as the differences in variability are moderate and the sample size is small. To allocate an unknown object to any one of the predetermined groups, the LDA classifier uses a pooled covariance in Bayes criteria. For classification of unknown objects, QDA uses the covariance of each group rather than pooling them in Bayes criteria for classification purposes (Naes et al., 2002; Singh et al., 2009a). Fisher's discriminant analysis (FDA) is a classical approach to metric learning which utilizes the pairwise similarity and dissimilarity for classification of images (Song et al., 2013).

Quadratic discrimination is the same as linear discrimination except that the boundary between the two regions is a quadratic surface. QDA is one among the most commonly used nonlinear techniques for pattern classification. The covariance matrices are different and are more flexible than LDA. QDA requires a huge sample size and performs better as the sample size gets larger.

3.3.1.2   Mahalanobis distance classifier

The Mahalanobis distance classifier determines the similarity of a data set from an unknown sample to a data set from known samples. Since Mahalanobis distance is determined based on standard deviation from the mean of the training samples, a statistical measure of how much the unknown sample resembles (or does not) the actual training sample could be determined. The main advantage of using Mahalanobis distance is that it is highly sensitive to the intervariable changes that occur in the training data (Pydipati et al., 2005). The Mahalanobis distance classifier is similar to maximum likelihood classification but is a faster method because it makes an assumption that all class covariances are equal. The Mahalanobis classifier could be stated as a simplified version of LDA with an assumption that known groups have equal posterior probabilities. The Mahalanobis classifier provides a good classification result when the data distribution is elliptically concentrated and also when an unknown sample is allocated to a group with minimum Mahalanobis distance (Naes et al., 2002; Singh et al., 2009a). The drawback of Mahalanobis distance is that when the feature is distorted by noise, due to squaring of the distances, a single feature due to its high values can cover up the information provided by other features, which may result in misclassification (Wölfel and Ekenel, 2005).

3.3.1.3   K-nearest neighbor

The *K*-nearest neighbor (KNN) classification separates the data into two sets: test and training set. For every row of the test set data, the *K*-nearest training set objects are determined and classified based on the majority rule. The KNN is a conventional nonparametric classifier that provides good classification performance for optimum *k* values. KNN classifies a pattern *x* by allocating it to the class that is very frequently represented among its *k* nearest patterns (Joshi et al., 2013).

To demonstrate the working of KNN, let us consider classification of a new object (query point) among a number of known objects. In Figure 3.6, the known objects are circles and plus sign, and the query point is a question mark. The task is to classify the question mark into either a circle or plus sign group based on the nearest neighbor. If we consider the case of 1-nearest neighbor, since the closest neighbor to the query point is a plus sign, it will be grouped in the plus sign class. If 2-nearest neighbors are considered, the second nearest neighbor is a circle; KNN will not be able to classify the outcome, since both the groups have similar score. If we consider the case of 5-nearest neighbors, the query point will be classified into the circle group, because in the nearest neighbor region of query point, three circles and two plus sign are present (StatSoft, Inc., 2013). KNN is a powerful algorithm for classification of objects depending on the closest training examples present in the feature space. An object is categorized based on the majority of its neighbors and is allocated to the class that is most common among its nearest neighbors (Patil et al., 2011).

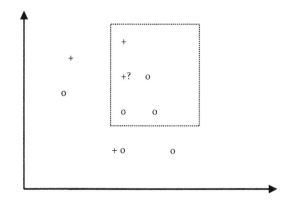

Figure 3.6 Classification by *K*-nearest neighbor.

The KNN classifier is a simple and efficient classifier based on distance. It does not require any training computations, but its testing time increases linearly with the size of the training set (Satti et al., 2013).

3.3.1.4 Support vector machine

A support vector machine (SVM) is a statistical learning theory used to classify unknown data by using training data as an input to create a decision function as an output. The SVM consists of linear and nonlinear classifiers (Pouladzadeh et al., 2012; Titova et al., 2013). The SVM classifies a group of samples into two different classes that are separated by a hyperplane that is defined in a suitable space. The basic concept of SVM is to construct a hyperplane that acts as a decision line that separates one class from the other in a binary classification. With a single SVM, it is possible to discriminate between only two different classes, but there are strategies that can be followed to adopt SVM for classification of more than two classes (Vapnik, 1998). When using a hyperplane to classify two possible classes, the objects nearer to the margin make a vector referred to as support vector (Figure 3.7). The optimization of margin is made easier with the support vector. The classification margin, which is determined by the hyperplane position, always corresponds to any changes in support vector but the hyperplane remains independent of any changes occurring to any item other than support vector. The main aim of the SVM method is to determine an optimum kernel function that can be used to represent the data to multidimensional feature space (Hassan and Al-Saqer, 2011).

The SVM is a superior machine learning statistical algorithm and it employs optimization algorithms to establish optimal boundaries between classes. The advantages of SVM are that it models nonlinear class boundaries, and overfitting is unlikely to occur. In SVM, the complexity of decision rule and the frequency of error are easy to control. The limitations of SVM are that the training is slow when compared to Bayes and decision trees. When the training data are not linearly separable, it is difficult to find optimal parameters and the structure of algorithm is difficult to understand. The training speed of the technique depends on the training data size, class separability, and kernel parameters, and the accuracy of the technique depends on the optimal hyperplane selection (Seetha et al., 2008).

For classification of more than two classes, the algorithm first collects data from each classifier and assembles the data to create a graph or tree consisting of many nodes such

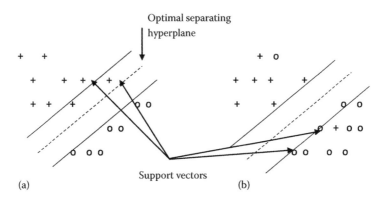

Figure 3.7 Support vector machine, an optimal hypersurface. (a) Linear and (b) nonlinear class separation.

that every node represents results from each binary classifier. Hence, it is possible to achieve classification of more than two classes by including more nodes on the trees (Nashat et al., 2011). The SVM models use a kernel function and act as an alternate method of training for classifiers such as linear, polynomial, and RBF in which the network weights are determined by solving a quadratic programming problem with linear constraints, instead of solving the unconstrained minimization problem as in neural network training (Palmieri and Fiore, 2010; Kaur and Singh, 2013).

3.3.2   *Potential of statistical classifiers for image classification related to food and agriculture applications*

Table 3.2 shows the applications of statistical classifiers for image classification in various research studies.

Luo et al. (1999a) studied the potential of machine vision for classification of sound wheat and six types of damaged kernels of Canada West Red Spring (CWRS). Different morphological and color features were extracted, and parametric and nonparametric (KNN) statistical classification methods were tested. The results of the study showed that the nonparametric method provided better classification accuracies of 93%, 90%, 99%, 99%, 99%, 98%, and 100% for healthy, broken, green-frosted, smudged, mildewed, heated, and fire-burnt kernels, respectively. They concluded that a nonparametric classifier, such as a KNN classifier, provided the best classification accuracies for wheat.

Mahesh et al. (2008) explored the possibility of near-infrared (NIR) hyperspectral imaging to distinguish between Canadian wheat classes and used LDA, QDA, and BPNN methods for classification purposes. The results of the study showed that classification accuracies for LDA and QDA models were 94% to 100% and 86% to 100%, respectively, for classification of various wheat classes. The classification accuracy of ANN models was 80% to 100% with greater than 90% accuracy for validation sets of ANN. Their study showed that both statistical and neural network classifiers have the potential to effectively classify various wheat classes.

Singh et al. (2009a) proposed an NIR hyperspectral imaging for detection of sprout- and midge-damaged wheat kernels. They used different types of statistical classifiers such as QDA, LDA, and Mahalanobis. The classification accuracy for healthy wheat kernels using LDA and QDA were more than 95%, whereas Mahalanobis accuracy was around 85%. The classification accuracy for sprout-damaged kernels were 100% for all three types of classifiers. The classification accuracy for midge-damaged kernels using LDA and QDA classifiers were lower in the range of 83% to 100%, whereas the Mahalanobis classifier had a higher accuracy of 91% to 100%. They concluded that statistical classifiers have the potential to classify sprout- and midge-damaged wheat grains with higher accuracy by LDA and QDA for healthy kernels, and the Mahalanobis classifier provides better classification accuracy for midge-damaged kernels.

Singh et al. (2012) examined the possibility of NIR hyperspectral imaging for identification of fungal damaged wheat kernels and used various statistical classifiers such as LDA, QDA, and Mahalanobis. The LDA classifier provided the highest classification accuracy of 97.3% to 100% for classification of sound and fungal damaged kernels. The QDA and Mahalanobis classifier had a classification accuracy of 97.3% to 99.3% and 98.0% to 99.3%, respectively.

Manickavasagan et al. (2010) proposed a thermal imaging method for classification of wheat classes and used QDA with bootstrap and leave-one-out methods for validation of

Table 3.2 Potential of Statistical Classifiers in Applications Related to Food and Agriculture

Type of statistical classifier	Application	Accuracy	Reference
SVM	Classification and grading of rice	86%	Kaur and Singh, 2013
LDA, QDA, Mahalanobis	Detection and classification of fungal damaged wheat	99% of fungal damaged and 96%–97.7% for healthy kernels	Singh et al., 2012
SVM	Classification of dried jujubes	98.15%	Lou et al., 2012
SVM	Classification of various food types	92.6%	Pouladzadeh et al., 2012
SVM	Classification of tomato		Fojlaley et al., 2012
SVM	Grading and classification of apples	100%	Suresha et al., 2012
SVM	Identification of pecan weevils in pecan nuts	97%–99%	Hassan and Al-Saqer, 2011
SVM	Quality inspection of biscuits	96%	Nashat et al., 2011
LDA, QDA	Classification of sprout-damaged wheat and barley	88.2% and 98.1% for LDA; 88.7% and 95.1% for QDA for healthy and sprout damaged, respectively	Vadivambal et al., 2010a,b
QDA	Classification of wheat classes	Ranging from 64% to 95% for different models	Manickavasagan et al., 2010
Not available	Classification of cereal grains, wheat and barley	76%	Douik and Abdellaoui, 2010
LDA, QDA, Mahalanobis	Classification of sprout- and midge-damaged wheat	LDA and QDA 95%, Mahalanobis 85% for healthy; 100% for sprout damaged by three; 83%–100% midge damaged by LDA, QDA; 91%–100% by Mahalanobis	Singh et al., 2009a
LDA, QDA	Classification of various wheat varieties	94%–100%, 86%–100% for LDA and QDA	Mahesh et al., 2008
LDA, QDA	To detect and classify insect infested and healthy wheat kernels	LDA, 77.6% and 83.0%; QDA, 83.5% and 77.7% for infested and sound kernels	Manickavasagan et al., 2008a
Discriminant analysis	Identification of citrus peel disease	96.7%	Qin et al., 2008

(Continued)

Table 3.2 (Continued) Potential of Statistical Classifiers in Applications Related
to Food and Agriculture

Type of statistical classifier	Application	Accuracy	Reference
Discriminant analysis	Quality monitoring of bakery products	88%	Abdullah et al., 2000
Non-parametric	Classification of barley, wheat, oats, and rye	85.1%–96.9%	Paliwal et al., 2003
LDA, QDA	Classification of poultry carcasses	91.4% and 75% for LDA and QDA, respectively, for unwholesome carcasses	Park et al., 2002
Parametric and nonparametric statistical classifier	Identification of healthy and damaged wheat kernels	90%–100%	Luo et al., 1999b
Discriminant analysis	Quality assessment and classification of edible beans	84.7%	Chtioui et al., 1999
Fisher's linear discriminant analysis	Quality inspection of potatoes	70.0%, 68.1%, and 76.7% for greening, shape detection, and bruise detection, respectively	Deck et al., 1995

discriminant function. Leave-one-out uses a single observation as a validation data from the original sample and the remaining observations are used as training data sets. This process is repeatedly performed until each observation is used as the validation data once. The bootstrap method is a resampling method used for estimating the distribution of statistics that are based on independent observations. The classification of the QDA model with bootstrap validation resulted in an accuracy range of 54% to 88%, whereas the leave-one-out method resulted in 40% to 84% accuracy. They concluded that bootstrap validation yielded higher accuracy for classification of eight classes of wheat. Manickavasagan et al. (2008b) evaluated the potential of thermal imaging to detect *Cryptolestes ferrugineus* in wheat kernels and used LDA and QDA statistical methods for classification of infested and healthy kernels. The classification accuracy for QDA was 83.5% and 77.7% for infested and healthy kernels, respectively, and for LDA was 77.6% and 83.0%, respectively.

Kaur and Singh (2013) proposed an algorithm for classification and grading of rice into premium quality, and grade A, B, and C using multiclass SVM. Eight hundred kernels were selected with 200 kernels from each group (chalky, broken, long and round, and sound) and were divided into two groups of 400 kernels for training and testing. Statistical characteristics, such as length, area, and perimeter, provided effective classification features. The SVM was able to classify different grades of rice with an accuracy of 86%.

Pouladzadeh et al. (2012) proposed a novel SVM-based method for recognition of various food types and extraction of nutrient information from the classified food. The data set comprised of 12 different food and fruit images of which 50% were used for training and another 50% for testing. From the acquired images, color, texture, size, and shape features were extracted and these characteristics were fed into the classification phase, where SVM was used as a classifier. A recognition rate of 92.6% was achieved based on the proposed algorithm. Fojlaley et al. (2012) proposed a neural network and SVM methods for classification of tomato and stated that performance of SVM classifier was better than the neural networks. Suresha et al. (2012) developed a SVM-based algorithm for grading of apples and showed that 100% accuracy could be obtained in grading apples using SVM.

Hassan and Al-Saqer (2011) evaluated the potential of SVM for identifying pecan weevils in the pecan nuts. To perform SVM, they selected polynomial function and radial basis function since these two functions provide better results for pattern-recognition problems. The database consisted of 205 images of pecan weevils with wide variation in the insects' age, size, and gender. The acquired images were processed to binary images. The proposed algorithm successfully identified 99% of pecan weevil and 97% of other insects using RBF and it required around 31 s for processing 75% of the data and the testing time was 0.15 s. They concluded that promising results were obtained in recognition of pecan weevil by using SVM.

Nashat et al. (2011) proposed a SVM approach for real-time quality monitoring of biscuits. The SVM was used to categorize biscuits into four classes: underbaked, moderately baked, overbaked, and significantly overbaked. The color inspection was composed of two steps: preprocessing and postprocessing. Preprocessing included image acquisition and smoothing, color transformation from RGB to HLS, and segmentation. Postprocessing involves dimensionality reduction and applying SVM to achieve classification of biscuits. A classification accuracy of 96% was achieved for stationary and moving biscuits. There was no significant impact on whether the biscuits were touching or not touching during the assessment of baking, but the processing time for biscuits in contact was higher, averaging 36.3 ms and 9.0 ms for touching and nontouching biscuits, respectively.

3.3.3 Studies involving both statistical and neural network classifiers

Seed classification is a critical process in seed production, quality control, and impurities identification. Pandey et al. (2013) performed classification of seeds using Euclidean distance and ANN classifiers. Images of seeds of wheat, rice, and gram were captured, and color and shape features were extracted from the images. Of the 200 images acquired, 150 were used for training purposes and 50 images were used for testing purposes. The classification accuracy of the Euclidean distance classifier was 84.4% whereas that of the ANN was 95% leading to conclusion that ANN provides more accurate results for classification of seeds.

Satti et al. (2013) developed a leaf recognition system for identification of plant species based on computer vision. A total of 1907 sample images of 33 different plant species were taken from a Flavia data set. Images were preprocessed, features were extracted, and classification was performed using ANN and KNN classifiers. The classification accuracy of ANN and KNN classifiers were 93.3% and 85.9%, respectively. The ANN performs better for the data set with a large number of images, whereas in a smaller data set KNN outperforms ANN. Also based on the time consumed by the classifiers, KNN performs faster in smaller data sets, whereas ANN is best suited for larger data sets.

Khoje et al. (2013) developed a fruit grading system based on skin defect identification, and performed the classification of images using SVM and PNN. Images of guava and lemon fruits were acquired and textural features were extracted. The overall classification accuracy of the SVM classifier was 91.41% and 91.72% for guava and lemon, respectively, and for PNN was 82.85% and 89.45%, respectively. Based on the results of the study, they concluded that performance of the SVM classifier was better than PNN, and the SVM method was recommended for skin defect identification and classification of fruits.

Mallick and Rout (2013) developed an ANN and SVM classifier for classification of food grains that look similar (such as finger millet and mustard, pigeon pea and soybean, cumin seeds and aniseeds, and split black gram and green gram). A block diagram for similar looking food grains classification is shown in Figure 3.8. The HSV components were separated from RGB components and 18 color features were extracted. A multilevel wavelet decomposition technique was used to extract information about the intensity variation of similar looking grains. The models were developed using BPNN and SVM, and the classification was performed using three types of feature sets such as color, wavelet, texture, and their combined model. The results showed that combined features provided better classification and ANN classification provided higher accuracy than the SVM model. But the time taken for training the SVM model was significantly less compared to ANN.

Citrus trees affected by disease result in an adverse effect on tree health, yield, and economic productivity. Early identification of disease symptoms is an important aspect of disease prevention and control. Pydipati et al. (2005) proposed a method for disease detection in citrus leaves using machine vision by applying statistical and neural network classifiers. Images of citrus leaves were acquired and preprocessed to remove unwanted noise, edge detection was performed to detect boundaries, and feature extraction was completed. Finally classification of images was performed using statistical (Mahalanobis classifier) and neural network (BPNN and RBF) methods. The overall classification accuracy of statistical classifier with Mahalanobis minimum distance classifier was 98% and BPNN was 98% followed by an RBF neural network method with an accuracy of 96% for classification of disease-affected citrus leaves. The authors concluded that they recommend Mahalanobis distance classifiers and BPNN classifiers for further studies involving disease-affected leaves in the actual outdoor scenario.

Hobani et al. (2003) developed an ANN classifier for classification of date fruits based on physical attributes. Seven varieties of date samples were imaged and seven classification models were developed based on physical and color attributes. A multilayer perceptron neural network model was used for classification of dates and an LDA was used for classification using a statistical technique. The result of the classification accuracy for ANN was in the range of 85.7% to 99.6% and for the statistical classifier in the range of 86.6% to 99.4%. ANN provided the best classification accuracy, although the accuracy of the statistical classifier was also close to ANN.

Ghazanfari et al. (1998) developed a machine vision technique for grading pistachio nuts. From the gray scale image of nuts, gray level histograms were obtained, and the mean of the histogram and area of the nut were features selected that were used as inputs for the

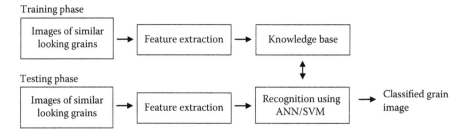

Figure 3.8 Block diagram showing methodology for classification of similar looking grains. (From Mallick, P.K., and S. Rout, *International Journal on Advanced Computer Theory and Engineering*, 1, 139, 2013. With permission.)

classifier. They used statistical (Gaussian, decision tree) and neural network (multilayer neural network) classifiers. The MLNN had higher classification accuracy compared to the other two classifiers.

Timmermans and Hulzebosch (1996) developed a grading system for potted plants using ANN and statistical classifiers. Two types of plants—saintpaulia (African violets) and cactus—were selected for the study. Saintpaulia plants were sorted on color, size, and flowering stage, and cactus plants were classified into six classes based on number of shoots and area of shoots. The classification of plants was performed using LDA, QDA, and the NN classifiers. In classification of saintpaulia plants, performance of NN was better followed by QDA and LDA. In sorting of cactus plants, the error in classification for LDA, QDA, and ANN was 9.6%, 6.6%, and 1.6%, respectively. Based on the study, they concluded that ANN provided better classification results for complex applications but the disadvantage of the NN classifier is the optimization of the process because there is no universal network that can solve all classification problems. Hence building and learning of the network is a challenging task.

Deck et al. (1995) compared the performance of a neural network and Fisher's discriminant classifier for quality evaluation of potatoes. Images were acquired using CCD cameras and RGB images were converted to an HSI image format. Three types of defects—shape, greening, and bruising—were tested. The results of the study showed that the back propagation neural network with three hidden nodes classified potatoes with greening with an accuracy of 74% compared to 70% accuracy for Fisher's method. The BPNN with seven hidden nodes resulted in a classification accuracy of 73.3% for shape classification compared with 68.1% accuracy of Fisher's method. The classification accuracy for bruised potatoes was higher for Fisher's method at 76.7% compared to the accuracy of BPNN at 56%. They concluded that BPNN performed better than Fisher's method except for the classification of bruised potatoes. The BPNN trained better than Fisher's method if the test data were represented closely by training data.

3.4   Comparison of statistical and neural network classifiers

Statistical classifiers are explained mostly in terms of equations and formulas, whereas neural networks are described mostly in terms of graphical representation. Neural networks are more often described in terms of their architecture and their learning algorithms, whereas statistical methods are defined in terms of mathematical models that are used and statistical properties of the results (Couvreur and Couvreur, 1997).

Researchers have agreed that with regard to classification accuracy, ANN outperforms statistical regression (Masters, 1994). As the dimensionality or the nonlinearity of the problem increases, the traditional regression procedures are unsuccessful in producing accurate approximation and the superiority of ANNs increases. In the polynomial approach, the limited ability of the statistical approach is clear because as the number of independent variable N increases, the number of polynomial parameter grows as N^m, where m is the order of polynomial. Whereas in ANNs, the number of parameters increases either linearly (as N) or quadratically (N^2) for m hidden units (Bishop, 1995). In solving a problem, the choice between statistical and ANN approaches depends on the choice of the problem to be solved. In solving problems of perception such as vision or speech, ANNs outperform the statistical approach, whereas for approximation of simple functions or modeling data of low dimensionality, statistical techniques should be used first to solve the problem, and ANN should be used only if higher accuracy is expected (Schalkoff, 1997; Basheer and Hajmeer, 2000).

In the statistical approach, the analysis is limited to a certain number of interactions, whereas in ANN many terms can be examined for interactions. Neural networks perform better for prediction, modeling, and optimization even if the data are not complete and are noisy. Neural networks are also suitable when the input or the output cannot be represented in mathematical terms or is qualitative in nature (Pandharipande, 2004). Unlike traditional methods, neural networks have an ability to learn about systems that need to be modeled without any knowledge of process parameters. Also, ANN has the ability to relearn according to new data and it is possible to add new data (Vassileva et al., 2000; Bhotmange and Shastri, 2011).

Multilayer neural network classifiers have the advantages of massive parallel processing, adaptivity, and fault tolerance. Jayas et al. (2000) stated that MLNN is best suited for classification of biological materials and it could be a potential tool for grading and sorting of agricultural products. Kim and Schatzki (2000) used ANN for sorting watercore-affected apples and stated that the algorithm can process 100 apples per second, which is a good processing speed to be implemented in a commercial apple grading facility.

The superiority of either the statistical or neural network method depends on the effort made during the design phase of the algorithm relevant to the choice of architecture, learning parameters, and so on. For instance, the superiority of KNN statistical or MLP neural network classifiers over one another depends on the efforts made for selection of most appropriate value for k in the KNN algorithm or selection of suitable architecture and learning parameters for the MLP network. Giacinto et al. (1999) suggested a combination of neural network and statistical classifiers to obtain higher accuracy values.

3.5   *Fuzzy logic*

Fuzzy logic is based on the concept of reasoning rather than in answering based on Boolean methods as computers do (i.e., yes or no or 0/1). Fuzzy logic theory explains the partial truth concept, that is, truth values between 0 and 1 (1 is completely true and 0 is completely false) and allows intermediate values that could be defined, which allows a more human way of thinking. The concept of fuzzy logic was introduced by Lotfi A. Zadeh in 1965 to model the complexity and vagueness in complex systems. To overcome the imperfections in analyzing data, fuzzy logic and probability theory are powerful tools. Fuzzy logic deals with representation and processing of vague and uncertain data, whereas probability is responsible for representation of uncertainty or randomness (Tizhoosh, 2012).

The applications of fuzzy logic are broad and provide an opportunity for modeling a variety of situations that are not precisely defined, and with the help of fuzzy logic many systems can be modeled and simulated (Brule, 1985). Variables are explained in fuzzy sets and rules are defined by combining the fuzzy sets logically. The fuzzy system is a combination of fuzzy sets together with fuzzy rules that relates input fuzzy set to an output fuzzy set (NATO, 1998).

Fuzzy image processing could be explained as a gathering of different approaches that represent and process the images and their features as fuzzy sets. The processing and representation depends on the chosen fuzzy technique. The basic structure of fuzzy image processing is shown in Figure 3.9. There are three main stages in fuzzy image processing: image fuzzification, membership modification, and image defuzzification (Tizhoosh, 1997).

Fuzzification represents the coding of image data and defuzzification is the decoding of results. These stages enable one to process an image with fuzzy technique. The intermediate step, the modification of membership, is an important step in which after the

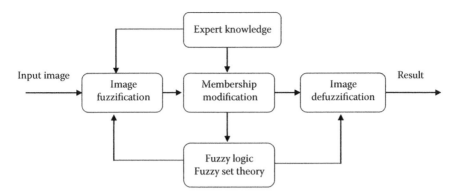

Figure 3.9 The basic structure of fuzzy image processing. (From Tizhoosh, H.R., *Fuzzy image processing: Introduction in theory and practice*, 1997. With kind permission from Springer Science+Business Media B.V.)

image data are converted from the gray level plane, fuzzy techniques like fuzzy clustering, fuzzy integration approach and fuzzy rule-based approach, are applied followed by defuzzification.

Kavdir and Guyer (2003) developed a fuzzy logic technique for grading and classifying apples based on external features and compared the results of the fuzzy logic approach with results from sensory evaluation by a human expert panel. In the fuzzy logic decision-making process, three main operations were involved: fuzzy input and output selection, formation of fuzzy rules, and deriving fuzzy inferences. Artificial defects were not forced on apples but those with naturally occurring defects were considered for the study. Quality features, such as color, defect, shape, size, and weight, were measured, and the apples were graded into three quality groups (good, medium, and bad). The fuzzy membership functions, fuzzification and defuzzification, were performed in MATLAB® and then the apples were graded by human experts. Grading of apples by the fuzzy logic technique had a good agreement (about 89%) with the results from the human expert panel. Shahin and Tollner (1997) classified apples based on watercore features using fuzzy logic and obtained a classification accuracy of 72%, and was suggested by authors that low classification accuracy could have been due to variations in the visual properties of fruit. The authors suggested that for grading of apples, although NN is a powerful tool for accurate classification of them it involves high computational cost, whereas fuzzy logic technique involves less computational cost.

Chacon et al. (2002) described the various approach of fuzzy logic in image processing and explained fuzzy binarization, fuzzy edge detection, and fuzzy geometry measurement. Yang et al. (2000b) used fuzzy logic decision-making for precision farming in recognizing weeds in the field. While processing the image, green objects were identified using the greenness method, which compares the red, green, and blue intensities. The RGB matrix was converted to binary form by assigning a value of 1 if the green intensity was greater than the blue and red intensities of the pixel; otherwise the pixel value was assigned 0. The greenness area of weed coverage was computed based on the resulting binary matrix and the values of weed coverage and weed patch were provided as inputs to the fuzzy logic decision-making system. The results showed that a fuzzy strategy could reduce herbicide usage by 5% to 24% and a further on/off strategy resulted in herbicide reduction by 15% to 64%.

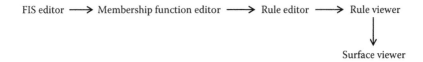

Figure 3.10 Fuzzy inference system (FIS).

Simonton and Graham (1996) developed a combined Bayesian pixel analysis using the color feature and fuzzy logic classifier using color and geometric features for structural analysis and identification of plant parts of geranium varieties. In pixel classification, the portion of the image associated with the plant is distinguished from the nonplant portion and employs Bayesian discriminant analysis. In fuzzy logic, plant part type was determined by first segmenting data and the decision process applied to classify the segments as stem, leaf, or petiole. The overall classification accuracy of leaf blades and petiole was 98% and 90% to 94% for the main stem.

Mustafa et al. (2009) developed a grading and sorting system for agricultural produce based on SVM and fuzzy logic. The automatic grading unit was designed to combine three processess: feature extraction, sorting, and grading. The features extracted were perimeter, area, major axis length, and minor axis length, and SVM was used for shape sorting. Fuzzy logic is an effective technique when human experience is required to be combined into the decision-making process and hence fuzzy logic was used for grading of the produce. The fuzzy inference system is shown in Figure 3.10 (Mathworks, 1998).

The grading was performed by first defining the number of system inputs and outputs, and further explaining the input and output membership function. The rules are based on if–then statements and in the rule editor, an expert knowledge is incorporated. The rule viewer was constructed from membership function and rules, and acts as a system diagnostic to display the rules that are active or how each membership function influences the result. The surface viewer exhibits the dependency of the output on the input and plots the system's output surface map. The grading system consists of three inputs (area, major length, and minor length) and one output (size of the produce). The classification accuracy was higher for apple, banana, and mango, whereas orange and carrot were wrongly classified as apple and banana. The grading accuracies for apple, banana, and mango were 98.85%, 98.75%, and 89.74%, respectively.

3.6   Conclusions

The artificial neural network is an efficient method for classification of images related to food and agricultural applications. When the neural network is properly structured with appropriate weights, the training of network is efficiently performed, which provides better classification accuracy. ANN can provide better solutions to problems involving nonlinearity, highly noisy, complex, and imperfect error prone sensor data (Rashmi and Mandar, 2011). Luo et al. (1999a) stated that multilayer neural networks were better than parametric classifiers in the classification of agricultural materials such as wheat. The performance of MLNN depends on the network architecture, especially the number of hidden layers and nodes in each hidden layer. In statistical classifiers, SVM was used for classification of various agricultural products such as rice (Kaur and Singh, 2013) and tomato (Fojlaley et al., 2012), and based on the results, it was concluded that SVM provided higher classification accuracies and could be used for classification purposes for online quality monitoring of various agricultural materials.

Roli et al. (1997) compared the performance of ANN and statistical methods for remote sensing applications and stated that no single algorithm is best suited for all applications. Appropriateness of methods depends on the selected data set and the efforts involved in the designing phase of the algorithm. The combination of two classifiers provided better accuracies than single classifiers. Deck et al. (1995) performed quality analysis of potatoes using BPNN classification and Fisher's linear discriminant analysis and concluded that each classifier performs better in classifying certain characteristics.

Regardless of the system's nonlinearity and the problem's dimensionality, the ability of ANN to learn the relationship between the input and output without explicit physical consideration and high tolerance for noisy data are the major reasons for the increased utilization of the ANN. But ANN is not the ultimate solution for all real-world problems because it has limitations. The limitations for use of ANN are that no defined rules or guidelines exist for the architecture design in ANN, and the inability to describe the procedure through which a final decision was made by the ANN (Basheer and Hajmeer, 2000). Other limitations of ANN are neural network models that are very complex for computation and need more training samples and the iterative training procedures converge slowly. Also, in classifying patterns that are not identical to training pattern, neural networks have difficulty compared to statistical methods. Hence, in classification of images, the performance of neural network models is based on having representative samples for training, while statistical methods need a suitable model for each class (Benediktsson et al., 1990). Vasighi and Kompany-Zareh (2012) stated that for certain types of data, simple linear discriminant analysis performs better than advanced, nonlinear techniques such as SVM and SOM methods, hence while dealing with various types of data, the proper selection of classification method is very critical for achieving higher classification accuracies.

The classification approach based on statistical and neural network methods have certain advantages and limitations. The selection of methods depends on the type of application and the type of image data to be classified. A combination of both approaches works well in some applications and also helps to increase the accuracy of classification.

chapter four

Imaging in the visible spectrum

4.1   Introduction

The origin of imaging technology started around 1960 and has seen a tremendous growth since its inception. The term *machine vision* is a popular term representing the wide range of technologies based on imaging, and provides automatic inspection and process control for various industrial applications. Computer vision is a technique of acquiring, analyzing, and processing of images to provide solutions for various product and process control operations in a wide range of industries. The optical imaging could belong to both machine vision and computer vision techniques, which provides solutions based on acquiring images in the visible range of spectrum.

Visible light falls in the range of 4×10^{-7} m (400 nm) to 7×10^{-7} m (700 nm) in the electromagnetic spectrum, which can be seen by the human eye (Figure 4.1). The visible spectrum is also termed the *optical spectrum* of light. The wavelength of the light determines the specific color and Table 4.1 lists the color corresponding to the specific wavelength in the visible spectrum.

Computer vision involving image processing has developed tremendously and is employed in many industries. Acquisition of images in the visible spectrum involves capturing images with analogue sensors followed by digitization or capturing images with digital sensors, which are then analyzed using image processing software. In many food processing plants, the quality evaluation is done manually by human inspectors. Manual inspection is laborious, tedious, inconsistent, and subjective. The role of computer vision and image processing has increased rapidly in the last two decades and many applications have gone beyond the research phase and are implemented in the commercial production line and in on-line quality monitoring applications. The sensors used for imaging in the visible spectrum, performance and comparison of sensors, and components of a visible imaging system and their applications are described in this chapter.

4.2   Image sensors and components of an imaging system

4.2.1   Sensors

Modern digital image sensors are solid-state image sensors mostly made of silicon. The major reason for using silicon is because it is a semiconductor and hence there exists an energy gap between its valence and conduction band known as bandgap. This bandgap is ideal for acquiring light in the visible region and near-infrared region. The bandgap for silicon is 1.1 eV. The visible light includes wavelengths between 400 and 700 nm, corresponding to photon energies of 2.75 eV and 1.9 eV, respectively. Depending on their energy, wavelength absorption occurs, and blue light (450 nm) is absorbed at the surface, while red light (650–700 nm) penetrates deeper into the silicon (York, 2011). Camera sensor technology is basically of two types: charge-coupled device (CCD) and complementary metal-oxide silicon (CMOS).

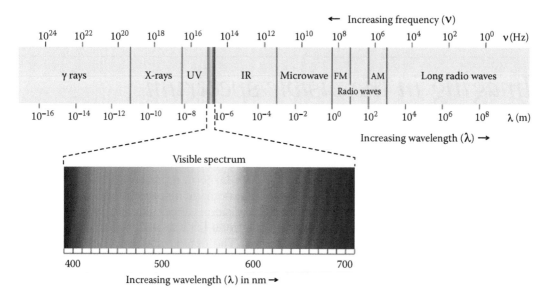

Figure 4.1 Electromagnetic spectrum showing the visible light region. (Wikipedia, 2013.)

Table 4.1 Colors Corresponding to the Wavelength in Visible Light Spectrum

Color	Wavelength (nm)
Red	625–740
Orange	590–625
Yellow	565–590
Green	520–565
Cyan	500–520
Blue	435–500
Violet	380–435

Source: Jones, A.Z., 2013, The visible light spectrum, http://physics.about.com/od/lightoptics/a /vislightspec.htm (accessed August 16, 2013).

4.2.1.1 *Charge-coupled device sensors*

Charge-coupled device (CCD) sensors were invented during the 1960s by researchers at Bell Labs, and these sensors were initially thought of as new types of computer memory circuit. But soon, other potential applications of CCDs, such as signal processing and imaging, were explored mainly due to the mild sensitivity of silicon that responds to wavelengths less than 1.1 μm. The ability of CCDs to detect light has made CCDs a premier image sensing technology. In CCD sensors, the charge is transferred from one pixel to another pixel until the end of periphery, which is then converted into voltage (York, 2011). CCD architectures are of three types, namely, frame transfer, interline transfer, and frame interline transfer. In frame transfer, the complete CCD image is shifted vertically in a column-parallel way. It takes only a millisecond to transfer the whole image and hence there are large smears. The interline transfer has a fill factor of around 20% or less but with microlenses, efficiency can be improved twice, with residual smear. A combination of both frame transfer and interline transfer approaches are used to reduce smear in frame inter-line transfer (Saleh and Aboulsoud, 2002).

CCD digital imaging sensors can acquire images in any of the three formats—point scanning, line scanning, and area scanning—each of these formats has specific applications. Point scanning uses a single pixel cell detector that scans an image sequentially through the X and Y coordinates and it is the simplest scanning technique. This kind of CCD detector is inexpensive and provides uniform measurement. However, the limitation of this system is that repeated numbers of exposures are needed to compose an entire image and registration errors can degrade images produced through the point scanning method. A line scanning detector scans along the linear axis to acquire a digital image, and each line of information acquired, stored, and then amplified before processing the next line. Linear scanners provide a higher rate of image acquisition and produce high resolution compared to single cell detectors. The scanning time is usually in the range of few seconds to minutes. Area scanning sensors use two-dimensional pixel array detectors that allow a whole image to be acquired with a single exposure. In area scanning, no movement of the image sensor is required and hence it does not require any costly translation devices. Of the three methods of scanning, image acquisition is fastest in area scanning with high registration accuracy between pixels. The limitations of area scanning are the lower resolution and reduced signal-to-noise performance compared to other devices, and it is generally expensive (Abramowitx and Davidson, 2010).

In traditional line scan cameras, an image is acquired line by line as the object moves past the sensor (Figure 4.2). Each line of reconstructed image is from a single short exposure; only a very little amount of light is collected and hence requires substantial illumination. This is overcome by time delay and integration (TDI) line scan cameras in which multiple linear arrays are placed side by side. After the exposure of the first array, charge is transferred to the next line and a second exposure is taken on top of the first and so on. Since each line of object is repeatedly imaged, cumulative exposure occurs, which reduces the noise thereby increasing the signal (Edmund Optics Inc., 2013).

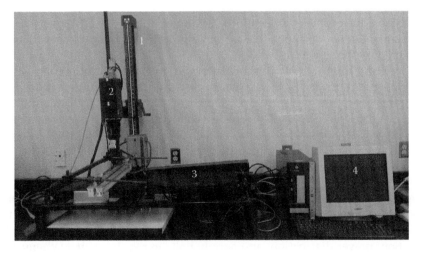

Figure 4.2 Line scan imaging system: (1) stand, (2) camera, (3) conveyor, and (4) image acquisition system. (Courtesy of Grain Storage Research Lab, University of Manitoba, Winnipeg, Canada.)

4.2.1.2 Complementary metal-oxide silicon sensors

Complementary metal-oxide silicon (CMOS) sensors sense the light the same way as CCD sensors, but there is a difference after the sensing of light. In CMOS sensors, the charge is not transferred along the pixel; rather each pixel has its own readout unit and light is converted at the pixel itself. In CMOS sensors, amplifiers are integrated directly into the pixel, which permits a parallel readout architecture in which each pixel can be individually addressed (York, 2011). CMOS sensors are classified as two main types based on pixel circuit architectures: passive pixel image sensor (PPS) and active pixel image sensor (APS). CMOS sensors have gained importance because of the demand for compact, low power, miniature digital imaging systems. Also CMOS offers submicron feature sizes and low junction leakage current. New circuit techniques permit a high dynamic range and low noise imaging that is on par with the best CCD sensors (Saleh and Aboulsoud, 2002).

4.2.2 Performance of image sensors

The common metric of image sensor performance is the pixel count, which is expressed in megapixels. In a sensor, the number of pixels depends on the chip area and the amount of chip dedicated for pixels versus digital logic and readout circuitry. Another performance metric is pixel pitch, which defines the amount of area each pixel in an array occupies. When the pitch is smaller, more pixels can be accommodated, but smaller pitches only acquire less light and hence are not suitable for higher frame rate imagers. Pixel fill factor describes how a pixel is physically laid out in a sensor. A pixel fill factor of 100% is ideal but not many sensors have a fill factor of 100% (York, 2011).

4.2.3 Comparison of CCD and CMOS sensors

In CCD sensors, the output analog signal needs to be converted to digital signal before it can be interpreted by the camera's image processing unit, whereas in CMOS sensors, digital output is directly obtained without the need for conversion. Compared to CCD sensors, CMOS sensors have lower power consumption and overheating does not easily happen (Esser, 2013). CMOS image sensors only consume about one-eighth power of CCD sensors, and the static power consumption of CMOS sensors is almost zero. Hence, CMOS sensors are more suitable for portable applications (Zhang et al., 2008). CMOS sensors are better than CCD sensors in responsivity, that is, for unit of input optical energy, the amount of signal delivered by the sensor (Litwiller, 2001).

Under identical illumination, the consistency of response of different pixels could be termed response uniformity. The uniformity of CMOS sensors under illumination and dark conditions are both worse than CCD sensors. The signal readout speed of CCD sensors is lower compared to CMOS sensors. Generally, signal readout speed is around 70 Mpixels/s for CCD sensors, whereas it reaches up to 1000 Mpixels/s for CMOS sensors. CMOS sensors could be integrated with various signal and image processing tools, whereas CCD sensors cannot be integrated with many digital control electronics (Zhang et al., 2008).

The light-sensitive area of pixels in CCDs is higher than in CMOS sensors, and the sensitivity is higher in CCD sensors compared to CMOS sensors. The focus of CCD sensor technology was on detector sensitivity and not much attention was provided to system integration, power dissipation, and supply voltage requirements. Whereas the focus of CMOS sensor technology was exactly opposite and the interest was focused on the fabrication processes with little attention to detector sensitivity (Carlson, 2002). Another difference between the two sensors is that a significantly smaller number of pixels is required to make CCD sensors than CMOS sensors, because the focal length scales with the pixel size (Carlson, 2002).

4.2.4   Line and area scan imaging

Line scanning is best suited for applications where continuously moving materials need to be inspected for faults or for quality monitoring. Line scan cameras have a single row of light-sensitive pixels that continuously scan the moving objects at a high line frequency (Figure 4.3). The resolution of line scan cameras varies between 512 and 12,888 pixels. It is necessary to synchronize the line rate of the camera to the moving object's speed to obtain the same resolution in the direction of motion (Y) as the resolution across the width of the object. Otherwise, if the line rate is fixed and the object speed varies, the object image will be elongated or compressed (Stemmer Imaging Ltd., 2013).

Line scan sensors build continuous images with a single line of pixels. Vertical resolution results from the object's own motion. Instead of a resolution of 1024 × 1024 in an area scan camera, line scan produces 1024 N, where N keeps increasing as long as the camera is working. Most applications using line scan imaging require synchronization between the camera and the moving object, which is achieved by the use of an encoder. A variation of line scan camera is the high sensitivity line scan camera, which is also called time delay and integration (TDI), and it is much more responsive to light compared to other line scan cameras. The increased sensitivity is due to the structure of the sensor and the timing method used to acquire images. In a typical line scan camera, a single line of an object is first integrated and then sent to the acquisition systems from the camera. Whereas in a high sensitivity line scan camera, each line of an object is integrated multiple times and the result is the sum of all line integration (Teledyne Dalsa Inc., 2014). Line scan cameras can be used for one-dimensional measurement, such as determining the width of a gap, or for acquisition of two-dimensional images when in combination with a scanning motion.

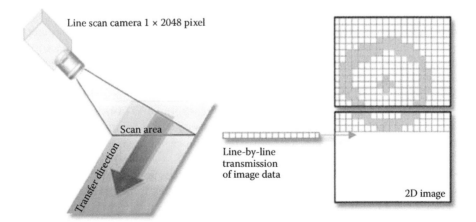

Figure 4.3 Working principle of line scan camera. (From Vision Doctor, 2009, Line scan camera basics, http://www.vision-doctor.co.uk/line-scan-cameras.html; accessed August 10, 2012. With permission.)

An area scan camera refers to the sensors that cover a whole area to form a rectangular array of pixels by creating a matrix of cells by a number of rows and columns. To acquire an image, an area scan camera uses either a square or rectangular sensor, and the resultant image has a width and height based on the number of pixels on the sensor, which provides different aspect ratios for different shapes of sensors.

4.2.5   Comparison of line and area scan imaging

Line scan cameras capture data using a single row of pixels, whereas area scan cameras capture an image of an area of interest with a matrix of pixels. Line scan cameras are best suited for imaging objects on a fast moving conveyor belt, whereas area scan cameras are ideal for stationary objects. A line scan camera can expose a new image while at the same time the previous image data are being transferred due to faster pixel readout, which does not occur in area scan imaging. Area scan cameras can image a fixed area quickly, whereas line scan cameras need to be moved over the area to produce a similar image. Line scan cameras provide much higher resolution and area scan cameras provide a fixed resolution (Newton Labs, 2013).

Line scan cameras are available in various technical specifications. Line scan cameras are also available as monochrome and color cameras suitable for various applications. With color cameras, different colors and shades can be detected thus giving color separation, which is useful for a variety of quality control applications. Color line scan cameras can be used in industrial applications including the food industry, paper and printing, mining and mineral, glass, plastic, and wood for the process and quality control applications. There are two types of color line scan cameras: one has color separation within the CCD sensor and the second has different color separation optics and has one sensor for each color channel. A line scan camera with three CCDs and color separation optics provides a better color separation performance than the other type of camera with a color line CCD (Lemström, 1995).

4.2.6   Components of line and area scan imaging

The basic components of a line or area scan imaging system are a line or area scan camera, lens, encoder, frame grabber, lighting, and trigger source.

Camera. A line scan camera is selected based on the application. The parameters to be considered in selection of a line scan camera are camera resolution, line rate, and output. If the line rate is too fast or too slow, it may result in geometric distortion of the image. The most common application of line scan technology includes photocopiers and flatbed scanners. Digital point and shoot cameras are examples of area scan cameras.

Lens. Line scan sensors are larger than area scan sensors and normally range from 5.12 to 57.37 mm wide. The lens used in line scan cameras is usually C-mount or F-mount. The F-mount lens is used for cameras with 2048 pixels or more, whereas a C-mount lens is used in cameras with lower pixels and are cost effective.

Frame grabber. A frame grabber captures digital still frames, and either stores, displays, or transmits in original raw or in compressed format. Frame grabbers can be classified into two categories: digital signal processing (DSP) and non-DSP. DSP frame grabbers can preprocess data (such as filtering, shading correction, scan delay compensation) to conserve the system resources, but they are very expensive. Non-DSP frame grabbers are comparatively faster and provide direct memory access functionality and are economic (Huang, 2013). A frame grabber for an analogue camera performs digitization, synchronization, formatting of data, and storage and transfer of data from camera to computer. In modern digital cameras, frame grabbers include many special functions such as acquisition control, input/output control, tagging of incoming images with time stamps, data formatting, image correction, and processing (Wu and Sun, 2013a).

Encoder. An encoder determines the line rate of the camera and is used to synchronize the total path covered and the pixel size. The encoder maintains the geometry of the image constant even when the rate of motion changes. An encoder is an electronic device or circuit that converts data into code. The synchronization of the scan rate of camera to the object movement is achieved by an encoder.

Illumination. The widely used light sources in digital imaging are fluorescent, incandescent, and light-emitting diode (LED) bulbs. There are other light sources such as electroluminescent (Wu and Sun, 2013a) and metal halide, high pressure sodium, and xenon lights which are used in areas requiring a bright light such as in large-scale industrial applications. Traditionally fluorescent and halogen incandescent lights are mostly used; however, recently, LED lighting has improved stability, intensity, and longevity (Martin, 2007). The proper selection and placement of the light source is an important step because nonuniform illumination may cause problems and complicate the process rather than simplify it.

The various illumination techniques used are incident light, dark field, and backlight illumination (Figure 4.4). Incident light illumination is the standard method of illumination for surface inspection using line scan imaging. The arrangement of camera and lighting is done in such a way that the camera is positioned at the reflection angle of the lighting so that maximum incident light is detected. In dark field, illumination is aligned flat so that the reflected light does not hit the camera and the image area appears dark. In this kind of illumination, the slots, elevations, and scratches appear bright, and this illumination is ideal to detect defects on the surface of materials. In backlight illumination, the position of the camera and illumination are exactly opposite and the sample is in between them. The contours of nontranslucent objects are visible and edge chippings can be detected by backlight illumination (Vision Doctor, 2009b).

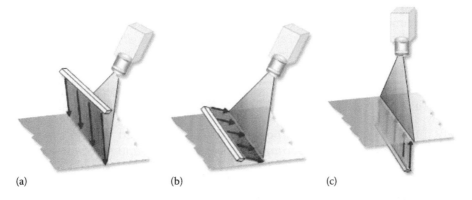

(a) (b) (c)

Figure 4.4 Illumination techniques. (a) Incident light illumination, (b) dark field illumination, and (c) backlight illumination. (From Vision Doctor, 2009, Illumination techniques for line scan cameras, http://www.vision-doctor.co.uk/illumination-techniques/illumination-line-scan-camera.html; accessed August 12, 2013. With permission.)

4.3   Applications of digital imaging in the visible spectrum

4.3.1   Agriculture

The applications of digital imaging have widely spread across the agriculture and related fields. Digital imaging could be used in assessing the viability of seeds, weed control by differentiating between weeds and plants, recognition of fruit to help in automatic fruit harvesting, identification of various types of fruits and vegetables for potential application in supermarkets, and classification of various types of cereal grains. The applications of digital imaging related to agriculture are discussed in this section. The potential applications of digital imaging in visible spectrum for agricultural activities are presented in Table 4.2.

4.3.1.1   Weed control

Weed management is very important in agriculture to improve the yield of the crop. Weed control is implemented by using huge quantities of weedicides or by use of tedious human laborers. Human labor is expensive and involves tedious work, and chemicals result in environmental and safety concerns. Weed control using digital images were used to distinguish between the type of weeds to enable application of weedicides at specific spots rather than over the entire area as proposed in precision agriculture. Many research works have been conducted using digital imaging to identify the weeds, differentiate between the crop and weeds, and to differentiate between the various types of weeds with the purpose of reducing the amount of chemicals applied on the field.

Ghazali et al. (2007) developed an image processing technique to differentiate between narrow and broad weeds based on combining color and textural information. The preprocessing of the image was performed by adopting a color filtering algorithm and two different feature extraction techniques were performed on the images: gray-level co-occurrence matrix (GLCM) and fast Fourier transform (FFT). Their results showed that using an excess color (Ex-C) filter, segmentation of the RGB (red, green, blue) color image was performed successfully. The classification accuracy using gray-scale level for GLCM and FFT were 85% and 89%, respectively, whereas using an EX-C filter the accuracies were 86% and 91%, respectively. An overall improvement in the weed classification was obtained using a color-based approach rather than the gray scale classification.

Ishak et al. (2009) developed a digital imaging technique for weed classification based on a combination of two techniques: Gabor wavelet (GW) and gradient field distribution (GFD). The common weeds found in oil palm plantations are broadleaf weeds (*Ageratum convzoides* and chromolaenaodorata) and grass weed (*Imperata cylindrical*). The color images were acquired using video camera in natural lighting conditions on sunny days around noon. The classification accuracies for broadleaf weeds using GW and a combination of GW and GFD techniques were 87% and 93%, respectively, and for grass weeds were 81.5% and 94%, respectively. The overall accuracy for GW and GDF was 84.25% and 93.75%, respectively, showing that a combination of GW and GFD techniques has good potential to classify different types of weeds. Bossu et al. (2009) proposed wavelet transform and Gabor filtering algorithms for discrimination between crop and weeds using synthetic and real images. Their results showed that wavelet transform provided more accurate results than Gabor filtering and also required less processing time.

Burgos-Artizzu et al. (2009) proposed a digital imaging method to assess the percentage of weed, crop, and soil in a digital image. Images were acquired using Nikon (Coolpix 5700) and Sony (DCR PC110E) cameras in a barley field. The most common weeds were *Avena sterilis* and *Papaver rhoeas*. The image processing involved different steps, including

Table 4.2 Potential Uses of Digital Imaging in Agriculture-Related Applications

Camera model	Material	Application	Average accuracy	Reference
MCA, mic-005 (Tetracam Inc., California)	Citrus	Detection of citrus greening disease	87%	Sankaran et al., 2013
Digital camera	Banana, beans, guava, jackfruit, lemon, mango, potato, sapota, tomato	Detection of leaf disease	94%	Arivazhagan et al., 2013
NA	Various plant leaves	Detection and classification of early scorch, cotton mold, ashen mold, late scorch, and tiny whiteness disease	83%–94%	Al-Hiary et al., 2011
NA	Various plants	Detection and classsification of leaf disease	93%	Bashish et al., 2011
NA	Grapefruit	Identification and classification of grapefruit peel disease; canker, copper burn, greasy spot, melanose, wind scar	96.7%	Kim et al., 2009
Color CCD camera	Tomato, cauliflower, lettuce seeds	To evaluate quality of germination	Imaging results were on par with human inspection	Ureňa et al., 2001
Weed detection				
Canon IXUS 330	Crop and weed	To differentiate between crop and weed using wavelet transform and Gabor filtering	73.4%–80.7%	Bossu et al., 2009
Color video camera	Broadleaf weeds (*Ageratum convzoides*) and grass weeds (*Imperata cylindrica*)	Weed classification using Gabor wavelet (GW) and gradient field distribution (GFD) technique	94%	Ishak et al., 2009
Nikon Coolpix 5700, Sony DCR PC110E	Barley field	To assess percentage of weed, soil, and crop	80%	Burgos-Artizzu et al., 2009

(Continued)

Table 4.2 (Continued) Potential Uses of Digital Imaging in Agriculture-Related Applications

Camera model	Material	Application	Average accuracy	Reference
NA	Narrow and broad weed	To differentiate between weeds using two feature extraction techniques, GLCM, FFT	86% and 91% using GLCM and FFT methods, respectively	Ghazali et al., 2007
Kodak DC260	Corn field	Herbicide application using site-specific locations	Herbicide application reduced by 11% to 16%	Yang et al., 2003a
Video camera XC-711P, Sony, Japan	Weed seeds	To identify different 57 seeds of weed	99%	Granitto et al., 2002
Kodak DC260	Corn field	Classification of crop and weed	100% for corn and 80% for weed	Yang et al., 2000a
Video camera Model 2222-1340 (Cohu Inc.)	Recognition of tomato plant and weed	To aid in selective herbicide application	73.1% tomatoes and 68.8% weeds	Lee et al., 1999
Wood				
Sony digital camera	Agarwood	Grade determination	80%	Abdullah et al., 2007
NA	Softwood lumber	Grading of lumber	81.3%	Silvén and Kauppinen, 1994
RS-170 camera	Red oak, cherry, maple, and yellow poplar	Grading lumber	Digital imaging combined with other techniques could be useful for grading lumber	Conners et al., 1992
Fruit recognition				
DSC-H5, Sony, Japan	Apple	Recognition of apple fruit on trees	83.33%	Lak et al., 2011
CCD camera	Melon	To identify melon in the tree for harvesting	93.57%	Edan et al., 2000
NA	Citrus fruits	To identify citrus fruit	100% accuracy when fruit is completely visible; 97% when 75% of fruit is visible; 90% accuracy when 50% of fruit is visible	Benady and Miles, 1992; Plá et al., 1993

(Continued)

Table 4.2 (Continued) Potential Uses of Digital Imaging in Agriculture-Related Applications

Camera model	Material	Application	Average accuracy	Reference
Solid state camera (Model TN2200) (General Electric, New York)	Apples and peaches	To locate fruits on trees	89%	Sites and Dewilche, 1988
3 CCD cameras	Apple	To detect apples from trees for harvesting	50%	D'Esnon et al., 1987
Canon PowerShot P1	15 different categories of fruit	To classify fruits and vegetables based on SVM, LDA, KNN algorithm at supermarkets and distribution centers	Classification error reduced up to 15 percentage points compared to single feature	Rocha et al., 2010
NA	Red apple, banana, durian, strawberry, lemon, watermelon, green apple	Fruit recognition in grocery store using KNN algorithm	90%	Seng and Mirisaee, 2009
NA	15 different categories of fruit	To classify fruits and vegetables	86%	Arivazhagan et al., 2010

segmentation of vegetation (crop and weed) and soil, elimination of crop area and calculation of crop cover, filtration of noise and errors, and finally calculating the percentage of weed in the image. They used a case-based reasoning (CBR) system that automatically determines the processing method suitable for each image based on previously experienced problems. The performance of the developed system was assessed based on processing images acquired at different field and controlled conditions such as varied lighting, different crop growth stage, and size of weeds, and the system achieved 80% correlation with the real data.

Yang et al. (2003a) developed a fuzzy algorithm based on digital image processing that could be used for herbicide applications in site-specific locations. A Kodak DC260 camera (Eastman Kodak, Rochester, New York) was used to capture the images of a cornfield under various lighting conditions that occur naturally. The weed coverage was determined by calculating the greenness ratio in which the intensities of red, blue, and green pixels were compared. A weed map was created by estimating the total coverage of weed and weed patchiness, and a fuzzy logic model was developed to determine site-specific herbicide application. Yang et al. (2000a) developed a digital imaging technique using an artificial neural network (ANN) for classification of crops and weeds. Back propagation neural network architecture was used in the study to differentiate between weeds and crops in the cornfield. The classification accuracy was 80% to 100% for corn and 60% to 80% for the weeds. The results indicated the potential of ANN for classification of weeds, and further studies need to be conducted to differentiate between different types of weeds in the field.

Lee et al. (1999) developed a weed control technique integrating imaging and robotic techniques. The system consisted of an RGB video camera (2222-1340, Cohu Inc.), illumination, computer, and a robotic cultivator. Two tests were performed: an outdoor test in a commercial tomato field and an indoor test using rectangular green targets to simulate tomato plants and circular targets to simulate weeds. The results of indoor tests showed that only 8% of rectangular targets simulated as tomato plants were sprayed and 100% of circular targets simulated as weeds were identified and sprayed. Overall the system correctly identified 73.1% of tomato plants and 68.8% of weeds in the outdoor field test. The results of indoor tests were better compared to outdoor tests, and the system needs significant improvement in speed and accuracy. The ideal speed of a robotic system should be around 3 and 8 km/h, and additional techniques need to be developed to improve the tomato plants recognition. They concluded that a real time robotic weed control unit with image processing capability was built and tested in real-time and the system needs further improvement for successful commercial applications.

4.3.1.2   Quality of seed germination

Germination is the most important quality characteristics of seeds and is the ability of a seed to produce a viable healthy seedling when they are placed in appropriate environmental conditions. In seedling nurseries, germination percentage is monitored by technicians who spend most of their time counting and grading. Ureña et al. (2001) developed an artificial vision system for evaluating the quality of seed germination. The image processing system consisted of a high-resolution CCD camera, frame grabber, computer, and image processing software. The seeds were sown in trays of 70×40 cm and the image of the tray was acquired by the image acquisition system. Seeds of tomato, cauliflower, and lettuce were used for the study. Seeds were sown in trays, kept in dark rooms, and transferred to green houses. Image acquisition began one week after seeds were sown and continued for one week. The detection of seedlings was based on the difference in color between the seedlings and the trays' rooting media. The segmentation algorithm based on the RGB components of the image helped in enhancing the contrast of the color between seedling and rooting media. Fuzzy logic algorithm was used for classification purposes. The seed germination detection was on par with the evaluations made by the technicians and hence digital imaging could be a useful tool for monitoring seed germination.

4.3.1.3   Disease detection in trees

Citrus greening or huanglongbing (HLB) is a serious disease that affects citrus trees and results in huge economic losses. Sankaran et al. (2013) explored the feasibility of detection of citrus greening disease using visible, thermal, and near-infrared imaging. Two camera arrays (MCA, MIC-005, Tetracam Inc., Chatsworth, California) were used to collect images at spectral bands of 440, 480, 530, 560, 610, 660, 690, 710, 740, 810, 850, and 900 nm. The data were collected from a total of 36 healthy and 38 infected trees. The spectral reflectance value assessment at visible and near-infrared regions indicated that compared to healthy trees, disease-infected trees had higher reflectance values in the visible region of the spectrum than in the near infrared region. Among all the visible and near-infrared bands evaluated, 560 and 710 nm showed maximum differences between healthy and HLB-affected trees. Classification using average spectral reflectance showed an overall classification accuracy, specificity, and sensitivity of 87%, 89%, and 85%, respectively. The results of the study demonstrated the potential of visible and near-infrared thermal imaging to detect disease-affected trees.

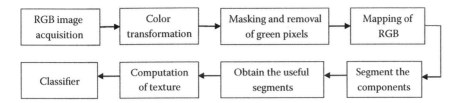

Figure 4.5 Basic approach to identify diseased leaf using image processing. (From Arivazhagan, S. et al., *Agricultural Engineering International*, 1, 90, 2013. With permission.)

Arivazhagan et al. (2013) developed a digital imaging algorithm to detect unhealthy leaves of plants and classify the leaf disease based on textural features. The procedure for detection of leaf disease is proposed in Figure 4.5. The algorithm was tested on 500 leaves of 30 different species of plants. The algorithm could detect and classify the diseases of leaves with an accuracy of around 94%. The authors stated that with this approach, the plant diseases could be identified at the early stages and hence by adopting proper pest control techniques, the diseases of plants could be contained. They also suggested that to improve the disease identification accuracy, training samples could be increased.

Bashish et al. (2011) implemented and evaluated an image processing technique for identification and classification of leaf diseases such as early scorch, late scorch, ashen mold, cottony mold, and tiny whiteness. The RGB color space was transformed into device independent color space, and *K*-mean clustering was used to partition the image into four clusters followed by the color co-occurrence method (CCM) for extracting the feature set. The accuracy of the technique was 93% and the authors concluded that the proposed method has a great potential to identify and classify plant leaf diseases. Kim et al. (2009) explored the potential of detecting grapefruit leaf disease (copper burn, greasy spot, canker, wind scar, and melanose) using image processing techniques. Images acquired in RGB color space were transformed to HSI (hue, saturation, intensity) color space. With 39 image texture features, algorithms were developed for selecting useful textural features. The classification models were developed based on reduced textural features and the classification accuracy of model based on 14 selected texture features resulted in an overall accuracy of 96.7% for classification of grapefruit peel disease.

4.3.1.4 Quality grading of wood

Agarwood (*Aquilaria malaccensis*), also known as eaglewood, has many applications including medicinal uses, perfumes, and incense. The grading of agarwood is done manually, which may result in subjective and inconsistent results. Abdullah et al. (2007) developed an image processing technique to determine the grade of agarwood. Images of grade A, B, C, D, and E were acquired using a Sony digital camera. The acquired images were then preprocessed using image filtering and threshold, and then image segmentation was performed. The results of the technique showed that the precision of grade determination was around 80% with lower detection accuracy for grade A agarwood. They stated that the system could be used to grade the agarwood except for grade A, which could be detected by the naked eye due to its darker color and intense fragrance.

Silvén and Kauppinen (1994) developed a color-vision-based technique for grading softwood lumber. About 2000 images of pine and spruce wood were analyzed using an image processing algorithm mainly utilizing the segemntation technique. The classification accuracy of the system was about 81.3%, which was on par with the human inspectors whose accuracy was normally be in the range of 75% to 85%. The resutls of the study showed that the digital imaging technique has a great potential for grading lumber.

The appearance of hardwood lumber varies significantly and grading the defects is very important in identifying the right type of wood for the specific application. Conners et al. (1992) explored the potential of a computer vision system for grading lumber. Four species of lumber—red oak, cherry, maple, and yellow poplar—were selected for the study. Images were acquired using a RS-170 solid-state camera. After color images of the samples were acquired, more samples of red oak lumber were soaked in water, and images were obtained at different surface moisture contents to determine the effect of surface moisture content. The initial results of the study showed that surface moisture content had a significant effect on the wood color. Higher surface moisture content resulted in very small color differences between clear wood and wood with surface defects. As the surface moisture of the wood dried, color difference was significant and hence Conners et al. stated that accurate grading could be obtained by analyzing dry woods. The primary focus of the research in monitoring surface defects of rough wood was difficult to solve using color imaging because dirty materials confused the segmentation procedure. The shadows produced by the rough surface also reduced the sensitivity of the results and even the knots had the same color as clear wood. Based on the study, the authors concluded that other imaging methods need to be supplemented with color imaging to detect defects in rough lumber and that color imaging alone is not sufficient to monitor wood defects.

4.3.1.5   Fruit recognition

The digital imaging technique for fruit recognition from tree branches and leaves was explored and experimented by many researchers. Jimènez et al. (1999) performed an extensive review on the research conducted for fruit recognition using automatic vision systems. Parrish and Goksel (1977) developed a computer vision system based on a black-and-white camera for detecting apples. D'Esnon et al. (1987) developed a color camera vision system for detecting apples, which was later modified by Rabatel (1988) with three CCD color cameras to detect apples. Levi et al. (1988) implemented a color-camera-based imaging to identify and locate oranges. Sites and Dewilche (1988) presented an imaging system with a black-and-white camera and three color filters in the range of 630 to 670 nm to increase the contrast of fruit and the background. A classification accuracy of around 80% to 90% was obtained for apples and peaches. More research studies were conducted on fruit harvesting of melon (Cardenas-Weber et al., 1991; Dobrusin and Edan, 1992) and citrus (Benady and Miles, 1992; Plá et al., 1993). Zhao et al. (2005) performed experiments to recognize apples in an orchard using the color data and texture properties.

In supermarkets, recognition of various kinds of fruits and vegetables including their variety is a challenging task for cashiers. To identify a particular produce, cashiers are provided with booklets with pictures and codes, but it is time consuming and makes the consumer impatient. Rocha et al. (2010) analyzed the color and textural features along with the appearance features to classify vegetables and fruits in a real-time supermarket scenario. A supermarket produce data set available online was used for the study. The supermarket data set images were obtained from a supermarket produce section comprising 15 types of fruits and vegetables (Agata potato, Fuji apple, Granny Smith apple, Asterix potato, cashew, peach, honeydew melon, kiwi, nectarine, onion, orange, plum, Spanish pear, Tahiti lime, and watermelon) using a Canon PowerShot P1 camera. The images were acquired at different days during various time periods to increase the variability of the data set and to create a more realistic situation. The analysis was based on color, shape, and texture descriptors, and various techniques such as linear discriminant analysis (LDA), support vector machine (SVM), classification trees, and *K*-nearest neighbor (KNN) were used. Rocha et al. proposed a fusion approach that combines features and classifiers, and validated the approach for classification of multiclass fruit and vegetables. They stated that the proposed fusion method was able to lower the classification error by 15 percentage points when compared with single features and classifiers.

Seng and Mirisaee (2009) proposed a fruit recognition technique based on color, shape, and size features to increase the accuracy of recognition. They developed a *K*-nearest neighbor (KNN) algorithm based on mean color value, roundness shape value, perimeter, and area (size) values of the fruit. Various fruits, including red apple, banana, durian, strawberry, lemon, watermelon, and green apple were selected for the study. They collected 50 fruit images out of which 36 images were used to train the system and the remaining 14 were used to test the system. There were five modules for fruit recognition: input selection, color computation, shape computation, size computation, and fruit recognition. The accuracy of the fruit recognition system was around 90%. Seng and Mirisaee stated that the system needs to be improved to recognize more variety of fruits other than those tested, and texture-based analysis could be combined with the existing size-, shape-, and color-based feature analysis techniques. They concluded that the fruit recognition is a potential technique that could be useful in grocery stores to automate the process of labeling and computing the price, and for plant scientists to conduct analysis on variations in morphology to understand the genetic and molecular features of the fruit.

Arivazhagan et al. (2010) developed a fruit recognition system based on color and textural features of fruits. They used a supermarket produce data set consisting of a total of 2633 images, out of which half were used for training and the other half for testing. To develop a solution for a real-time situation, it was essential to accommodate illumination variations, specular reflections, sensor artifacts, background clutter, and shading. The complexity was reduced by a preprocessing technique of background subtraction for segmenting the object of interest. The accuracy of recognition rate for fruits using color features was 45.49% and using texture features was 70.8%, whereas the accuracy using color and texture features was 86.0%. Arivazhagan et al. concluded that the proposed method for classification of fruits can analyze and recognize fruits, but the accuracy could be further improved by including the shape and size features and by increasing the total number of images used for classification.

4.3.1.6 *Cereal grain*

Cereal grain classification using machine vision had been explored by many researchers. Cereal grain classification based on morphological features (Barker et al., 1992; Sapirstein and Kohler, 1995; Paliwal et al., 1999; Majumdar and Jayas, 2000a); textural features (Majumdar and Jayas, 2000c); color features (Neuman et al., 1989a,b; Luo et al., 1999b; Majumdar and Jayas, 2000b); and a combination of morphology, color or textural features, or wavelet features (Majumdar and Jayas, 2000d; Paliwal et al., 2003; Visen et al., 2004b; Choudhary et al., 2008) were studied. Table 4.3 highlights the potential applications of digital imaging in classification of various cereal grains. Figure 4.6 shows an area scan imaging setup for classification of cereal grains.

Silva and Sonnadara (2013) developed a digital imaging technique using ANN to classify nine varieties of rice. The images of 50 grains from each variety were acquired using a Sony (DSC-W270) digital camera. Silva and Sonnadara developed algorithms to extract morphological (13), textural (15), and color (6) features, and neural network models were developed. The classification accuracy was higher by textural features compared to morphological and color features, and an overall accuracy of 92% was obtained. Silva and

Table 4.3 Potential Uses of Digital Imaging in Classification of Cereal Grains

Camera model	Material	Application	Accuracy	Reference
Sony DSC-W270	Rice	Classification of nine varieties of rice	92%	Silva and Sonnadara, 2013
DXC-3000A, Sony, Japan	Barley, oats, rye, CWRS, CWAD wheat	Classification of various types of cereal grains	98.5%, 99.93%, 100%, 99.97%, 100% for barley, oats, rye, CWRS, CWAD wheat, respectively	Mebatsion et al., 2013
BenQ D E520	Wheat and barley	Classification of wheat and barley	99%	Guevara-Hernandez and Gomez-Gil, 2011
DFK31AU03, The Imaging Source, Germany	Maize	Classification based on color and shape	90% for color classes, 73% for shape classes	Mladenov et al., 2011
Color camera	Corn	Detection of fungal infection	81%–89%	Tallada et al., 2011
VIVITAR color camera, New Jersey	Wheat and barley	Classification of wheat and barley	93.83% (fuzzy logic and statistical), 98% (ANN)	Douik and Abdellaoui, 2010
XCD-X700, Sony, Japan	Wheat	Classification of eight different classes of wheat (CPSR, CPSW, CWAD, CWES, CWHW, CWRS, CWRW, and CWSWS)	89.8% and 85.4% for QDA and LDA, respectively	Manickavasagan et al., 2008b
DXC-3000A, Sony, Japan	CWRS, CWAD wheat, rye, oats, barley	Classification of wheat, barley, rye, and oats	99.4%, 99.3%, 98.6%, 98.5%, and 89.4% for CWRS, rye, barley, oats, and CWAD wheat, respectively	Choudhary et al., 2008
DXC-3000A, Sony, Japan	Barley, oats, rye, wheat, durum wheat	Classification of various types of grain	98%	Visen et al., 2004b
DXC-3000A, Sony, Japan	CWRS, CWAD wheat, rye, oats, barley	Classification of cereal grain using length, shape, and color features	100%, 94%, 93%, 99%, 95% for CWRS, CWAD wheat, rye, oats, barley, respectively	Paliwal et al., 1999

(Continued)

Table 4.3 (Continued) Potential Uses of Digital Imaging in Classification of Cereal Grains

Camera model	Material	Application	Accuracy	Reference
DXC-3000A, Sony, Japan	CWRS, CWAD wheat, rye, oats, barley	Comparison of neural network and statistical classifier for cereal grain classification	Neural network classification was better with more than 96% accuracy for all cereal grains	Paliwal et al., 2003
Area scan, DXC-3000A, Sony, Japan; Line scan, Trillium TR 2K Dals, Ontario, Canada	Barley, oats, rye, CWAD, CWRS wheat	Compare the variability in grain due to random orientation of kernel, different growing region, and variability due to line scan and area scan camera	Variability due to length, color, and textural features was low, whereas coefficient of variation for width related features was high during random orientation; for different regions, highest variability was observed in color features followed by area of kernel in morphological features; no significant variation in features due to different camera	Paliwal et al., 2005
DXC-3000A, Sony, Japan	CWRS, CWAD wheat, barley, oats, and rye	Classification based on morphology, color, and texture	98.9%, 91.6%, 97.9%, 100%, and 91.6% for morphology; 95.7%, 94.4%, 94.2%, 97.6%, and 92.5% for color; 87%, 95.7%, 100%, 100%, and 81.8% for texture	Majumdar and Jayas, 2000a,b,c,d
DXC-3000A, Sony, Japan	CWRS wheat	Identification of damaged kernels	93%, 90%, 99%, 99%, 99%, 98%, and 100% for healthy, broken, green frosted, smudged, mildew, heated, and burnt wheat, respectively	Luo et al., 1999b

(Continued)

Table 4.3 (Continued) Potential Uses of Digital Imaging in Classification of Cereal Grains

Camera model	Material	Application	Accuracy	Reference
Monochrome WV-CD50, Panasonic	CWRS wheat	Measurement of grain uniformity in commercial samples	Coefficient of variation (CV) for cargo samples less than CV of rail car samples by 58%, 63%, and 64% for grade 1, 2, and 3, respectively	Sapirstein and Kohler, 1995
DXC-M2, Sony	CWRS, CWRW, CPS (Canadian prairie spring), CU (Canadian utility), CWAW (Canada Western Amber Durum), CWSWS (Canada Western Soft White Spring)	Color attributes of different classes were examined	Significant color differences were observed between different classes and some varieties within the same class of wheat	Neuman et al., 1989a,b

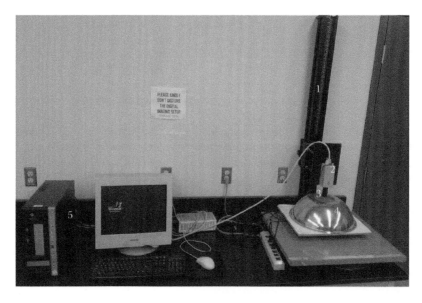

Figure 4.6 Area scan imaging setup for classification of cereal grains: (1) stand, (2) camera, (3) lens, (4) illumination, and (5) data acquisition system. (Courtesy of University of Manitoba, Winnipeg, Canada.)

Sonnadara concluded that the preliminary results obtained by the experiments could be further improved by using different preprocessing techniques and other neural network models to suit the requirements of the rice processing industry.

Guevara-Hernandez and Gomez-Gil (2011) presented a machine vision classification of wheat and barley grains. The images were acquired using a BenQ D E520 digital camera and a total of 545 wheat and barley grain kernels were used for the study. From the images, 99 features were extracted (21 morphological, 6 color, and 72 textural features) and analyzed using a discriminant analysis (DA) and *K*-nearest neighbor (KNN) algorithm. The results showed that higher classification accuracy of 99% was achieved when color, morphological, and textural features were used rather than using one feature set only. Guevara-Hernandez and Gomez-Gil stated that using more than three feature sets may reduce the classification accuracy and increase the computational cost.

Mladenov et al. (2011) developed an imaging classification method for grain samples based on color and shape properties. Maize grain variety Kneja-433 was used for the study and a CCD camera (DFK31AU03, The Imaging Source, Germany) was used to acquire the images of the sample. The classification accuracy based on color features was 90% and based on shape features was 73% when the impurities were not included in the testing. The classification accuracy decreased when nongrain impurities were added to the samples. Mladenov et al. concluded that classification error decreased when proper procedures were adopted for fusion of color and shape features.

Douik and Abdellaoui (2010) studied the grain classification by analyzing the morphological, color, and wavelet features. The cereal grains selected for the study was Tunisian hard wheat, Tunisian tender wheat, and Tunisian barley, and a high-resolution camera was used to capture the images. A total of 152 parameters were extracted for each type of grain (18 color, 122 morphological, and 12 wavelet features). Douik and Abdellaoui implemented statistical classification, fuzzy logic, and ANN classification methods. The classification accuracy for the statistical method was 76%, the fuzzy logic method was 85.7%, and the accuracy for the combination of statistical and fuzzy logic was 93.8%. But the best classification accuracy of 98% was achieved using ANN classification.

Choudhary et al. (2008) explored the potential of cereal grain classification based on wavelet, morphological, color, and textural features. The cereal grains used for the study were Canada Western Red Spring (CWRS), Canada Western Amber Durum (CWAD) wheat, rye, oats, and barley. The images were acquired with an area scan color camera (DXC-3000A, Sony, Japan). They extracted 93 color, 51 morphological, 56 textural, and 135 wavelet features from each kernel of grain. The classification was performed using single-feature, two-feature, three-feature, and all four feature sets. Their results showed that the wavelet feature improved the accuracy of classification when used along with color, morphological, and textural features, but classification accuracy was lower when used alone. Choudhary et al. concluded that four feature sets model provided the best classification accuracy.

Fungal contamination of grain results in significant economic losses to farmers, grain handlers, and processors and results in deteriorated quality of the final product, which may even result in food safety and health issues for the consumers. Tallada et al. (2011) evaluated the potential for detection of fungal infected corn using digital color imaging. Samples of corn hybrid Burrus 794sRR grown in a commercial field (Kilbourne, Illinois) were used for the study. Fungal-infected corn kernels were graded into four levels: level 1 (no visible sign of damage except minor discoloration), level 2 (tiny spots of fungal growth on surface and slightly discolored), level 3 (moderate infection, visible fungal infection on 30% to 70% of surface), and level 4 (severely infected over the entire surface of corn). Images acquired using a digital camera were used to develop models using linear discriminant analysis (LDA) and neural networks. Better classification accuracies of around 81% to 89% were achieved at higher levels of infection, whereas when the entire data set was considered, the classification accuracy was 75% for both control and infected samples. When the results of digital imaging were compared with near-infrared reflectance spectroscopy, the classification accuracy of digital imaging was lower and less attractive.

4.3.2   Applications of visible imaging for fresh produce and other food products

The quality of produce and the presence of any defects are traditionally monitored by human inspectors. Human inspection is subjective and inconsistent, and lack of trained personnel has led to an effort to develop automated inspection. Many researchers have explored quality monitoring of various fresh produce using digital imaging. The results of various research works are summarized in this section. Table 4.4 highlights the potential applications of digital imaging in quality monitoring of fresh produce.

4.3.2.1   Potato

Potato (*Solanum tuberosum* L.) is the fourth most important food crop after wheat, rice, and maize around the world. Potato is sensitive and is affected by bacteria, viruses, fungi, and nematodes. Potato grading is commonly performed by human inspectors, which could give inconsistent results and is time consuming. Much research has been conducted using machine vision techniques for grading potatoes. Hassankhani et al. (2012) developed a machine vision unit for detection of surface defects in potatoes. The system consisted of four fluorescent lamps, a CCD camera, and a computer. The potatoes were graded into six classes: healthy, cracked, rotting, cutting, greening, and rhizoctonia fouled. For sorting of potatoes with various defects, an algorithm was developed to check for existence of defects and then the percentage of each defect in a potato was calculated and classified based on the highest percentage of defect. An average classification accuracy of 97.67% was obtained for potato classification with various defects and was comparable with the results of other studies. Hassankhani et al. concluded that the system could be used for on-line grading of potatoes.

Ebrahimi et al. (2011) developed an algorithm based on machine vision for detecting potatoes with green skin, which has a negative impact on human health. Images were acquired using a CCD camera for 25 potatoes affected with greening surface, and preprocessing was performed for segmentation of potatoes from the background. An algorithm was developed in RGB and HSI space and tested by comparing the green area estimated by the algorithm to the actual green area in the potatoes. The average error between estimated green area and actual greening was 5.26% and concluded that the digital imaging has a potential to detect greening defects in potatoes. Rios-Cabrera et al. (2008) developed an ANN algorithm to classify misshapen potatoes using three models: backpropogation, perceptron, and Fuzzy ARTMAP (FAM). Images were acquired using a Basler F602C camera and potato surface defects were classified as scab, greening, and cracks. The results of the study showed that FAM outperformed the other two algorithms and required less than 1 ms per pattern for training and testing. Rios-Cabrera et al. stated that due to the fast processing time, the FAM algorithm was best suited for defect detection and quality monitoring in commercial production lines. Zhou et al. (1998) developed a computer-vision-based imaging system to classify potatoes based on weight, diameter, shape, and color. The classification accuracy was 91.2% for weight, 88.7% for diameter, 85.5% for shape, and 78.0% for color-based classifications. The overall classification accuracy was 86.5% based

Table 4.4 Potential Uses of Digital Imaging in Quality Monitoring of Fresh Produce

Camera model	Material	Application	Accuracy	Reference
CCD (Proline, UK)	Potato	Detection of surface defects	97.6%	Hassankhani et al., 2012
GA4162PF (CNB, Korea)	Potato	Detection of greening defects	Average error between estimated and actual greening was 5.26%	Ebrahimi et al., 2011
Basler F602C	Potato	To classify misshapen potatoes using Fuzzy ARTMAP, backpropogation, and perceptron algorithm	93.8%, Fuzzy ARTMAP outperformed other models with lower processing time of 1 ms per pattern	Rios-Cabrera et al., 2008
CCD line scan camera	Potato	Classification based on shape, size, and defects	93.2% by LDA, 94.9% by MLF-NN	Noordam et al., 2000
Not available	Potato	Classification based on weight, diameter, shape and color	86.5%	Zhou et al., 1998
XC-711 (Sony)	Potato	Automatic grading of potatoes	97.3% for stationary and 81.6% for moving potatoes	Heinemann et al., 1996
CoolPix L3 (Nikon)	Apple	Maturity grading in apples	66.2%	Garrido-Novell et al., 2012
UC610 (Uniq, United States)	Apple	To monitor bruises, insect bites, and rot defects using 3 cameras	Classification error reduced from 15% using 1 camera to 11% by using 3 cameras	Xiao-bo et al., 2010
SSC-DC58AP (Sony)	Apple	To monitor surface defects	96%	Puchalski et al., 2008
CCD video camera	Apple	Grading based on surface color	95%	Nakano, 1997
EOS 400D (Canon, United States)	Artichoke	Measurement of post-cutting changes in color	Good correlation coefficient of 0.9 was observed between L^* and visual appearance score	Amodio et al., 2011
WV-CP470 (Panasonic)	Strawberry	Automatic grading	Accuracy by color sorting was 88.8%, accuracy by shape sorting was 90%	Liming and Yanchao, 2010
Video Hi8, CCD-TRV128E PAL	Raisins	Grading of raisins	96%	Omid et al., 2010

(*Continued*)

Table 4.4 (Continued) Potential Uses of Digital Imaging in Quality Monitoring of Fresh Produce

Camera model	Material	Application	Accuracy	Reference
Digital camera	Cantaloupe	To determine the volume of cantaloupe	Average difference in volume determination by imaging and water displacement method was 7.6%	Rashidi et al., 2009
Progressive scan camera	Mandarin	To sort mandarin segments	93% for sound segments and 83% for broken	Blasco et al., 2009
PowerShot A70 (Canon, United States)	Banana, red pepper	Color measurement	Correlation coefficient of 0.97 was obtained between computer vision and colorimeter method	Mendoza et al., 2006
Nikon Coolpix 900	Lettuce	Evaluation of shelf-life and acceptability	Correlation coefficient of 0.9194 to 0.9941 was obtained between imaging and human inspection	Zhou et al., 2004
CCD-XC003P (Sony)	Orange, peach, and apple	Quality grading of fruits	86% and 93% for blemish and size detection, respectively	Blasco et al., 2003
Color camera	Tomato	Quality grading based on color, size, shape, and defects	Good correlation between imaging parameters and maturity of tomato	Jahns et al., 2001
KY-F30B (JVC)	Tomato	Quality grading using color and maturity	79%	Edan et al., 1997
TVC-6200-2 (Kayo International, New York)	Cucumber	To determine the chlorphyll content	Good corelation obtained between gray level of image and chlorophyll content	Lin et al., 1993

on all the criteria, and the conclusion was that the system can be incorporated along with manual inspection to reduce the time of sorting.

Barnes et al. (2010) developed an automatic method using digital imaging to detect blemishes in potatoes (Figure 4.7). The setup consisted of a color camera (Sony DSLR-A350K) placed above the tubers. The potatoes were kept inside a white cylinder covered with white board with four daylight bulbs around the cylinder. Experiments were conducted on white and red potatoes with blemishes. Segmentation of potato from the background was performed after image acquisition, and a pairwise classifier was used to detect blemishes. An adaptive boost algorithm was used to discriminate between potatoes with

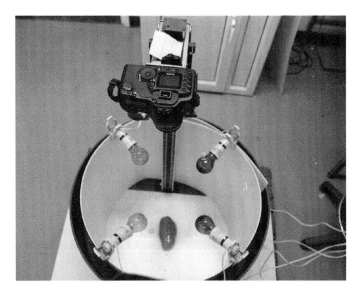

Figure 4.7 Imaging setup for defect detection in potatoes: (1) camera, (2) bulb, (3) white cylinder, and (4) potato. (From Barnes, M. et al., *Journal of Food Engineering*, 98: 339, 2010. With permission.)

blemishes and healthy ones. The results of the study showed that an accuracy of 89.6% and 89.5% was achieved for white and red potatoes, respectively.

Noordam et al. (2000) developed a machine-vision-based grading system using three CCD line scan cameras to classify potatoes based on shape, size, and defects, such as mechanical damage, common scab, cracks, and greening. They used LDA along with a Mahalanobis distance classifier for color segmentation and Fourier-based shape classification techniques. An average classification accuracy of around 90% was obtained for LDA and multilayer feedforward neural network (MLF-NN) classification. They concluded that the imaging system was robust and classification of potatoes was robust and was able to classify 50 potatoes.

Heinemann et al. (1996) developed a vision-based automated inspection unit for grading of potatoes using imaging. A 9.1 kg box consisting of 65 U.S No. 1 potatoes were used as samples and three runs with the same sample set were conducted. The automated unit consisted of an imaging chamber, camera (Sony XC-711), conveyor, sorting unit and computer. The classification accuracy of the system was 80%, 77%, and 88% for the moving potatoes during three replications at the speed of 3 potatoes/min, whereas the classification accuracy was 98%, 97%, and 97% when the potatoes were kept stationary. During movement, shape analysis was affected, which contributed to the classification error. Heinemann et al. concluded that there are certain limitations, such as slow speed and misclassification error during movement, that need to be addressed before it could be used commercially.

4.3.2.2 Apple

The external appearance of apple is one of the most critical factors in the economic value and quality grading. Postharvest quality grading of apple is a laborious process and use of computer vision has been explored by many researchers for quality assessment of apples. Although many types of defects may occur on the apple surface, identification of defects at the stem end and calyxes is a challenge due to the complexity involved in the assessment of such defects. Xiao-bo et al. (2010) evaluated the potential of a digital imaging technique to monitor defects, such as bruises, insect bites, and rots at the stem end and calyx. The image acquisition system consisted of three color CCD cameras (UC610, Uniq, United States), six lighting tubes, a frame grabber and a computer. Fuji apples were used for the study and out of 318 apples selected, 199 apples were classified as accepted grade and 119 apples were rejected due to blemishes. The image analysis for defect detection consisted of initial segmentation where blemishes were coarsely segmented and in refinement, an active contour model was used to refine the segmentation, which enables the blemishes to be detected accurately. The classification error of accepting apples with blemishes was lowered from 21.8% with one camera to 4.2% with three cameras, whereas the rejection of good quality apples increased 11% to 15.07%. They concluded that the defect detection algorithm should be improved to reduce the rejection of good quality apples. Another limitation of the system was that the algorithm was not able to differentiate between different defects such as fungal growth, bruises, scabs, and disease-affected apples.

Puchalski et al. (2008) developed an image processing system to monitor defects on the surface of apples. Six varieties (Golden Delicious, Gala, Jonagold, Fiesta, Ligol, and Melrose) with different surface defects were selected, and after harvest and before testing the apples were stored at 0°C. Bruises were artificially created on some of the apples by dropping them on the surface of wood. The various defects that were analyzed were bruising, punches, fungi attack, frost damage, insect holes, and scabs. Images were acquired using a CCD camera (Sony, SSC-DC58AP) and eight images of each apple, which was oriented vertically and rotated, were obtained. Since multiple images were acquired during rotation and combined for analysis, defects seen such as dark areas appeared with the same shape in at least three or more frames, which reduced the false positives and improved the accuracy of classification. The results of the study showed that classification accuracy was 96% for determining various defects.

4.3.2.3 Strawberry

The grading of strawberries is based on size, shape, maturity, color, and presence of any defects. The grading of fruits using computer vision techniques is nondestructive, objective, and can simultaneously detect multiple quality characteristics. Liming and Yanchao (2010) explored the potential of developing an automatic grading system for strawberries using an image processing technique. The automatic grading system consisted of a mechanical unit (conveyor belt, platform, gripper, and motors) and the image processing unit consisted of a camera (WV-CP470, Panasonic), image collecting card, and computer. The results of the experiment showed that for size analysis, the error between the measured size and the actual size was less than 5%. The color sorting was based on three classifications: light red, bright red, and black-red. The color grading by imaging resulted in 88.8% accuracy when compared with manual grading by color. Liming and Yanchao concluded that when using an imaging technique, size grading error was less than 5%, color sorting accuracy was 88.8%, and the accuracy of shape classification was above 90%, and hence a digital imaging technique could be a useful tool for grading strawberries.

4.3.2.4 Raisins

Manual sorting and evaluation of raisin quality is subjective and unreliable, and manual error may reduce the value of the product. A digital-imaging-based automatic sorting system can reduce the inconsistencies in sorting, improve the grading, and reduce the dependence on manual labor. Omid et al. (2010) developed an image processing algorithm for accurate grading of raisins. The grading system consisted of a conveyer belt, induction motor, light source, video camera (Video Hi8, CCD-TRV128E PAL), and capture card. A feature extraction algorithm was developed that could classify raisins based on color and size features into two categories: desirable and undesirable. The accuracy of classification of raisins into desirable and undesirable categories was 96% when compared with the human expert classification. The digital imaging technique seems to be a potential tool for grading of raisins and this could be extended for grading and sorting of other agricultural materials such as lentils and almonds.

4.3.2.5 Cantaloupe

Cantaloupe (*Cucumis melo*) is an important fruit due to its high nutritive value. Size of the fruit is the most important quality parameter, however, volume-based sorting may be more efficient than mass-based sorting. Rashidi et al. (2009) determined the volume of cantaloupe using image processing techniques. Fifteen fruits of various sizes free from any visual defects were randomly selected from storage. The imaging system consisted of a digital camera, fluorescent ring light, and computer. Two images were captured one before and one after manually rotating the fruit 90°, and a disk approximation technique in image processing was used to calculate the volume of cantaloupes. Volume determination by image processing showed an average percentage difference of 7.6% when compared with the volume determination by the water displacement method. Rashidi et al. concluded that image processing provides a simple, accurate, and noninvasive method to determine the volume of cantaloupes and could be useful for monitoring and sorting in postharvest operations.

4.3.2.6 Mandarin

Mandarin segments are canned and sold to many industries and consumers. In Satsuma (*Citrus unshiu*) processing, preliminary tasks such as peeling and separation of segments are done automatically, but the final inspection and sorting are performed only manually to ensure the quality of the product. Blasco et al. (2009) tested an automatic machine for inspecting and sorting mandarin segments using image processing. The proposed prototype consisted of the feeding unit, inspection unit, and sorting, which included a conveyor belt, fluorescent lamps for illumination, a camera, and the outlet. The prototype was installed in a commercial mandarin processing facility for industrial testing and two tests were performed. The first one consisted of on-line testing of 10 replicas of 3 kg mandarin segments that were inspected by the prototype model. An industrial quality expert analyzed the results of the machine output to compare the actual performance of the prototype. The second test included acquisition and analysis of 15,000 images of raw material and segments. The segments were classified by the algorithm and the results of the classification were compared to the one conducted by the human experts. The classification accuracy for sound segments was 93%, whereas for the broken ones it was 83%. The prototype developed was able to handle 1000 kg/h, which was an acceptable speed for commercial processing. Blasco et al. concluded that the developed prototype and the image processing technique could be useful for automatic sorting of mandarin segments in commercial facilities.

4.3.2.7 Tomato

Quality grading of fruits and vegetables is done based on visual appearance. Jahns et al. (2001) performed quality grading of tomatoes based on attributes like color, size, shape, and defects using image analysis. The experimental setup consisted of a standard color camera, frame grabber, illumination, and computer. Size was measured as the largest diameter, the major axis, and area of the tomato. Maturity of tomato based on color was measured with an RGB image. Using color calibration data, the RGB image was transformed to a standardized CIE/XYZ image. The shape and curvature was measured by estimating the perimeter, area, and major and minor axes. They provided a fuzzy model based on optical characteristics, which showed a good correlation with respect to maturity parameters. Jahns et al. proposed that contact and destructive quality measurement could be reduced to a minimum by adopting imaging techniques.

4.3.3   Color measurements

Color is one of the basic measures of quality indicator of agricultural and food products. Color plays a major role in determining the physical, chemical, and sensory quality of many agricultural products. Many studies have been conducted to evaluate the potential of determining the color characteristics of products using digital imaging. There are many advantages of computer vision techniques for color measurements compared to traditional techniques. A color digital image is expressed in RGB form with these three components per pixel in the range of 0 to 255. In research with food materials, color is mostly represented by L*a*b* in which L* represents the luminance or lightness component that ranges from 0 (black) to 100 (white), a* ranges from –120 to +120 (green to red), and b* ranges from –120 to +120 (blue to yellow). L*a*b* is defined based on an international standard developed by Commission Internationale d'Eclairage (CIE) in 1976 for color measurement. The illumination is important and standard illuminants are defined by CIE and the widely used illuminants in food research are A (2856 K), C (6774 K), D_{65} (6500 K), and D (7500 K) (Yam and Papadakis, 2004).

Garrido-Novell et al. (2012) studied the RGB color imaging for grading maturity levels in apples. Forty apples from cultivar Golden Delicious without any physical defects were selected for imaging. The imaging system consisted of a digital camera (Nikon, Coolpix L3) with halogen lamps for illumination. Linear discriminant analysis (LDA) was used to classify RGB values of apple images and the leave-one-out method was used to validate the classification model. The values of red were between 89 to 168 and green values were in the range from 91 to 146 while the blue component did not provide any significant information and was the least important channel among the three resulting in red and green values being used as input to LDA. The classification accuracy of the model was 66.2% and they compared RGB imaging to hyperspectral imaging and stated that the classification accuracy was better in hyperspectral imaging.

Fresh-cut artichokes (*Cynara scolymus* L.) are more convenient but postcut browning is a major quality problem. Amodio et al. (2011) evaluated the color measurement of postcutting changes in artichokes that were treated with anti-browning agents using digital image analysis. Artichoke (cv. Catanese) in batches of 48 was washed, trimmed, and cut into quarters, and the control group was dipped in water while other groups were dipped in antibrowning solution for one minute. These were then dried, and at 3, 24, 48, and 120 h of storage, the appearance of samples were evaluated and images were immediately acquired. Image acquisition was performed by a digital color camera (Canon EOS 400D, United States) and four fluorescent lamps were used for illumination. A standard regression was performed to find the correlation between color parameters (L*a*b*) obtained on whole surface and areas of browning by image analysis and the appearance score based on human eye. The results of the experiment showed that cysteine was the most effective antibrowning agent in preventing browning in artichokes. The color index (L*a*b*) for the whole artichoke and the browned area had good correlation with the appearance score, specifically L* values showed the highest correlation and were used as the predictors of appearance to validate the method. Amodio et al. concluded that digital imaging is a rapid technique to assess the appearance color and quality of fresh produce.

Mendoza et al. (2006) studied the color measurements of fruit and vegetables using an image analysis technique. Bananas (*Musa Cavendish*; green, yellow, and yellow with brown spots) and red pepper (*Capsicum frutescens*), were selected for the study. The computer vision system consisted of two fluorescent lamps and a color digital camera (PowerShot A70, Canon, United States) that was connected to a computer. To avoid any kind of external light and reflections, the camera and illuminators were covered with a black cloth. The sensitivity analysis of imaging system demonstrated that lightness L* values were significantly affected when the background color was changed from black to white. Mendoza et al. stated that computer-vision-based image analysis could be a useful technique to quantify the color of any food material.

Yam and Papadakis (2004) presented a very simple digital imaging method to measure the color of food surfaces. These measured the color of microwaved pizza with a 2.1 Mp digital camera (Olympus C-2000Z) and the illumination source was two D65 lamps. Once the images were acquired, these were analyzed using Photoshop. Three color models were used in this study to define color: RGB (red, green, blue), CMYK (cyan, magenta, yellow, black), and L*a*b*. In qualitative analysis, darker, lighter, and more appealing were the terms used to compare pizza samples. In quantitative analysis L*a*b* was used due to the fact that it is device independent and also covers a larger range compared to RGB and CMYK. The authors concluded that analysis of food surface color could be performed by a simple digital imaging method. Although, imaging it is not a replacement for other color measurement techniques, it could be an attractive alternative owing to its simple, versatile, and low-cost attributes.

Segnini et al. (1999) performed a video image analysis to assess the color of potato chips. Commercially manufactured potato chips (Lättsaltade, OLW, AB, Sweden) were used as samples and a colorimeter (Dr. Lange, Germany) was used to measure the color. Using a video camera (NV-G1, VHS-C, Panasonic) images were acquired and two fluorescent lamps were used for illumination. Chips were categorized into acceptable chips (no visible spots), chips having spots (with acceptable color but not acceptable due to spots), and nonacceptable chips (darker, browner, and not acceptable). Ten chips from each category were imaged and color was expressed in L*a*b*. The analysis showed that there was a statistically significant difference between the three categories and acceptable chips were lighter compared to the chips-with-spots category, and they were lighter than nonacceptable chips. To evaluate the sensitivity of the video camera, 40 chips were taken randomly and sorted into 10 categories ranging from lightest to darkest color. Using video image analysis, colors were measured. The results showed that a clear relationship existed between L*a*b* values and scale of the human eye. The results of the study showed that sensitivity of the technique correlated with the human eye and have some advantages, such as no sample preparation, and quantification of characteristics, such as spots on the chips surface.

Minimally processed and ready to use (RTU) vegetables are popular with consumers. Lettuce is a RTU vegetable, and its color and appearance are useful to assess the shelf life and consumer acceptance. Zhou et al. (2004) evaluated the shelf life and acceptability of lettuce using digital image analysis. The lettuce samples for the study were bought from Pride Pak Canada Inc. (Mississauga, Ontario). The lettuce was shredded and treated with or without chlorinated warm water (48°C) and then washed with chlorine water at 4°C, dried by centrifugation, packed in plastic bags, and maintained at 4°C for 24 h before shipping. The received samples were kept at 4°C or 10°C up to 18 days. The images were acquired using a digital camera (Nikon Coolpix 900) on 1, 4, 6, 8, 11, 14, and 18 days after the samples were packed. To assess and grade the sample based on acceptability (McKellar et al., 2004), a human sensory of 12 panelists assessed visual qualities of color, texture, and dryness, and rated them on scale of 1 to 5 (1, acceptable; 2, mostly acceptable; 3, somewhat acceptable; 4, mostly unacceptable; 5, unacceptable). The images were examined for percentage of brown area, and changes in the color and percentage brown area were a good indication of lettuce quality. The correlation coefficient between the shelf life and percent of brown area was in the range of 0.9194 to 0.9941 and high correlation was obtained between visual evaluation and percentage of brown area. The authors concluded that digital image analysis is a potential tool to monitor the quality and shelf life of lettuce.

Nakano (1997) evaluated the potential of digital imaging and neural network for grading of apples by assessing the surface color. The system consisted of a turntable, CCD camera, image processor, and neural network model. The apple variety San-fuji was used in the study. The apples were sent directly to the laboratory from the field. After acquiring images, two neural network models were applied: model A was to assess if the color of the apple was normal or abnormal red; the second model B was to grade the apples into five categories (superior, excellent, good, poor, and injured). The results of the analysis showed that model A was able to classify a pixel with 95% accuracy into normal red, injured red, poor red, vine, and background color. Model B was able to classify 92.5% of superior apples, 33.3% of excellent, 65.8% of good, 87.2% of poor, and 75.0% of injured apples. The classification accuracy was lower for excellent and good apples, and hence a clear input data or other methods of output treatment are required to increase the classification efficiency of the model.

The maturity of fruits and vegetables are related to color change. Lin et al. (1993) explored the potential of video imaging to determine the chlorophyll content of cucumbers. The imaging equipment consisted of a video camera (TVC-6200-2, Kayo International Inc., Hanpange, New York) with a wavelength specific filter at 550 nm. Cucumbers of five age groups (17, 19, 21, 23, and 25 days after anthesis) were harvested. The image of the whole cucumber was first obtained and then a disk was separated from the midsection of the cucumber. The results of the study showed that depending on the age at harvest, green color of the cucumber varied significantly and the most intense color appeared on cucumbers harvested at 20 to 23 days after anthesis, which was shown by the lowest gray value. Also, storage of cucumbers for 1 week resulted in significant loss of green color, which was observed by increasing gray levels. They stated that an imaging technique could be useful for product sorting and shelf-life prediction of cucumbers.

Color is one of the vital quality characteristics of meat and a critical sensory characteristic that affects the final quality of the product and the price factor of raw meat. Girolami et al. (2013) evaluated the quality of beef, chicken, and pork using a computer vision system. Muscle samples were collected from 15 animals of each species: chicken (*Pectoralis major*), beef (*Longissimus dorsi, Semimembranosus,* and *Semitendinosus*), and pig (*Longissimus dorsi*). Images were acquired using a CMOS sensor EOS 450D digital camera (Canon). L*a*b* was also measured with CR-400 colorimeter. The color characteristics displayed by both methods were evaluated by 15 trained panelists. The results showed that a digital imaging method provided a valid measurement that resembled the real one rather than the colorimeter method.

Valous et al. (2009) evaluated the color quality of presliced hams using a computer vision system. Four varieties of commercial ham samples made from pork (cooked, smoked), chicken (roasted), and turkey (smoked) were bought from a market in Dublin,

Ireland. The computer vision system consisted of an illumination source with four fluorescent lamps, and a color digital camera (Canon PowerShotA75, Canon, United States) connected to a computer. After the computer vision system was calibrated and overall images of ham were segmented, a color segmentation algorithm was developed for identification and segmentation of fat-connective tissues and pores. Average color values of L*a*b* and RGB components calculated from ham surfaces were analyzed statistically. The results of the study showed that a computer vision system can be used to identify regions of interest such as pores and fat-connective tissue and quantitative information can be extracted from the ham surface with high levels of accuracy. Thus a computer vision system could be used as a tool to quantify and evaluate the presliced hams.

Larraín et al. (2008) evaluated the digital imaging technique to estimate L*a*b*, hue angle, and chroma of beef, and compared it to results from colorimeter. Twenty-one Angus crossbred steers were used for the study and right strip loins were aged for 14 days at 4°C and steaks were made from the *longissimus lumborum* muscle. Color readings were obtained from colorimeter (Minolta Chromameter CR-300, Osaka, Japan), and digital images were acquired using a digital camera (Canon PowerShot A70). The RGB values obtained from digital images were transformed to CIE L*a*b* color space. The color readings from the images could be used to predict a*, hue angle, and chroma from the color coordinates measured with a colorimeter. They concluded that digital imaging is a potential tool to detect color changes in beef and other meat products.

The quality of seafood is assessed based on freshness, which can be determined by various physical, sensory, chemical, and microbiological methods. But chemical and microbiological methods are sensitive only in the advanced stage of deterioration. Dowlati et al. (2013) determined the freshness of fish using digital imaging based on color changes of gills and eyes. Wild gilthead sea bream (*Sparus aurata*) from a local market (Valencia, Spain) were used for the study and all fish were stored in ice for 17 days. Images were acquired every 24 h. The images were captured using a color digital camera with two fluorescent lamps for illumination and the color parameters L*a*b*, total color change (ΔE), and chroma (c*) were assessed. From the images, it could be seen that the color of the eyes (pupil) looked white and cloudy during the storage time due to chemical changes resulting in organoleptic changes such as appearance and color. Regression equation developed to evaluate the color parameters during the storage time fitted well with values of R^2 greater than 0.96. The authors concluded that image processing has the potential to assess the fish eye and gill color changes, and regression models can be developed to predict fish freshness. Dowlati et al. (2012) presented a detailed review on machine vision techniques for quality assessment of fish and fish products.

Color is an important quality attribute of pork and is difficult to assess because the color is not uniform even within the same muscle. Lu et al. (2000) evaluated the color of fresh pork loin using computer vision techniques. The imaging system consisted of a Sony CCD camera (XC-711), frame grabber, monitor, and computer. The samples were 44 randomly picked pork loins and the muscle color was evaluated by a sensory panel. The color evaluation was based on a score of 1 to 5 (1, pale purplish gray; 2, grayish pink; 3, reddish pink; 4, purplish red; 5, dark purplish red). Neural network and statistical models were used to determine the color scores. Prediction error (difference between average sensory and predicted color score) of 0.6 or lower was acceptable for practical purposes. The results showed that out of 44 samples, 93.2% of samples had a lower than 0.6% prediction error based on neural network, and 84.1% of samples showed an error lower than 0.6 in statistical modeling. Lu et al. concluded that an imaging technique along with a neural network could be a potential solution for prediction of fresh pork color.

Many other researchers have evaluated the quality of meat using digital imaging. Gerrard et al. (1996) evaluated the beef quality with respect to beef marbling and color score using digital imaging techniques. Jeyamkondan et al. (2000) developed a video image analysis for quality grading of beef and stated that the grading based on imaging was equivalent to the grades provided by human inspectors. Chen and Qin (2008) and Jackman et al. (2009) developed a segmentation method for beef marbling and stated that the performance of the proposed model was robust and comparable to assess meat by visual inspectors. Faucitano et al. (2005) developed an imaging technique to measure pork marbling characteristics.

4.3.4 Quality evaluation of other food products using digital imaging

4.3.4.1 Ready-to-eat meals

Consumption of ready-to-eat meals is rapidly growing, but the challenge is to automate the production. Munkevik et al. (2007) developed an automatic computer-based method for sensory evaluation of complex meals. The components of the meal consisted of potatoes, vegetables, meatballs, jam, and sauce placed on white plates. The images were acquired using a Philips camera (TOUCAM PCVC740K) and stored at a resolution of 1280 × 960 pixels, and the color representation used was RGB. Five experienced judges performed quantitative sensory analysis. Seventy-two attributes divided into four categories (amount, shape, placement, and component spatial relation) were identified as the important sensory qualities. The image analysis included image preprocessing, segmentation, feature extraction, and a three-layered artificial neural network was used to transform the image features to sensory attributes developed by the sensory panel. The component classification was good with 99.1% for potato, 99.0% for peas, 98.6% for plate, and 97.8% for carrots, and lower than 95% for meatballs, sauce, and jam. The results of the study showed that a computer vision system has great potential to perform automatic sensory evaluation and achieve almost the same results as that of a human sensory panel and hence could be used for automatic online sensory evaluation in food industry.

4.3.4.2 Egg

The quality monitoring of eggs is largely done by human graders, which results in two types of errors: good quality eggs are graded as defective or defective ones graded as good quality, both of which results in economic loss. An automatic grading system that could detect blood spots, cracks, dirt, and stains would reduce the dependence on human graders, improve the quality of egg grading, and increase the profitability. Patel et al. (1998) developed a digital imaging system with artificial neural network for defect monitoring in poultry eggs. The imaging system consisted of a CCD video camera (Sony DXC-930), frame grabber, and an incandescent lamp to back illuminate the egg. The images were analyzed by applying a neural network model to detect crack, blood spot, and dirt stain in eggs. The blood spot detection in eggs had an average classification accuracy of 92.8%, average classification accuracy for dirt stained eggs was 85.0%, and for crack detection was 87.8%. These classification accuracies exceeded the accuracy level required by the U.S. Department of Agriculture for grading eggs. Patel et al. concluded that defect detection in eggs could be achieved by applying computer vision and neural network techniques.

4.3.4.3 Beef

Tenderness is an important quality attribute of beef, but the attributes that define the grading criteria do not have sufficient information about tenderness. Many research studies have been conducted to evaluate the quality of meat using textural features. Shiranita et al.

(1998, 2000) evaluated the quality of beef meat using marbling score and textural analysis. They performed neural network analysis and multiple regression analysis, and stated that the results were in agreement with the results of the human inspectors, and that the imaging technique could be used for quality evaluation of beef. Basset et al. (2000) classified meat slices according to the age, breed, and muscle type based on texture analysis using digital imaging and stated that digital imaging has great potential to classify meat samples. J. Li et al. (2001) evaluated the ability of image analysis using textural features to classify tough and tender beef. Fifty-nine cross steers were slaughtered and after 72 h of aging, 59 short loins from the carcasses were taken in two sets. One set was used for imaging and the other set was used to perform sensory evaluation. The imaging system consisted of a Sony CCD camera (XC-711), frame grabber, and computer. The captured images in RGB format were then transformed into HSI format (hue refers to the type of color, i.e., red or yellow; saturation is the relative purity or amount of white, i.e., red vs. pink; intensity refers to the brightness). The features were extracted using a wavelet-based decomposition method. The results showed that classification accuracy of 83% was obtained using image texture analysis to classify beef tenderness and hence they concluded that texture feature alone was not sufficient to classify beef products, but it can be an important indicator for tenderness prediction. Ballerini and Bocchi (2006) developed an image processing technique to measure the fat content in beef. After the images were acquired, image processing was applied in three stages; meat extraction, removal of connective tissue, and fat segmentation. The results were compared with the results from chemical analysis and the digital imaging technique had a good correlation with the chemical analysis results, and hence the authors concluded that imaging could be used as a potential tool to determine fat content in beef.

4.3.4.4   Yeast biomass
Fermentation of food was one of the earliest developed food technologies and yeast was used for fermentation of food and beverages. Biomass production during fermentation was quantified by direct counting under microscope or by destructive methods, but there are limitations in each method. Acevedo et al. (2009) developed a digital imaging method based on RGB analysis to predict yeast biomass. The images were acquired using a digital color camera (Nikon Coolpix 4300, Nikon, Japan) with white light illumination. Yeasts (*Saccharomyces cerevisiae* spp.) were immobilized in alginate capsules and images of 10 capsules were captured. Multivariate data analysis was performed with the partial least square method. The yeast growth in alginate hydrogel was evident from the change of color on the surface of the capsule. The surface color of the capsule before and after yeast growth was quantified by histogram intensity, and significant differences in capsule colors were observed from RGB histograms. The first and second principal components explained around 85% of variation with the yeast concentration determined by PC1 and cell viability was determined by PC2 values. They concluded that digital imaging could be used to quantify immobilized biomass in a simple, fast, and reliable manner.

4.3.4.5   Bakery
Bakeries constitute a major segment of the food industry and real-time inspection of quality monitoring is very important. Since biscuits are produced in huge quantities, quality evaluation by human inspectors is very tedious. Nashat et al. (2011) developed an imaging technique based on a support vector machine to monitor the quality of stationary as well as moving biscuits on the conveyor belt. Unlike other products, no standards exist for color grading of biscuits. The color of biscuits depends on each brand and product, but consumers expect the color in every biscuit in each packet to be exactly the same.

The authors categorized the biscuits into four categories: underbaked, moderately baked, overbaked, and significantly overbaked due to difference in temperature within the oven. The imaging system consisted of a CCD SONY camera (XC-003P), color frame grabber, and illumination system. The digital images of biscuits acquired by CCD camera were represented in RGB color space, which is device dependent. Hence, RGB information is transformed into HLS (hue, lightness, saturation) color space. The accuracy of classification of the system was greater than 96% for stationary biscuits and those biscuits moving at a speed of 9 m/min. But the image processing time for biscuits in contact was significantly slower compared to nontouching biscuits and the average time was 36.3 ms and 9.0 ms for touching and nontouching biscuits, respectively. Nashat et al. concluded that a digital imaging technique could be a potential tool for quality inspection of biscuits in real time.

The quality inspection of muffins is performed by trained people, but an automatic system to standardize the quality monitoring would reduce the subjective and inconsistent results produced by human evaluators. Abdullah et al. (2000) examined the classification of light- and dark-colored muffins using a digital imaging system. The imaging system consisted of a CCD color camera (TMC-7RGB, Pulnix America Corp., California), frame grabber, fluorescent light, and computer. Muffins were prepared by baking the mixture (flour, baking powder, eggs, sugar, and water) at 300°C and displayed upside down. To classify muffins according to their color a multivariate discriminant algorithm was developed and tested on 200 muffins (100 light colored and 100 dark colored). The results of the study indicated that muffins were classified with an accuracy of 88%, whereas classification by quality inspectors resulted in 20% to 30% variation between them. They concluded that digital imaging could be a potential technique to classify bakery products with an accuracy rate better than manual inspection.

Researchers at the Georgia Institute of Technology and Flower Bakery in Villa Rica, Georgia, developed a digital imaging system to monitor the quality of sandwich buns (Britton, 2003). The fresh buns are scanned using a digital camera. When the buns pass along the conveyor belt, the color, shape, and size of the buns are monitored through computer vision, which removes buns that do not fit in the defined criteria.

4.3.4.6 Pasta

Pasta is one of the most important foods consumed globally and the pasta quality has always been of concern to processors. To meet the demands of consumers, pasta processors should avoid defects like crumbling, unevenness, and cracks that occur due to extra hydration, and the pasta must not stick together. Mokhtar et al. (2011) evaluated the imaging technique to monitor pasta during production. Two kinds of pasta—Spätzle, ribbon cut egg noodles (with cracks, broken pieces, unevenness, and stickiness); and bucatini, hollow spaghetti (cracks occur because of unbalanced drying conditions)—were used for the experiment. Images were acquired using a CCD camera and flat LED lights were used as illumination. Images were analyzed, and size, shape, and color features were evaluated. The results showed that error in determining stickiness, crumple, and unevenness were 1%, 5%, and 13%, respectively. The study showed that digital imaging could monitor quality evaluation in pasta production.

4.3.5 Inspection of packaging of food components in bottles

In the food and beverage industry, bottling is an important method of packaging the materials. Proper closure of bottle and perfect level of filling are the two most important criteria in quality monitoring of packaging bottles. Much research has been conducted to implement an automatic visual inspection system to monitor bottle fill level and perfect cap closure.

Abdelhedi et al. (2012) designed and tested an automatic vision monitoring system for inspection of olive oil bottling for detection of any defects in oil level and cap. The experimental setup is shown in Figure 4.8. The conveyor belt had a sensor that sent signals to the computer, triggering the CCD camera (SVCam-ECO line eco424, AIA, Michigan) interfaced with the computer to capture the bottle image, which was then processed by the computer. Image processing techniques such as local thresholding, edge detection, and area calculation were used. The image processing techniques for detection of bottle cap and level of oil fill was tested, and the results showed good precision to qualify for implementation of a system in real-time monitoring of bottles in the production line. Yazdi et al. (2011) developed an automatic visual inspection system (AVIS) to check the integrity of cap closure in bottles and to perform liquid level checks in bottles to ensure that the liquid is not over- or underfilled. The system was based on digital imaging using feature extraction techniques, and the algorithm would only accept proper cap closure and correct liquid level in the bottle and reject all other possibilities.

Prabuwono et al. (2006) explored the detection of cap closure with a webcam placed at 15 cm from the bottle with the conveyor speed at 106 rpm. They obtained an accuracy of 94.3% for a moving bottle. Zhu (2009) monitored the correct content level in fusion bottles. They applied image binarization to determine the threshold value, and a filtering method was performed. Sobel's algorithm was applied for the edge detection method and obtained an accuracy of 100% when infusion bottles were tilted. Pithadiya et al. (2009) compared the performance of various edge detection algorithms (Canny, Log, and ISEF) for inspection of liquid levels in bottles.

Duan et al. (2004) implemented a machine vision system for inspection of bottle finish using digital imaging. The Hough transform algorithm was used for detecting the region of interest and two neural network algorithms were used for low- and high-level inspection. They concluded that the proposed design and algorithm were efficient for automatic inspection chink defects and bottle finish. More research was conducted by Wang et al.

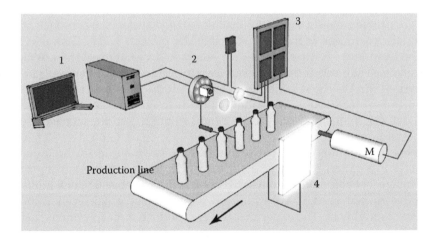

Figure 4.8 Design of a machine vision system for monitoring fill level and cap in bottles: (1) computer, (2) camera, (3) electrical control panel, and (4) backlight. (From Abdelhedi, S. et al., *International Journal of Computer Application*, 51, 39, 2012. With permission.)

(2005) using a fuzzy support vector machine and they obtained an accuracy of 98% in detecting bottle finish defects.

4.3.6 *Engineering applications of digital imaging in the visible spectrum*

Quality control of objects in the industrial environment is traditionally performed by human experts. An industrial computer vision system could be a better replacement for human experts because manual inspection is slower, subjective, and requires training of humans to acquire the skills. Malamas et al. (2003) performed a detailed survey and study of vision systems and applications in the industrial environment. They stated that most industrial applications are based on one of the four types of inspection: dimensional accuracy, quality of the surface of object, accurate assembling of parts or structural quality, and the accuracy of operation of a process. Monitoring the dimensional quality involves checking the dimension, roundness, corners, shape, positioning, alignment, and orientation of the object. The surface quality of the objects is inspected by monitoring the scratches, wear and tear, cracks, proper finishing, roughness, and texture of the product. The structural quality is monitored by checking for any missing parts such as rivets or screws, or detection of the presence of foreign objects. The operational quality relates to the monitoring of operations according to the manufacturing standards and specifications.

Computer vision or machine vision in the industrial and manufacturing sector tackles the computerized image interpretation to monitor and solve quality-related issues. The major limitations of human inspection are fatigue, subjective nature, lower output, and higher cost, whereas computer vision systems have consistency, repeatability, and accuracy compared to human inspection. Rao (1996) analyzed the potential of machine vision in semiconductor manufacturing processes. One of the most important criteria in circuit inspection is the early detection of process problems, and patterned wafer inspection is the critical problem in semiconductor manufacturing. The author examined the classification of automatic defect in wafer inspection. Rao analyzed the choice of algorithm based on variability in defects, variability in defect samples, and complexity of patterns. The performance was tested over a period of one year and over 100,000 images were acquired during the first two stages. The performance of the system was based on type of defect and process variation, and classification accuracies were between 80% and 99%. They stated that the major problems associated with machine vision systems are the lack of standardization and lack of images at the early stages of the project. A.D.H. Thomas et al. (1995) reviewed the techniques related to real-time automated visual inspection (AVI) in industrial applications. They stated that there are two major areas of automated visual inspection applications: first is the rejection of defective product to ensure quality control and second is to gather statistical information that helps to provide feedback to the manufacturing process. The first is known as feedforward solution, and the second case is known as feedback solution.

One of the important quality control measures in the manufacturing industry is surface roughness evaluation. Many inspections are currently performed using a stylus, but the disadvantage is that it requires physical contact with the object, which limits the speed of the process. Kumar et al. (2005) evaluated digital image magnification for measurement of surface roughness. The experiments were conducted on specimens made by various machining processes, such as milling, grinding, and shaping. The imaging system consisted of a CCD camera, computer, video monitor, and image processing software. A gray scale analyzing technique was used for analyzing the acquired images. The analysis showed that a good linear relationship was observed between average surface roughness

(R_a) and gray level average (G_a) values with high accuracy. Based on their results, Kumar et al. stated that digital imaging techniques could be a promising tool to evaluate the surface roughness of specimens obtained by various machining operations.

Aluze et al. (2002) developed an imaging system for defect detection and characterization of defects of 3D objects. The design of lighting is important to evaluate mirror-like 3D objects, and the algorithms were tested on cosmetic products such as lipstick lids and perfume caps. The experimental setup consisted of a camera, light source, and object. The imaging system tries to generate images of product defects referred to as defect signatures. The defect signatures should not be dependent on system parameters and multiple signatures of a single defect imaged from different viewpoints should be identical. The system designed by the authors generated defect signatures independent of system parameters, and the system was reliable and effective. A number of images acquired from different light stripe locations were summed up to optimize and increase the contrast between defects and flawless regions. They tested the system on objects of various shapes (including planar, spherical, and cylindrical) and conducted two experiments. The objects inspected by human operators were tested with an imaging system and classified as either accepted or rejected. Then the results were compared with human evaluations. Objects that were accepted by human evaluators but rejected by computer vision were tagged as false alarms. The results of the study showed that false alarm and undetected defects were very low, and hence the authors concluded that the imaging system is very reliable for detecting surface defects on 3D objects.

Technology advancement has resulted in significant reduction in the size of electronic products that are more powerful and require intensive inspection processes. In a manufacturing industry, 30% of the tasks are inspection and monitoring, out of which 60% are done manually. Of the defects identified in visual inspection, 30% are part defects, 50% of defects are related to assembling of parts, and 20% are defects due to soldering (Hata, 1990). Edinbarough et al. (2005) developed a vision- and robot-based monitoring system for on-line inspection of electronic products. The vision system consisted of a CCD camera, computer, and neural network software. The developed system was able to monitor integrated circuits (ICs) of printed circuit boards (PCBs), and the performance was also tested on several electronic products.

Straightness is a critical parameter to ensure the quality of screw threads in seamless steel pipes. Straightness inspection is performed by human inspectors, which results in low speed and is subjected to human error. Although many methods were explored, none of them is suitable for on-line measurements of straightness of pipes. Lu et al. (2001) explored the machine vision technique for straightness measurement of seamless steel pipes. The measurement was performed by laser sensors placed along the axis of pipes and the laser beam emitted by sensor was magnified by the lens resulting in an arc during intersection of the axes' external surface. CCD cameras capture the images of the steel pipes, which are transmitted to frame grabber, digitized, and stored, and the straightness is estimated by the imaging algorithm. Lu et al. stated that the imaging technique is successful in measuring the straightness of screw threads in steel pipes, but at least a minimum of three sensor groups should be used. The authors suggested that for seamless steel pipes of 1500 mm, more than five sensors are better to produce high-precision results. They concluded that laser visual measurement techniques along with machine vision are an important tool for on-line measurement of straightness in seamless steel pipes with high measurement precision.

Electric contacts are electrical components used in electrical devices to connect or disconnect electrical circuits. Sun et al. (2010) explored the potential of machine vision using digital imaging to inspect electric contacts. Electric contacts are classified into three groups: buttons, rivets, and tips, and are mainly made of two parts: head and shank. The system acquired the images from three views and they inspected the top, bottom, and side surfaces of electric contacts to monitor different types of defects, such as extra metal, deckle edge, and edge break from the top view; side cracks from the side view; and eccentricity and back cracks from the bottom view. Different preprocessing and feature extraction methods were used for detecting defects from different views. The system monitored a total of 229 samples from the production lines and the results showed that the proposed digital imaging system was effective in inspection and monitoring of defects in electric contacts.

In the electronics manufacturing industry, especially printed circuit boards (PCBs), solder joint is a critical process that provides the electrical connection. The quality of solder joint is an important factor that determines the quality of the electronic component and also maintains the product reliability. Many researchers have explored the quality of solder joints in electronic components using image analysis (T.H. Kim et al., 1999; Lee and Lo, 2002; Acciani et al., 2006; Lin et al., 2007). Mar et al. (2011) developed a computer vision system for inspection of solder joints on PCBs. The inspection procedure for solder joints includes image acquisition, segmentation of image, feature extraction, and classification. The region of interest from the image is extracted by Hough transform, and an illumination normalization technique is used to eliminate the effect due to uneven illumination conditions. Mar et al. developed two inspection modules: front end and back end for automatic solder joint classification. They classified five different types of solder joints: good joint, excess joint, less solder joint, no joint, and bridge solder joint. The authors concluded that the Log-Gabor filter technique resulted in high recognition rates.

In the machinery industry, various machine parts are connected by bearings to reduce friction. The quality of bearings has a major influence on the performance of machines and hence strict inspection procedures have been adopted in the bearing production process to maintain the quality of bearings. Bearing inspection is mostly performed by human inspectors under bright lights. Manual inspection is highly subjective and inconsistent. Research studies have been conducted to explore the potential of machine vision to inspect bearing defects. Wu et al. (2010) monitored the tapered roller bearing using machine vision. They inspected missing rollers in tapered roller bearings and roller bearings installed in the opposite direction of standard procedure. The automatic inspection system consisted of mechanical and electrical parts, illumination, CCD camera, and computer. The authors stated that the defect inspection system is reliable, effective, and stable. Deng et al. (2010) developed a machine vision system for defect detection of the surface of bearings using a CCD camera. They utilized least square fitting to locate the region of interest, and contrast enhancement and low pass filtering was used to improve the image quality. Their results showed that the digital imaging system was highly efficient, accurate, and could be used at ease to detect the surface defects in bearings. H. Wang et al. (2011) proposed a system for inspection of character defects in bearing production by imaging through CCD camera and stated that imaging techniques could improve productivity and replace the manual inspection process. Shen et al. (2012) proposed a machine vision technique to inspect cover defects in bearings. The cover of bearings is comprised of the inner ring, seal, and outer ring. The defects to be monitored include cracks and rusts on the outer and inner rings; cracks, rusts, deformation and scratches on seals; and dimensions of chamfers. The imaging system consisted of an area scan camera, lens, LED lights for illumination, and light shield. Two tests were performed: In the first test, the number of samples analyzed by machine vision was 805 and the accuracy of detection was 98.2% by imaging, whereas accuracy of human inspection was 98.9%. In the second test, accuracy of machine vision system was 98.7%, whereas that of human inspection was 98.8%. The authors concluded that a novel inspection algorithm can detect bearing defects with high accuracy and efficiency, and it could be implemented in the production line for automatic detection of defects replacing human inspectors.

4.4 Advantages, limitations, and future of imaging in the visible spectrum

4.4.1 Advantages

The digital imaging system is simple, and easy to setup, upgrade, and replace. Digital cameras are available at many specifications at lower prices compared to any other advanced imaging system. Compared to other imaging techniques such as X-ray, X-ray CT, MRI, or thermal imaging, optical imaging is the simplest and easiest to operate in the imaging system and does not require any special training for personnel. Digital imaging techniques provide consistent and accurate results, and eliminates subjectivity as compared to manual inspection. Digital imaging provides high speed of operation and could be incorporated in on-line production lines and for quality monitoring throughout day and night without any interruption. The fatigue and slowness in the process associated with manual inspection does not occur in imaging techniques. Optical imaging is a noncontact measurement and does not pose any health hazard. Imaging in the visible spectrum could be used for quality assessment of many food materials, agricultural products, cereal grains, and fresh produce.

Imaging techniques reduce production costs in manufacturing facilities by identifying defective parts at early stages of the process and the defects can be rectified and reintroduced or rejected based on the defect. This greatly reduces the cost of production rather than the defective part being removed at the end of the process. Imaging techniques allow inspection of the whole lot of a product produced rather than sampling of batches or random sampling of the product. Imaging systems can be installed in environments that are hazardous for humans to work.

4.4.2 Limitations

With numerous advantages, digital imaging techniques also have certain limitations. Components of the imaging system need proper installation for optimal performance. Illumination plays a major role in digital imaging, which could significantly affect the results. The system requires proper illumination to reduce the time on image processing; otherwise the images require more advanced processing techniques and sometimes may also affect the accuracy of the results. During the processing of acquired images, segmentation is done to extract the region of interest from the background during which color and shape are considered as the critical features, but both color and shape can be affected by illumination. Hence, proper type and position of illumination is very critical to obtain good quality images.

Digital imaging systems work well in controlled environments, but performance is still lacking in many real-time situations. In certain applications, machine vision cannot be a substitute for human vision because judgment of the human eye is often better at evaluating the very subtle nuances that contribute to the quality of the product. The capacity of the human brain to process the image visualized by the eye and make decisions based on human judgment is still unique and to duplicate this ability by machine vision is still challenging (Fabel, 1997).

There is no unique system and software to solve all industrial problems. Each problem requires a specific setup and software component. Systems require advanced software components for processing of images and require skilled personnel to write algorithms for each application based on the specific needs. In many applications, it was not possible to obtain 100% accuracy in defect detection or classification. It is also important to calibrate the system, and the algorithms need to be tested and compared with the results from traditional instruments (Leta et al., 2005). Compared to other advanced imaging techniques such as X-ray, X-ray CT, hyperspectral, and thermal imaging, digital imaging has its own limitations and cannot compete with the advanced imaging modalities. For instance, internal structures cannot be detected with images in the visible spectrum. Various internal quality defects in fruits and vegetables such as internal breakdown, internal browning, and watercore cannot be detected by digital cameras, and special imaging techniques such as X-ray CT, MRI, or ultrasound are essential to detect such internal defects.

4.4.3   Future

Regarding the components of optical imaging in machine vision, CCD sensors are currently widely used and CMOS sensors could grow in the future. A significant market for special types of cameras with increased speed and resolution could boost the development of 3D cameras, which may include integrated optics, illumination, and processing. Frame grabbers may be replaced by smart cameras or imaging computers for mainstream applications (Alper, 2012). Most color cameras use colored filters, which are inexpensive but make errors during color measurements. In the future, new color camera technology with higher accuracy, and using programmable filters to acquire red, green, and blue images sequentially may be available in the market at a competitive price (Dawson, 2011). Manufacturers of machine vision components have understood the market needs and are adopting newer technology to boost the performance of imaging systems so as to promote the technology to the next level.

Applications of optical imaging in the visible spectrum are widely expanding in the agriculture, food, and beverage industries. With the installation of a basic imaging setup, the industries are seeing an increased accuracy, speed, and reduction in the dependence of manual inspection for maintaining the quality of the products and processes. In the future, any industry that requires precise, fast, and continuous repetitive measurement of product specification and quality could benefit by imaging the technique.

The industrial image processing division in Germany alone has reported record sales of €1.5 billion for 2011, which was not foreseeable when the technology was introduced around 25 years ago. Significant development in microelectronics and image sensors has led to improved performance of industrial digital cameras and increased the range of functions. Technology improvement has also resulted in compact size and decreased price range (Marofsky, 2012). An increase in adoption of imaging technology has resulted in a decrease in the price trend of imaging components, which has further made the technology available even to small-scale industries. In the mid-1980s, a machine vision system cost was $40,000 to $60,000, whereas the cost of the machine vision components have reduced significantly and today is available for as low as $5000 (Fabel, 1997). A group of image processing experts who participated in a roundtable discussion in Pullach, Germany, stated that only 10% of potential applications of image processing have been explored and there remains a huge area that has not yet been explored to adopt image processing techniques.

chapter five

Hyperspectral imaging

5.1 Introduction

Hyperspectral imaging is a combination of spectroscopy and imaging techniques to acquire the spectral and spatial information of an object. Hyperspectral imaging, also called imaging spectrometry or imaging spectroscopy, provides physical and geometrical features of products such as size, shape, appearance, and color, along with the chemical composition of the product through spectral analysis. A spectral image obtained from hyperspectral imaging is a stack or pile of images of the object of interest at various bands of spectrum. An imaging technique provides intensity at each pixel of an image $I (x, y)$; a spectrometer gives a single spectrum $I (\lambda)$; and a hyperspectral image gives a spectrum at every pixel, that is, $I (x, y, \lambda)$. A hyperspectral image is a 3D block of data, comprising two spatial dimensions (x rows $\times$ y columns) and third spectral dimension (λ wavelength) that can be seen as a collection of many images where every image is measured at various wavelengths or can be seen as a group of many spectral values at every pixel (Garini et al., 2006). The three-dimensional hyperspectral data is called a hypercube. A schematic representation of a hypercube is shown in Figure 5.1. The image element is called a pixel in a two-dimensional image at a single wavelength; in the three-dimensional hypercube, the image element is called a voxel.

The initial application of hyperspectral imaging was in remote sensing for observation of targets without physical contact. The invention of charged-coupled device (CCD) by G. Smith and W. Boyle in 1969 was an important factor in the progress of hyperspectral imaging technology (Gomez, 2002). Alexander Goetz and his colleagues at NASA's Jet Propulsion Laboratory (JPL), California Institute of Technology, developed the airborne imaging spectrometer (AIS) in the 1980s and then developed the Airborne Visible/Infrared Imaging Spectrometer (AVIRIS). In 1987, AVIRIS was the first imaging spectrometer that measured the reflected solar spectrum ranging from 400 nm to 2500 nm with 10 nm intervals (Goetz, 1995). The success of this instrument resulted in the development of various sensors and data acquisition systems that introduced multispectral and hyperspectral imaging instruments for ground based and airborne remote sensing applications. Further improvements in the system resulted in the application of hyperspectral imaging in various fields including agriculture, geology, medical, pharmacy, and food.

5.2 Hyperspectral imaging

5.2.1 Principle

The basic principle underlying hyperspectral imaging is that all kinds of materials reflect, scatter, emit, and absorb electromagnetic energy in different patterns at specific wavelengths because of the difference in their chemical composition and inherent physical structure. This characteristic is known as the spectral signature or spectrum, and is unique for every object (ElMasry et al., 2012a,b). Spectral resolution could be described as an ability to resolve the spectral features or a measure of the smallest spectral feature

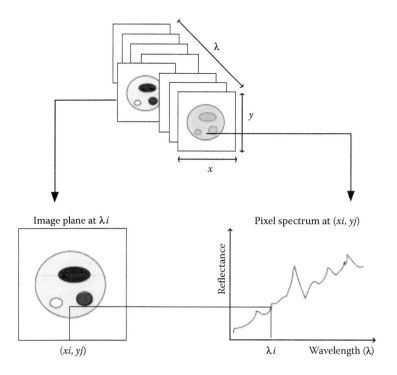

Figure 5.1 Schematic representation of a hypercube showing the relationship between spatial and spectral dimensions. (From Gowen, A.A. et al., *Trends in Food Science and Technology*, 18, 590, 2007. With permission.)

a spectrometer can resolve. For instance, if during hyperspectral imaging, a sensor collects data from 500 to 1100 nm, which is spread over 50 spectral bands, then the width of each spectral band is about 12 nm, and this band width is called spectral resolution (Space Computer Corporation, 2007). Spectral sampling interval is the interval between data points, which occurs in the measured spectrum specified in wavelength units.

Spectral imaging could be classified as hyperspectral, multispectral, and ultraspectral imaging. Hyperspectral imaging is different from multispectral imaging in the number of spectral bands and spectral resolution. In multispectral imaging, the number of bands is very few (usually less than 10), whereas hyperspectral imaging has hundreds of contiguous and regularly spaced bands. Also, in every pixel, multispectral imaging does not provide a real spectrum, whereas every pixel in hyperspectral image provides a full spectrum (Ariana and Lu, 2008). Ultraspectral images are those images with more than 100 to 500 bands and with a resolution power higher than 0.001 (Giallorenzi, 2000; Kung et al., 2012). Ultraspectral imaging is developed to meet the growing demands for increased spectral resolution and have spectral resolution to allow molecular absorption that can be presented in two dimensions (Meigs et al., 2008).

Based on the method by which spatial information is achieved, the hyperspectral image can be acquired using any of the three common ways: whiskbroom (point scanning), pushbroom (line scanning), or tunable filter (area scanning) where the hyperspectral image could be obtained either one spectrum at a time, or one line or one image at a time, respectively (Figure 5.2). In the whiskbroom method, a complete spectrum of a single point or pixel is obtained at a time and then the sample is moved to obtain another spectrum.

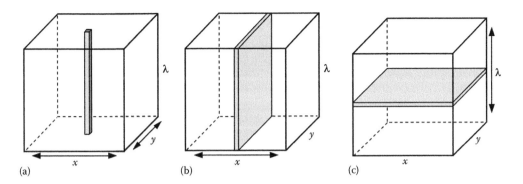

Figure 5.2 Three approaches to generate hyperspectral image. (a) Whiskbroom (point) imaging, (b) pushbroom (line) imaging, and (c) tunable filter (area scan) imaging. (From Qin, J., Hyperspectral imaging instruments, in *Hyperspectral imaging for food quality analysis and control*, ed. Sun, D.W., 2010. With permission.)

In the pushbroom or line scanning method, a whole line of an image is recorded at a time using two-dimensional dispersing elements and a two-dimensional detector array. The tunable filter method is called area scanning or wavelength scanning because the sample is kept fixed and images are obtained one wavelength after another for the whole object (ElMasry et al., 2012b).

A hyperspectral imaging system can provide information in a wide range of electromagnetic spectrums from approximately 200 nm (ultraviolet) to around 2500 nm (nearinfrared [NIR] range). For application in food analysis, hyperspectral imaging is used in the very near infrared and visible regions having a spectral range of 900 to 1700 nm and 380 to 800, respectively. Hyperspectral imaging can be grouped in two regions: shortwave infrared region (SWIR) from 700 to 1100 nm and long wave infrared region (LWIR) from 1100 to 2500 nm. Hyperspectral imaging could be carried out in different modes, such as reflectance, emission, and transmission. Of the three modes, reflectance is the most commonly used method in the visible NIR (400–1000 nm) or NIR (1000–1700 nm) range. Reflectance hyperspectral imaging is widely used to identify various defects and contaminants, and to monitor the quality characteristics of food and agricultural materials (Gowen et al., 2007). In fluorescence imaging, light absorption by a chromophore at a specified wavelength is followed by light emission, usually at longer wavelengths. Fluorescence emission characteristics of food materials are altered by many factors, such as fecal or pathogenic contamination, and intrinsic changes in product quality due to contamination may result in the variation in the fluorescence emission characteristics of the product (Kim et al., 2001). Transmission hyperspectral imaging is mostly used for identification of internal defects and online estimation of internal characteristics of biological materials.

5.2.2 Instrumentation for hyperspectral imaging

The basic parts of a hyperspectral imaging unit are a camera; spectrograph; detector; filter; illumination; and a computer for acquisition of data, storage, and processing. A schematic representation of a hyperspectral imaging unit is shown in Figure 5.3.

Hyperspectral detectors record the reflectance and transmittance spectra of samples. An array of detectors called focal plane arrays (FPAs) are most widely used in hyperspectral imaging rather than point detectors. The advantages of using FPA detectors are to obtain

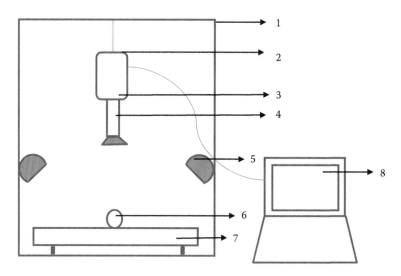

Figure 5.3 Schematic of a hyperspectral imaging system: (1) frame, (2) camera, (3) spectrograph, (4) lens, (5) illumination, (6) sample, (7) translation stage, and (8) computer (data acquisition and storage).

uniform or constant background, high signal-to-noise ratio, decreased scanning time, and less distortion of the image. A linear detector array is utilized in line scan imaging and 2D detector arrays are utilized in area scan imaging systems. Commercially available FPAs are platinum silicide (PtSi), indium antimonide (InSb), germanium (Ge), indium gallium arsenide (InGaAs), mercury cadmium telluride (HgCdTe), and quantum well infrared photodetectors (QWIPs). Of these detectors, the most widely used detectors are InSb, InGaAs, HgCdTe, and QWIP (Tran, 2003). InSb detectors are very sensitive and provide good quality images, but need cryogenic cooling to work at room temperature, which makes this detector highly expensive. HgCdTe detectors are highly sensitive and have the ability to work efficiently in a broad infrared region (2000 to 26,000 nm). These detectors can work well at room temperature, but the limitations of using HgCdTe detectors are the instability and nonuniformity of pixels (Tran, 2003). QWIPs are suitable for long wave infrared imaging applications and the performance of QWIPs is superior to HgCdTe detectors at lower temperature (45 K) but with an increase in temperature the dark current increases. InGaAs detectors are widely used in 900 to 1700 bands of wavelength and are best suited for monitoring the quality of agricultural and food materials. The advantages of InGaAs detectors are higher sensitivity, low noise, broad range of spectra, and quick response in the NIR region, but the major limitation is their lower sensitivity for wavelengths greater than 1700 nm range (Singh, 2009).

Spectrographs are optical components that convert a camera to a hyperspectral imaging device with high spectral resolution. Spectrographs are one of the most important components that help in generating a spectrum of every point present on the scanned line. The spectral resolution of any hyperspectral imaging system is dependent on the ability of the spectrograph to analyze features in the electromagnetic spectrum. The spectrograph's slit width, and size of the entry and exit apertures determine the magnitude of the spectral resolution (ElMasry et al., 2012b).

The filters are selected depending on the type of hyperspectral imaging. Grating devices are used for pushbroom hyperspectral imaging and tunable filters are ideal for area scan hyperspectral imaging. The spectral transmission of tunable filters can be regulated by application of acoustic and voltage signals. An ideal filter should have minimum time for tuning, minimum out-of-band transmission, minimum thickness, less utilization of power, not sensitive to the environment and the incidence angle of incoming light, large aperture, and infinite spectral range. In practice, each type of filter has certain advantages and disadvantages, and selection must be made based on the application (Gat, 2000). The most commonly used electronically tunable filters are liquid crystal tunable filters (LCTFs), acoustic optical tunable filters (AOTFs), and interferometers.

Illumination is an important factor in acquiring good quality images. The most important properties of an illumination system are spatial, spectral, and angular uniformity, which indicates that the light that illuminates the samples should have the similar spectrum across the full sample. When the spectrum of light illumination in one region of the sample varies from the other parts of the sample, the spectral analysis algorithm may provide less accurate results. Hence, the light illuminating the sample should be spectral, spatial, and provide angular uniformity (Katrašnik et al., 2013). If the images are obtained using a nonuniform illumination system, the images may have specular reflections, shadows, and shading effects that could significantly hinder the performance of the imaging algorithm (Katrašnik et al., 2011). An ideal illumination for hyperspectral imaging should possess the following characteristics: homogeneous illumination, polarized light with known Stokes parameters, controlled reflection from the sample, deep transmission through samples, and no radiation damage to the sample being imaged (Mahesh, 2011). But in real time, no illumination system is ideal and certain compromise is made based on the specific application. In NIR applications, quartz halogen lamps, tungsten halogen lamps, tunable lasers, light emitting diodes (LEDs), and heated xenon lamps are employed as sources of illumination. Among these, tungsten halogen lamps are widely used in hyperspectral imaging because they are durable, stable, and capable of emitting 400 to 2500 nm light.

After acquiring hyperspectral images, the data are sent to a high-speed computer for storage and further image processing. Numerous techniques are available to analyze hyperspectral data and these techniques are used to decrease the data dimensionality and retain the significant spectral information. Effective algorithms are developed to analyze the voluminous data and to extract important spatial and spectral features.

The major challenge in hyperspectral imaging is the high dimensionality of the data generated, which should be reduced to lower dimension of data without affecting the original information. There are two types of dimensionality reduction methods: feature extraction and feature selection. Of these two, feature selection is preferred because feature extraction requires most of the original data representation for extraction and critical information may be distorted due to transformation in feature extraction, whereas in feature selection most of the original information is preserved (Sohaib et al., 2012).

Dimensionality reduction can also be classified into two other branches: linear and nonlinear. The most widely used linear transformation technique for dimension reduction is the principal component analysis (PCA). In PCA, orthogonal projections are computed, which maximizes the variance of data and yields the data set in an uncorrelated coordinate system (Plaza et al., 2005). Nonlinear techniques include Laplacian Eigenmaps, local tangent space analysis (LTSA), local linear embedding (LLE), and diffusion maps (Doster, 2011).

5.3   Applications of hyperspectral imaging techniques

5.3.1   Agriculture

Hyperspectral imaging was initially developed and used for applications in remote sensing. But the potential of hyperspectral imaging was explored in other fields such as agriculture to monitor soil conditions and soil nutrients, to monitor characteristics and quality of wood, and to monitor quality of cereal grains. In Table 5.1, details of spectral imaging systems along with their applications related to agriculture are presented. Yang et al. (2003b) examined the potential of hyperspectral imaging for airborne and stationary agricultural and natural resource applications. The airborne imaging system consisted of a digital camera, spectrograph, and lens, whereas the stationary imaging system, in addition to the aforementioned parts, had a focal plane scanner that was connected between the spectrograph and front lens. The images were obtained during a calm and sunny

Table 5.1 Details of Hyperspectral Imaging Systems Used in Agricultural and Grain Applications

Spectrograph/ camera model	Company	Spectral range (nm); spectral resolution (nm)	Application	Reference
HySpex VNIR-1600	Norsk Elektro Optikk, Lørenskog, Norway	400–1000; 3.7	To monitor wood moisture content	Kobori et al., 2013
ImSpector V10	Spectral Imaging Ltd., Oulu, Finland	380–1030	To detect micronutrient content in oilseed rape leaves	Zhang et al., 2013
ImSpector V10	Spectral Imaging Ltd., Oulu, Finland	360–1010; 10	Spatial distribution of botanical composition	Suzuki et al., 2012
EO1 Hyperion, pushbroom	NA	400–2400; 10	To detect soil salinity	Rekha et al., 2012
NA	Sensors Unlimited Inc., Princeton, New Jersey	1000–1700; 5	To determine density and moisture content of wood	Mora et al., 2011
Specim ImSpector N17E/VDS Vosskühler NIR300PSCL	Spectral Imaging Ltd., Oulu, Finland	900–1700; 3.6	Determine the chemical composition of wood	Thumm et al., 2010
ImSpector V10; Teli8310CS B/W	Spectral Imaging Ltd., Oulu, Finland	400–1000; 5	To determine wood compression	Duncker and Spiecker, 2009
ASD FieldSpec® Pro FR	Analytical Spectral Devices Inc., Boulder, Colorado	350–2500; 3–11	Monitoring nutrient enrichment	Siciliano et al., 2008
ImSpector V10	Spectral Imaging Ltd., Oulu, Finland	400–1000; 10	Automatic weed detection	Okamoto et al., 2007
ImSpector V9/ SensiCam	Spectral Imaging Ltd., Oulu, Finland/The Cooke Corp. Ltd., United States	457.2–921.7	Airborne remote sensing applications for agriculture	Yang et al., 2003b

period from agricultural plots, rangelands, and waterways in south Texas. Various factors such as variation in speed, altitude, and pitch affected the image quality. The images acquired from the system had geometric distortion problems and the authors developed procedures to rectify geometric distortions of the images. The presence of geometric distortion was owing to the movement in across-track direction and variation in roll was because an aircraft possesses six degrees of freedom while moving. In the images, the highway and road on two sides of the agricultural plot became wiggly lines but they were supposed to be straight lines. These distortions were rectified by moving every line in an across-track direction to the reference line so that the highway and the road could be seen as straight lines in the corrected image. Thus, based on the reference line method, correction procedures were formulated to rectify the geometric distortion in across-track direction.

Suzuki et al. (2012) developed a hyperspectral imaging technique to map the spatial distribution of plant species and herbage growth for pastures. The field mainly had pasture of perennial ryegrass (*Trifolium perenne* L.), with some cover of white clover (*Trifolium repens* L.). Images were acquired using the ImSpector V10 imaging system and the interpretation of the collected data required optical correction due to changes in illumination, such as sunshine or cloudy periods, at the time of image acquisition. During the mapping process, plant species were extracted from the image by differentiating between plants and nonplants using normalized difference vegetation index (NDVI) thresholding. Perennial ryegrass was estimated using partial least square regression (PLSR). The overall classification accuracy was 91.6% for plants and the results of the study demonstrated the ability of hyperspectral imaging for determining the botanical composition and herbage mass of perennial ryegrass. Okamoto et al. (2007) developed a hyperspectral imaging technique for automatic weed detection in the field. A portable imaging unit ImSpector V10 was used to differentiate between sugar beet and four different types of weed species by differentiating between the spectral characteristics of the various species of plants. The discriminant analysis provided a classification accuracy of 90% for plant species and weeds and concluded that hyperspectral techniques have great potential for monitoring and detection of weeds in the field.

In soil salinization, the dissolved salts accumulate on the top layers of the soil. Rekha et al. (2012) examined the ability of hyperspectral imaging to detect soil salinity in coastal areas. They selected two locations, the first region (A) being near a shrimp farming site (four locations) and the second site (B) was near a perennial brackish water creek (two locations) where there was no shrimp farming, and both the sites were located between 11.47 and 11.45 North latitude and 79.72 and 79.73 East longitude of Chidambaram Taluk, Tamilnadu, India. The hyperspectral images were collected from the EO1 Hyperion pushbroom sensor. The electrical resistivity survey was conducted on both sites to validate the results obtained by hyperspectral analysis. The hyperspectral analysis showed that the two regions have various wavelength and reflectance, and site B showed higher reflectance. The results of the experimental study showed that at site A, soil properties and reflectance were similar at all four locations and high resistivity values indicated that there was no salinization. But in region B, near the brackish water creek, salinization was observed, which was confirmed by low resistivity data. Hence this study showed that salinization issues owing to shrimp farming is site specific, which was also stated by the National Environmental Engineering Research Institute (1995) that found that magnitude of salinization issues occurring due to shrimp farming is low and does not occur at all the sites.

In wetland ecosystems, eutrophication and nutrient enrichment are of major concern and there is a need for a fast and efficient way to monitor the nutrients in wetlands and other coastal areas. Siciliano et al. (2008) evaluated hyperspectral imaging for detecting and monitoring nutrient enrichment in wetlands. The experiments were conducted at Coyote Marsh on Elkhorn Slough National Research Reserve (Central California). The study was conducted based on three approaches: (1) a long duration water monitoring program; (2) a study to determine nutrient and spectral responses of wetland plant, common pickle weed, *Salicornia virginica* (Fern. & Brack); (3) a hyperspectral imaging system (ASD FieldSpec® Pro FR) for assessment of the wetland ecosystem of Elkhorn Slough. The results showed a consistent positive relationship between levels of nitrogen and plant response. The two spectral indices—derivative chlorophyll index (DCI) and photochemical reflectance index (PRI)—had significant correlation with water nutrients. They concluded that hyperspectral imaging is an effective tool to detect nutrient enrichment and suggested that with further research of the physical mechanism linking water capacity, plant characteristics, and spectral imaging features, more information and knowledge of nutrient enrichment could be obtained.

5.3.2   Wood

The moisture content of wood is an important quality factor in the wood industry. Gravimetry is the simplest method to determine moisture content of wood among the available methods, but it does not allow detection of fine spatial moisture content distribution. Kobori et al. (2013) explored visible-NIR hyperspectral imaging for monitoring wood moisture content. Scots pine (*Pinus sylvestris* L.) and European beech (*Fagus sylvatica* L.) were selected for the study and each sample set consisted of 10 samples per species. HySpex VNIR-1600 (Norsk Elektro Optikk, Norway), a pushbroom line scanning system, was used for the study. Wood samples were air-dried and their weights were determined before and after hyperspectral images were obtained. After seven cycles, samples were dried at 103°C for 72 h and weighed. Moisture content maps obtained at initial and final stages of drying showed opposite tendencies. Partial least square regression (PLSR) prediction of moisture content was performed and the validation showed high prediction accuracy, and standard normal variate (SNV) treatment provided the best results for visualizing the moisture content distribution in wood.

For a given volume of wood, weight can be determined based on moisture content and density, which are the two most important properties of wood that influence the physical and mechanical characteristics. Great variation exists among both the properties with respect to location, between trees, and within trees. Accurate measurement of density and moisture content are provided only by the oven-drying method, which is time consuming, hence Mora et al. (2011) determined the moisture content and density of wood using NIR hyperspectral imaging. The samples (125 wood disks of 4 cm thickness) were collected from 63 loblolly pine trees (*Pinus taeda* L.). The hyperspectral imaging unit consisted of a tunable filter with InGaAs camera (Sensors Unlimited Inc., Princeton, New Jersey). Due to the presence of noise, spectra were collected only from 1005 to 1645 nm. The hyperspectral images revealed several features, such as knots, resin defects, and growth rings, with clearly distinguishable early wood and latewood bands. The images also showed an abrupt transition in reflectance from wood to bark. Based on hyperspectral imaging data, successful models were obtained for density ($R^2 = 0.81$) and moisture content ($R^2 = 0.77$). Mora et al. concluded that hyperspectral imaging could be a potential tool to determine the density and moisture content of wood samples.

Wood is a heterogeneous matrix and this heterogeneity results in poor wood characteristics like warp due to crook, twist, or bow. These characteristics occur because of spatial variation in characteristics such as microfibril angle, density, and shrinkage. Hence, understanding of spatial distribution is essential to improve characteristics of products made from wood. Since determination of chemical properties of wood using traditional methods are expensive, lack spatial selectivity, and are destructive, Thumm et al. (2010) determined the chemical composition of wood samples using NIR hyperspectral imaging. Clonal trees from Esk forest (New Zealand) were used for the study, and samples with 25 to 30 mm thickness were used. Samples were dried in a kiln for a period of two weeks to avoid cracks and check formation, and conditioned at 25°C and 65% relative humidity before acquiring images. Images were obtained using a Specim ImSpector N17E prism-grating-prism spectrograph attached to a VDS Vosskühler NIR300PSCL line scan camera (VDS Vosskühler GmbH, Osnabrück, Germany). Images were obtained between 900 and 1700 nm at 3.6 nm intervals. The results of the study showed that NIR hyperspectral imaging could be used to create chemical maps of wood, although many data processing steps were essential to process raw data to obtain chemical maps. The ability to visualize the distribution of wood properties is useful in the overall understating of heterogeneity of wood properties.

Compression wood formation is a reaction that occurs because of an external stress creating a strain on the tree and formation of compression wood is an undesirable reaction. Duncker and Spiecker (2009) developed a methodology based on reflected light to detect compression wood in Norway spruce (*Picea abies* L.), using hyperspectral image analysis. Reflected light from the cross-section of the stem surface was recorded with an imaging spectrograph ImSpector V10 (Spectral Imaging Ltd., Oulu, Finland) in the spectral range of 400 to 1000 nm with 5 nm spectral resolution (121 bands). The hyperspectral image analysis was able to identify severe and moderate compression wood from other wood tissues with an overall accuracy of 91%. The various research experiments have proven the possibility of hyperspectral imaging in determining various properties such as moisture content, density, and chemical composition of wood, which shows that hyperspectral imaging may become an important technology in the wood processing industry.

5.3.3   Grain

The hyperspectral imaging technique was used to study the various quality parameters of grain. Table 5.2 presents the list of hyperspectral imaging systems used in the grain applications and the details of the imaging system.

5.3.3.1   Sprout- and midge-damaged kernels

Sprouting is the process of germination of kernels that occurs by absorbing water. Preharvest sprouting occurs in the field before harvest and significantly reduces the wheat yield, and an enzyme α-amylase produced in sprouted kernels deteriorates the baking quality of wheat resulting in lowering the value of the grain. Traditional falling number and rapid visco-analyzer methods to determine sprout-damaged kernels are time consuming and destructive. Pregermination of cereal grain results in reduced viability of grain, and hence determination of preharvest sprouting is important for producers and manufacturers. The methods of pregermination detection such as falling number, tetrazolium tests, germination, and visual inspection currently used are destructive or subjective. McGoverin et al. (2011) explored the capability of near-infrared hyperspectral imaging (NIR-HIS) to determine nonviability in wheat, barley, and sorghum. The images were acquired using a SisuCHEMA infrared hyperspectral imaging unit and the kernels were placed with germ up position. Spectra were obtained from

Table 5.2 Details of Hyperspectral Imaging Systems Used in Grain Applications

Spectrograph/ camera model	Company	Spectral range (nm); spectral resolution (nm)	Application	Reference
ImSpectorN17E™/ NIR spectral camera	Spectral Imaging Ltd., Oulu, Finland	1000–1700; 7	To detect Fusarium damaged, yellow berry and vitreous kernels	Serranti et al., 2013
(a) ImSpector N25E/XEVA CL 2.5 320 TE4 camera	Spectral Imaging Ltd., Oulu, Finland	1100–2400; 6.3	To detect undesirable materials in cereal	Fernández Pierna et al., 2012
(b) MatrixNIR™ Whiskbroom	Malvern Instruments, Analytical Imaging, Columbia, Maryland	900–1700; 10		
VNIR 100E, Pushbroom	Lextel Intelligence Systems, Jackson, Mississippi	400–1000; 2.75	To detect Fusarium damage in wheat	Shahin and Symons, 2012
Pushbroom spectrometer	NA	400–1000; 2	To image the ears of sprouting wheat	Wu et al., 2012b
SisuCHEMA	Spectral Imaging Ltd., Oulu, Finland	1000–2498; 6.3	To determine viability in barley, wheat, sorghum	McGoverin et al., 2011
ImSpector V10/ PCO 1600 Monochrome camera	Spectral Imaging Ltd., Oulu, Finland/Cooke Corporation, United States	400–1000	To detect sprout damage in wheat	Xing et al., 2010
ImSpector V10	Spectral Imaging Ltd., Oulu, Finland	400–1000	To detect fungi infection in maize	Del Fiore et al., 2010
C7042/ SU640-1.7RT-D	Hamamatsu Photonics, Hamamatus, Japan/Sensors Unlimited Inc., Princeton, New Jersey	700–1100 nm	To detect sprout- and midge-damaged wheat; to detect insect infestation; to detect fungal infestation	Singh et al., 2009a,b, 2012
SisuCHEMA	Spectral Imaging Ltd., Oulu, Finland	1000–2498; 6	To determine maize kernel hardness	Williams et al., 2009
SU640-1.7RT-D	Sensors Unlimited Inc., Princeton, New Jersey	960–1700; 10	To identify wheat classes	Mahesh et al., 2008

1000 to 2498 nm at an interval of 6.3 nm, producing images of 320 (*x*) × 583 (*y*) × 239 (λ) dimensions. Partial least squares discriminant analysis (PLS-DA) was used to distinguish between nonviable and viable kernels. Principal component analysis (PCA) was able to distinguish between viable and nonviable classes in higher components such as fifth principal component (PC5) for sorghum and barley and in sixth principal component (PC6) for wheat, whereas other chemical and topographic information were presented by lower principal components.

Midge damage is caused by orange wheat blossom midge (*Sitodiplosis mosellana* [Gehin]) larvae, which results in shriveled, cracked, and deformed kernels. Singh et al. (2009b) examined the potential of hyperspectral imaging for determination of sprout and midge damage in wheat. Sound kernels, artificially sprouted kernels, and naturally midge-damaged Canada Western Red Spring (CWRS) wheat kernels were used for the study. The imaging unit (Figure 5.4) consisted of image sensor (Model no. C7042), with InGaAs camera and a liquid crystal tunable filter in the wavelength range of 1000 to 1600 nm. The images of healthy and midge-damaged kernels were acquired with crease-down and crease-up positions, whereas sprouted kernels were imaged only in crease-down orientation. Multivariate image analysis was performed using PCA, and algorithms for classification were developed using statistical discriminant analyses. They identified three specific wavelengths—1101.7, 1132.2, and 1305.1 nm—as critical and used in the feature extraction. The highest and consistent classification accuracy was obtained by Mahalanobis classifier for damaged kernels, whereas LDA and QDA provided good classification results for healthy kernels. One hundred percent accuracy in classification of sprout-damaged kernels was obtained by LDA, QDA, and Mahalanobis classifiers. The accuracy of classification for kernels with crease-up position was 95% to 100%, which was little higher than samples with crease-down orientation, which provided 91.7% to 100% accuracy. Xing et al. (2010)

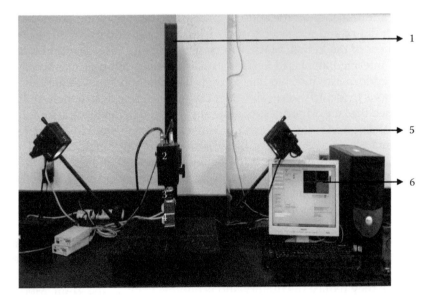

Figure 5.4 Near infrared hyperspectral imaging system: (1) stand, (2) NIR camera, (3) lens, (4) liquid crystal tunable filter, (5) illumination, and (6) data processing system. (Courtesy of University of Manitoba, Winnipeg, Canada.)

determined the effectiveness of using visible NIR hyperspectral imaging to assess sprout damage in wheat kernels. The imaging system consisted of a 14-bit monochrome camera with a spectrograph (ImSpector V10). Images were acquired, PCA was performed, and the healthy kernels displayed a lower spectral reflectance in the 720 nm region as opposed to the sprouted kernels. The average spectra showed that reflectance ratio at 878 nm to that at 728 nm could be a potential indicator for classifying healthy and sprouted kernels. By using both spectral and spatial features in the classification procedure 100%, 94%, and 98% of healthy, sprouted, and severely sprouted kernels, respectively, were correctly classified. Xing et al. concluded that hyperspectral imaging could be a potential technique in the future for identification of sprout-damaged kernels.

Singh et al. (2009a) and Xing et al. (2010) examined the ability of hyperspectral imaging to determine sprouting in individual wheat grains, and Wu et al. (2012b) applied hyperspectral imaging to obtain imaging spectra of sprouting wheat ears. The spectral characteristics of sprouting and nonsprouting wheat ears were extracted to explore the feasibility to determine the sprouting of whole ears of wheat. A pushbroom imaging spectrometer developed by the Beijing Agricultural Information Technology Research Center and University of Science and Technology of China had a spectral range of 400 to 1000 nm with a spectral resolution of 2 nm. Hyperspectral images of individual wheat ears and wheat kernels were collected and PCA was performed. Preharvest sprouting could be reflected by spectral characteristics specifically at 675 nm where sprouting parts of wheat showed absorption valley, and lower spectral reflectivity was observed at 450 to 500 nm as more serious sprouting occurred. The authors' results showed that only in cases of advanced sprouting, images of wheat ears could be used to determine sprouting occurrence. At the initial stages of sprouting damage, hyperspectral images of wheat grain alone could be used to identify sprouting occurrence.

5.3.3.2 *Kernel hardness and wheat class identification*

Maize kernel hardness is an important quality factor to producers and processors because it has a significant influence on the end-use processing quality of the grain. Maize kernel constitutes both floury and glassy endosperm, but the ratio of the two is the key to determine the hardness of the kernel. Maize can be grouped into three levels of hardness, i.e., soft, hard, and intermediate. Hard kernels possess glassy endosperm, whereas soft ones possess floury endosperm; intermediate kernels have both in equal quantities. Currently employed methods to identify kernel hardness require sample destruction. Williams et al. (2009) determined the kernel hardness of maize by infrared hyperspectral imaging. Images were obtained using a MatrixNIR camera (Malvern Instruments Ltd., United Kingdom) and a sisuChema SWIR (shortwave infrared) hyperspectral imaging unit. The spectral range was between 960 and 1662 nm at increments of 6 nm. PLS-DA models were used to differentiate between floury and glassy endosperm, and it was possible to determine with two to three principal components. Williams et al. concluded that hyperspectral imaging is a potential technique to classify maize kernels as hard or soft based on glassy or floury endosperm.

Cereals are one of the most essential sources of raw material for food to feed the world. Cereals are more often contaminated with various products, such as damaged or spoiled grains, straw, other cereal grains, small plastics, and stones, which although many of them are not harmful, they reduce the quality and economic value of the grain. Moreover, processors will have to use additional operations for cleaning the grain. Hence, Fernández Pierna et al. (2012) examined the use of NIR hyperspectral imaging for detection of undesirable substances in cereal grain. The study included 112 samples of wheat, barley, and spelt and the contaminants included broken grain, straw, grains from other crops, insects, plastics, stones, weeds, wood pieces, and animal feces. The images were collected in the 1100 to 2400 nm spectral range with a 6.3 nm resolution. Initially, PCA was applied to distinguish some group of impurities, and based on results from PCA, discriminant models for various categories of impurities were developed. Due to the ability of a support vector machine (SVM) in solving pattern recognition issues, SVM was used to classify contaminants in five categories: animal contaminants (insects), cereal contamination, botanical impurities, cellulose waste (wood, straw), and other contaminants (plastics, stone, paintings). Results showed that classification accuracy of 95% or higher was obtained. The authors stated that NIR hyperspectral imaging could be a potential tool to detect contaminants in agricultural products and these techniques combined with chemometric tools could be used for online or offline detection of contamination and quality control of agricultural products.

Different wheat classes have different chemical compositions and are suited for different end-use products. Visual inspection for classification of wheat classes has many drawbacks, such as low throughput, inconsistency, and labor intensive. Mahesh et al. (2008) studied the possibility of NIR hyperspectral imaging to distinguish various wheat classes. The imaging system (Figure 5.4) consisted of an InGaAs camera (SU640-1.7RT-D) with liquid crystal tunable filter. The models for classification were developed using QDA and LDA methods and two back propagation neural network (BPNN) architectures were utilized for developing artificial neural network (ANN) models. The classification accuracies for LDA and QDA models were 94% to 100% and 86% to 100%, respectively. In ANN, overall classification accuracies were around 90%. In conclusion, Mahesh et al. stated that NIR hyperspectral imaging combined with ANN and statistical classifiers have the ability to distinguish Canadian wheat classes.

5.3.3.3 Insect and fungal damage detection

Insect infestation is a major issue in the grain industry, which results in reduced weight, reduction of nutrients, lower germination potential, and higher risk of contamination by fungi. Conventional insect detection methods include visual inspection, Berlese funnel, insect traps, and flotation. The disadvantages of these conventional methods are that they are time consuming, subjective, inaccurate, and fail to identify internal insect infestation. Hence Singh et al. (2009b) explored the capability of hyperspectral imaging to detect insect-damaged wheat kernels. Healthy samples and samples infested with species of rusty grain beetle (*Cryptolestes ferrugineus* [Stephen]), rice weevil (*Sitophilus oryzae* [Linnaeus]), red flour beetle (*Tribolium castaneum* [Herbst]), and lesser grain borer (*Rhyzopertha dominica* [Fabricius]) of CWRS wheat were used for the experiments. Images were obtained in crease-down and crease-up orientations for 300 healthy and 300 insect-damaged kernels. Multivariate image analysis was performed using PCA, and algorithms were developed using linear, quadratic, and Mahalanobis statistical analyses. The classification accuracy was in the range of 85% to 100% using linear and quadratic discriminant analyses for healthy and insect-damaged kernels. The results of the experiment showed that NIR hyperspectral imaging could be a promising technology to detect insect-damaged grain kernels.

Fusarium head blight, a common fungal disease, deteriorates the quality of cereal grains such as barley, oats, and wheat. Fusarium head blight is caused by *Fusarium graminearum* (Schwabe) due to wet weather conditions at flowering, and infection at an early stage results in heavy damage to the seeds resulting in production of mycotoxins such as deoxynivalenol (DON). Visual inspection of grain is a common method, but it is time consuming and early infection cannot be easily detected by the naked eye. Other laboratory methods for detection of molds and mycotoxin, such as chromatography, mass spectrometry, and enzyme-linked immunosorbent assay, are not suitable for rapid online detection. Shahin and Symons (2012) explored the possibility of visible/near-infrared hyperspectral imaging for detection of fusarium infection in wheat. Seven major Canadian wheat classes were selected and samples from each class contained healthy, mildly affected, and severely affected kernels, which were individually assessed and ranked by trained grain inspectors. A pushbroom hyperspectral imaging system (VNIR 100E) in the visible-NIR wavelength range was used for the experiments. Images were obtained by placing individual wheat kernels in a crease-down position on a board in batches of 24 to 36, and the images were acquired in the diffuse reflectance mode. The detection accuracy of sound kernels was 91%, and accuracy was 99% for severely damaged kernels. But for the mildly damaged kernels, the detection accuracy was only 80% to 82%. Of the seven wheat classes tested, the best fungal damaged kernel detection was for Canada Eastern Red Spring (CERS) with 92% to 95%, and the lowest detection accuracy was for the Canada Western Amber Durum (CWAD) with 83% to 85% accuracy. Shahin and Symons concluded that hyperspectral imaging could be used to detect sound and fungal-damaged wheat kernels with an accuracy rate of 90% and false positive of 9%.

Several fungi infect cereal grains in the field and during postharvest storage conditions, and the early detection of toxigenic fungi could be useful to prevent the contaminated grain from entering the supply chain. Maize (*Zea mays* L.) is an important cereal crop and is mainly infected by fungi belonging to *Fusarium* spp. and *Aspergillus* spp. Traditional methods to identify fungi are time consuming and expensive. Del Fiore et al. (2010) explored the hyperspectral imaging technique to detect fungi infection on maize at an early stage of infection. Twelve commercial maize hybrids infected with *Aspergillus* strains (*A. parasiticus, A. flavus, A. niger*) and two *Fusarium* strains (*F. graminearum, F. verticilloides*) were used for the experiments. Hyperspectral images were obtained using the ImSpector V10 imaging system in the visible-NIR spectral range. The assays made with kernels of various moisture content showed that spectral differences were caused due to fungal contamination. The results of the study indicate that hyperspectral imaging can be used to distinguish fungi-infected maize kernels from healthy ones after 48 h of inoculation.

Mycotoxins are toxic carcinogens that are produced by fungal species *Penicillium*, *Aspergillus*, and *Fusarium*. Mold or fungal growth in cereal grain causes loss of germination, discoloration, loss of dry matter, higher levels of free fatty acid, and production of mycotoxins. Singh et al. (2012) studied the possibility of detecting fungal infection in wheat kernels using short-wave NIR hyperspectral imaging. The imaging unit comprised of a 532 × 256 pixel size FFT-CCD area scan image sensor (Model no. C7042) working in the visible (400–700 nm) and NIR region (700–1100 nm). The samples consisted of wheat grain affected with storage fungi such as *Penicillum* spp., *Aspergillus glaucus* group, and *A. niger* (Van Tieghem). Five samples were randomly selected and placed on a black paperboard and images were acquired in the wavelength region of 700 to 1100 nm. The algorithms for classification were developed using statistical discriminant analysis classifiers (quadratic, linear, Mahalanobis). Based on the results, it was concluded that NIR hyperspectral imaging resulted in high classification accuracy of 97.3% to 100% for healthy and fungal-damaged wheat kernels using linear discriminant analysis.

Serranti et al. (2013) developed a hyperspectral imaging technique for detection of three different types of wheat kernels: *Fusarium* damaged, yellow berry, and vitreous kernels. *Fusarium* species causes fungal infection, which causes food safety concerns and results in reduced price for the grain. Yellow berry wheat kernels have undesirable yellowish and soft kernels, which affect the flour quality. Nonvitreous kernels have an opaque and starchy appearance, whereas vitreous kernels are characterized by a hard, glassy, and translucent appearance, which is required by the industry. These three types of wheat kernels are often found in a lot and it is essential to develop a sorting procedure to eliminate the affected kernels, which reduce the overall quality of the batch. The hyperspectral imaging unit was a pushbroom type, which consisted of an ImSpectorN17E™ spectral camera. Analysis of spectral data was performed using different techniques such as PCA and partial least square discriminant analysis (PLS-DA) and a model was developed to distinguish between different types of kernels. The classification was obtained between 1013 and 1650 nm by selecting three ranges of wavelengths (1209–1230 nm, 1489–1510 nm, 1601–1622 nm). The classification error was 1% for vitreous, whereas 4% for yellow berry, and *Fusarium* damaged kernels in the first model; and 1% for vitreous, and 6% for yellow berry and *Fusarium*-damaged kernels in the next model. The results of the study showed that hyperspectral imaging could be a potential method for classification and real-time monitoring of the quality of grain.

5.3.4 Food

5.3.4.1 Fruits and vegetables

Hyperspectral imaging is emerging as a potential technique in determining the various quality characteristics of fresh fruits and vegetables, nuts, beans, and various types of meat. Researchers in the food industry are testing the various aspects of hyperspectral imaging to incorporate the technique in the on-line quality monitoring system. The various potential applications of hyperspectral imaging in the food industry are discussed in this section. In Table 5.3, applications of hyperspectral imaging related to fresh produce and other food materials along with the details of corresponding spectral imaging system are provided.

The grape harvest is currently based on the sugar content in the fruit pulp. The composition of fruits changes during maturity of the fruit. The different types of sensory and chemical methods available to assess the maturity of the fruit are destructive in nature and time consuming. Rodríguez-Pulido et al. (2013) examined the possibility of NIR hyperspectral reflectance imaging to characterize grape seed based on variety and maturity level. Two varieties of red (Tempranillo and Syrah) and one variety of white (Zalema) fruit were selected for the study. NIR hyperspectral images were obtained in the reflectance mode with a pushbroom imaging unit comprised of a spectrograph (ImSpector N17E) CCD camera and two tungsten halogen lamps. To analyze and minimize the noise and retain useful information from the data, preprocessing techniques were applied, and partial least square regression (PLSR) was applied to raw spectral data. The results of the analysis showed that the PLRS model has the ability to predict the maturity level of a sample based on spectral features. PCA and GDA (general discriminant analysis) methods were able to characterize grape seeds based on their varieties. The authors concluded that hyperspectral imaging has great potential for assessment of grape quality during postharvest applications.

Most of the analytical techniques used to evaluate the sensory and physicochemical qualities of grapes are destructive, time consuming, and require complicated equipment. Baiano et al. (2012) assessed the possibility of hyperspectral imaging for determination of sensory attributes and physicochemical qualities of table grapes. Four varieties of white grapes (Thompson seedless, Baresana, Italia, and Pizzutello) and three red/black grapes varieties (Crimson seedless, Michele Palieri, and Red globe) were obtained from the market.

***Table* 5.3** Details of Hyperspectral Imaging Systems Used for Applications Related to Fresh Produce and Food Materials

Spectrograph/ camera model	Company	Spectral range (nm); spatial resolution (nm)	Application	Reference
ImSpectorN17E	Spectral Imaging Ltd., Oulu, Finland	897–1753; 3.34	To assess microbial contamination in meat; grading and classification of pork	Barbin et al., 2012b, 2013
SU640-1.7RT-D	Sensors Unlimited Inc., Princeton, New Jersey	900–1700	To detect infestation in mung bean	Kaliramesh et al., 2013
ImSpectorN17E™	Spectral Imaging Ltd., Oulu, Finland	897–1752; 3.34	To characterize grapes according to maturity	Rodríguez-Pulido et al., 2013
SisuCHEMA	Spectral Imaging Ltd., Oulu, Finland	920–2514; 6–7	Quality control of star anise	Vermaak et al., 2013
ImSpector V10	Specim Ltd., Haarlem, The Netherlands	400–1000; 5	To determine physico-chemical and sensory qualities of grapes	Baiano et al., 2012
ImSpectorN17E	Spectral Imaging Ltd., Oulu, Finland	897–1753; 3.34	To predict Enterobacteriaceae loads in chicken fillet	Feng et al., 2012
ImSpectorN17E	Spectral Imaging Ltd., Oulu, Finland	897–1753; 3.34	To identify and authenticate red meat species/to assess the quality attributes of lamb meat	Kamruzzaman et al., 2012a,b
SU640-1.7RT-D	Sensors Unlimited Inc., Princeton, New Jersey	960–1700	To determine bruises in strawberries	Nanyam et al., 2012
ImSpector V10E	Spectral Imaging Ltd., Oulu, Finland	400–1100; 2.8	To determine downy mildew in cucumbers	Tian and Zhang, 2012
Specim V10E	Spectral Imaging Ltd., Oulu, Finland	400–1000; 5	To analyze the texture of salmon	Wu et al., 2012a
ImSpector V10E	Spectral Imaging Ltd., Oulu, Finland	890–1750; 6	To determine water-holding capacity of fresh beef; classification of cooked turkey hams	ElMasry et al., 2011a,b

(Continued)

Table 5.3 (Continued) Details of Hyperspectral Imaging Systems Used for Applications Related to Fresh Produce and Food Materials

Spectrograph/ camera model	Company	Spectral range (nm); spatial resolution (nm)	Application	Reference
ImSpector V10	Spectral Imaging Ltd., Oulu, Finland	400–1000; 5	To detect *E. coli* contamination in spinach	Siripatrawan et al., 2011
Specim V10E	Spectral Imaging Ltd., Oulu, Finland	400–1000	To identify freeze damage in mushrooms	Gowen et al., 2009b
ImSpector V10E/ IPX-2M20	Spectral Imaging Ltd., Oulu, Finland/Imperx Inc., United States	400–1000; 2.8	To predict beef tenderness	Naganathan et al., 2008
ImSpector V10E	Optikon Corporation Ltd., Ontario, Canada	400–1000	To determine the quality attributes of strawberries	ElMasry et al., 2007
ImSpector V9	Spectral Imaging Ltd., Oulu, Finland	425–775; 4.5	To differentiate walnut shell and pulp	Jiang et al., 2007
ImSpector	Spectral Imaging Ltd., Oulu, Finland	400–1000; 5	To predict sweetness and amino acid content in soybean	Monteiro et al., 2007
ImSpector V9/ C4880-21	Spectral Imaging Ltd., Oulu, Finland/ Hamamatsu Photonics, Hamamatus, Japan	500–1040; 1.65	To assess quality of apples	Noh and Lu, 2007
ImSpector N17E/ SU320MX-1.7RT	Spectral Imaging Ltd., Oulu, Finland/Sensors Unlimited Inc., Princeton, New Jersey	900–1700; 4.4	To monitor mechanical damage in cucumbers	Ariana et al., 2006
ImSpector V9/ C4880-21	Spectral imaging ltd., Oulu, Finland/ Hamamatsu Corp., Japan	500–1000	To determine firmness of peach fruit	Lu and Peng, 2006
ImSpector/ SU640-1.7RT-D	Spectral Imaging Ltd., Oulu, Finland/Sensors Unlimited Inc., Princeton, New Jersey	900–1700	To measure bitter pit in apples	Nicolaï et al., 2006
ImSpector V9	Spectral Imaging Ltd., Oulu, Finland	447.3–951.2; 4.5	To determine chilling injury to cucumbers	Cheng et al., 2004
ImSpector 1.7/ SpectraVideo™ camera	Spectral Imaging Ltd., Oulu, Finland/ PixelVision Inc., United States	424–899	To detect surface defects in apples	Mehl et al., 2004

For building the PLSR model, 80 white berries and 60 red/black grapes (20 from each cultivar) were selected. The lab-scale hyperspectral imaging equipment consisted of a CCD camera attached to a spectrograph (ImSpector V10) coupled with a lens. After images were obtained, soluble solid content (SSC), pH, and titratable acidity (TA) were determined for the berries. PLSR models were calibrated to determine the correlation between spectral response and the quality characteristics (i.e., SSC, pH, and TA). Good correlation was found between spectral information and physiochemical indices. For titratable acidity, the coefficient of determination was found to be 0.95 and 0.82 for white and red/black grapes, respectively. The coefficient of determination for SSC was 0.94 and 0.93, and for pH were 0.80 and 0.90 for white and red/black grapes, respectively. The authors concluded that good correlation was found between spectral information and quality indices, and hyperspectral imaging is a promising technique to evaluate the physicochemical qualities of table grapes.

The quality of cucumbers is often affected by various types of pests and diseases. Downy mildew affects the cucumber at different stages and at maturity cucumbers are often severely affected. Traditional methods used for monitoring the quality of cucumbers are slow and cannot be used in real-time monitoring. Tian and Zhang (2012) explored the hyperspectral imaging to determine downy mildew in cucumber leaves. Ten infected leaves and ten healthy leaves were collected from a cucumber greenhouse in Shenyang Agricultural University and the images were obtained using a hyperspectral imaging system (ImSpector V10E). PCA was applied to the spectral data and then a image fusion technique was adopted. Image fusion is the technique of merging certain images from various sensors to obtain a more complete picture and to improve the reliability and clarity of images by removing the unwanted information. Other image processing techniques, such as image enhancement, binarization, and dilation treatments, were applied to detect downy mildew in cucumber leaves. The results of the study provided an accuracy rate of 90% for detecting disease-affected leaves and the authors concluded that hyperspectral imaging techniques could be a potential tool to detect downy mildew in cucumber.

Severely injured cucumbers could be easily identified during sorting or manual inspection, whereas mechanical injury results in internal damages to pickling cucumbers. Internal damage reduces the quality of the cucumbers and results in bloating during brining which causes major loss to pickle processors. Currently available methods to detect internal damages are destructive and time consuming, and hence are not ideal for automatic sorting and grading of cucumbers in a commercial setup. Ariana et al. (2006) studied the effectiveness of hyperspectral imaging to identify and segregate mechanically damaged cucumbers. The imaging system consisted of an InGaAs area array camera (Model SU320MX-1.7RT), a spectrograph (ImSpector N17E) connected to a camera, lens, frame grabber, and a computer. Ninety "Journey" cucumbers selected for the study were grouped into three categories. One group was bruised by dropping; another group by rolling under load to stimulate stress, which occurs due to mechanical harvesting system; and no injury was made to the third group. Images were acquired at 0 to 3 and 6 days after samples were exposed to mechanical stress. PCA was carried out to lower the spectral dimensions and enhance image features. Maximum reflectance variation between healthy and bruised tissue was in the wavelength range of 950 and 1350 nm. The reflectance of healthy tissue remained constant over time, whereas the reflectance of bruised tissue increased over a period of time, and then reached the reflectance value closer to that of healthy tissue, which may be due to healing of the wound. The classification accuracies were between 93% and 82% for the band ratio of 988 and 1088 nm. Ariana et al. concluded that NIR hyperspectral imaging has potential to detect mechanical bruises in pickling cucumbers in a commercial setting.

Chilling damage to cucumbers occurs when they are stored at low temperatures for a prolonged period of time. The chilling damage is difficult to detect at early stages and the symptoms normally appear after the produce is moved to a warm environment. Cheng et al. (2004) tested a hyperspectral imaging method to determine chilling injury to the cucumbers. Freshly picked cucumbers were segregated into 30 groups of 3 cucumbers each, kept in plastic bags punched with holes. Fifteen bags were stored at 0°C and another 15 bags were stored at 5°C. For the following 15 days, one bag from each cold storage temperature was moved to a laboratory maintained at 18°C to 20°C. Images were acquired for the 6 newly moved cucumbers and for the cucumbers previously moved. Analysis was performed using a combination of PCA and FLD (Fisher's linear discriminant) methods. The results of the study showed that integration of both methods provided good performance, and classification accuracy was improved. They concluded that integration of the PCA–FLD method for hyperspectral imaging could be applied for the quality inspection applications of agricultural products.

Strawberries are very frail and easily susceptible to mechanical injury resulting in bruises and spoilage. Nanyam et al. (2012) assessed the ability of hyperspectral imaging to detect bruises in strawberries. The specific objective of the study was to calculate the ratio of bruised to unbruised regions to evaluate the quality of the strawberries. Strawberries were purchased from local stores and 30 were bruised with a spherical impactor. A day after bruising, images were acquired using a NIR camera (SU640-1.7RT-D), with LCTF and lens, and two halogen lights for illumination. A multiband segmentation algorithm was developed to create a mask for extraction of the pixels from the edible area of the sample. Uniband univariate classifiers are used to categorize unbruised and bruised pixels, and a decision fusion strategy was developed that could increase the classification accuracy of bruised and unbruised pixels. The study provided an effective algorithm to determine bruise damage in strawberries using NIR hyperspectral images. The developed method estimates the ratio of bruised to unbruised regions in strawberries, but the decision fusion strategy developed was general and hence could be used for any other biological material for quality inspection.

Sorting and quality monitoring of fruits is mostly performed manually or using automatic methods based on the outer surface quality characteristics. However, characteristics such as total soluble solids (TSS), dry matter content, sugar content, and juice acidity are critical internal qualities. Most of the techniques to determine the internal quality indices are destructive and labor intensive. Development of a nondestructive method to determine these quality indices will be very helpful for all those involved in the production, processing, and distribution of fresh produce. ElMasry et al. (2007) explored hyperspectral imaging techniques to determine quality characteristics such as TSS, moisture content (MC), and acidity (pH) of strawberry. Strawberries were obtained from retail stores and fruits without any bruises, diseases, or damages were selected for the study. To generate variation in the properties of selected fruits, some were maintained at room temperature for 2 and 3 days, while some were maintained at lower temperature (5°C) for 3 and 5 days, thereby resulting in fruits of varied ripeness and other quality attributes. The hyperspectral imaging system consisted of a fruit holder, illumination unit, a spectrograph (ImSpector V10E), and a CCD camera. PLS analysis was used to construct a model between spectral response and their quality attributes. Multiple linear regression (MLR) models were developed with the optimal wavelength and the performance of the model was determined by the standard error of prediction (SEP), standard error of calibration (SEC), and correlation coefficient (r) between the predicted and measured values of the attribute. The correlation coefficient for the complete spectral range for MC, TSS, and pH were 0.90, 0.80, and

0.87 with SEC of 6.085, 0.233, and 0.105 and SEP of 3.874, 0.184, and 0.129, respectively. Using MLR models, the correlation coefficient for predicting MC, TSS, and pH were 0.87, 0.80, and 0.92, with SEC of 6.72, 0.220, and 0.084, and SEP of 5.786, 0.211, and 0.091, respectively. The authors concluded that based on the results a nondestructive hyperspectral imaging technique could be developed to determine the quality attributes of strawberries.

The shelf life and consumer satisfaction of peach fruit is based on the firmness of the fruit. Firmness, one of the important textural attributes, is tested by the Magness Taylor (MT) method, which is destructive and prone to operational error. Nondestructive firmness testing would ensure quality characteristics and consistency of fruit, thereby increasing consumer acceptance and industry profits. Lu and Peng (2006) explored hyperspectral scattering to determine the firmness of peach fruit. Visually inspected peach fruit without any defects were selected for the study. A total of 450 Red Haven and 440 Coral Star varieties were used for the study. The imaging system had a CCD camera (Model C4880-21), a spectrograph (ImSpector V9), a quartz tungsten halogen lamp, and a sample holder. The 677 nm wavelength, which corresponds to chlorophyll absorption, showed maximum correlation with fruit firmness and was useful for determining firmness of both peach varieties. The coefficient of determination (r^2) for Red Haven and Coral Star was 0.77 and 0.58, respectively. The authors concluded that hyperspectral imaging is a potential tool to nondestructively determine the firmness of peach fruits.

The contamination of apples with *E. coli* occur when apples come in contact with the ground, which may contain fecal substances or ingesta of an animal's gastrointestinal tract. Apples with fungal-contaminated surfaces, skin scratches, or cuts and bruises may result in bacterial growth, and ultimately decays. Hence, detection technologies to determine apple surface defects and contaminants are important to ensure the quality and grade of the apples supplied to the consumers. Lu (2003) developed a NIR hyperspectral technique to detect bruises on apples. Imaging was performed in the spectral region between 900 and 1700 nm, and concluded that 1000 to 1340 nm was the most effective spectral region for bruise detection in apples. Mehl et al. (2004) explored the ability of hyperspectral imaging methods to determine surface defects and contaminants in apples. Red Delicious, Gala, Golden Delicious, and Fuji apples were chosen for the study, and the apples were free of anti-fungal or wax protection treatment. Defective and contaminated apples were collected from the trees or gathered from the ground and comprised of those with bruises, scabs, side rots, molds, and flyspecks. Apples were kept in plastic bags and the temperature was maintained between 0°C and 4°C. The imaging system was comprised of a CCD camera (SpectraVideo™ Camera), a spectrograph (ImSpector 1.7), a focus lens, and two halogen lamps. Analysis was performed using an asymmetric second difference method, which is an analytical technique to separate defects or contaminants in various apple cultivars, and then compared with the results from PCA methods. PCA methods utilized a spectral range of 682 to 900 nm and detected bruises and contaminated apples from four cultivars. The study showed that PCA and asymmetric second difference method gave similar results for identification of bruises, disease, and fungal contamination in apples. However, PCA was complex and required longer time for data processing, whereas the second difference method required less computational time and only three wavelengths for processing.

Bitter pit, a physiological disorder that develops in apples postharvest, affects the quality of fruit and reduces the economic value of the fruit for the producers. Currently available methods to determine bitter pit are destructive and hence there is a lack of nondestructive method to determine bitter pits in apples. Nicolaï et al. (2006) assessed the capability of NIR hyperspectral imaging for identification of bitter pit in apples. Apples harvested from trees were stored for a period of 5 to 6 weeks in a cold temperature to enhance bitter pit development. The imaging system consisted of an InGaAs camera (SU320-1.7RT-V), a spectrograph (ImSpector), small moving platform, and halogen lamps. A discriminant PLS calibration model was developed to distinguish between bitter pit lesions and healthy apple skin. The results of the study showed that hyperspectral imaging could detect bitter pit lesions although invisible to the naked eye, but could not distinguish between corky tissue and bitter pit. The reason for misclassification errors may be the lowered luminosity at the image boundary, hence it was proposed to obtain multiple images to cover the entire surface of apples to avoid boundary artifacts.

The maturity of apple is a crucial factor to decide the time of harvest and the postharvest quality characteristics. Apple maturity is evaluated by various quality characteristics such as skin color, fruit firmness, sugar content, titratable acid, and ethylene production. Most of the methods used to measure these quality traits are destructive, time consuming, and have operational error. Noh and Lu (2007) determined the apple quality using hyperspectral laser-induced fluorescence imaging. Four hundred Golden Delicious apples were placed in a controlled atmosphere prior to experiment. The imaging system was comprised of a CCD camera (C4880-21), a spectrograph (ImSpector V9), a zoom lens, a long pass filter, and a computer. Fluorescence scattering images were acquired at 0, 1, 2, 3, 4, and 5 min of illumination. To determine the fruit quality attributes, the standard tests were conducted. PCA and neural network was used to develop models to predict the various fruit quality. The results of the study showed that good predictions were obtained for apple skin hue, with a correlation coefficient of 0.94. For skin chroma, fruit firmness and flesh hue, a good correlation coefficient greater than or equal to 0.74 was obtained for 1 min of illumination. For soluble solids, titratable acid, and flesh chroma, poorer correlations were obtained. Noh and Lu concluded that hyperspectral fluorescence imaging is a potential method to determine the quality characteristics of apples and further work is required to increase the efficiency of the current technique for assessment of fruit quality.

Presence of pits or pit fragments in cherries poses a serious threat to consumers and results in economic losses to the producers and processors. The current techniques to remove pits from cherries although effective cannot guarantee that the final product contains no pits or pit fragments. Qin and Lu (2005) presented a hyperspectral transmission imaging technique for detection of pits in cherries. The imaging system was comprised of a CCD camera, a spectrograph covering a wavelength range of 400 to 1000 nm, a lens, lighting arrangement, and a computer. Montmorency tart cherries were grouped into three categories according to their weight: small (less than 4.0 g), medium (between 4.0 and 5.5 g), and large (greater than 5.5 g) and grouped into two color classes: dark and light red. A neural network algorithm was developed to classify cherries with and without pits. The size of the fruit and defect played a major role in the classification of cherries with and without pits, whereas orientation or color showed a small or negligible effect on pit classification. When the neural network classifier was trained and tested with the same size, color, or defective fruit, lower classification error (3% or less) was achieved. Based on the study, the authors concluded that hyperspectral imaging has potential to detect pits in cherries.

Fresh vegetables are considered healthy food, but when they are consumed raw, there is a risk of pathogen contamination. Fresh spinach especially has been associated with outbreaks of *E. coli* O157:H7, *Salmonella* spp., and *Listeria monocytogenes*. Many of the current techniques now used to detect pathogens are complicated and expensive, and hence a simple, nonexpensive detection method is needed. Siripatrawan et al. (2011) examined the possibility of hyperspectral imaging to detect *E. coli* contamination in spinach. Spinach

(*Spinacia oleracea* L.) leaves were purchased from the market and fresh leaves without cuts, decay, or bruises were selected and contaminated with a nonpathogenic strain of *E. coli* K12 (NBRC 3301). A hyperspectral imaging system was used to obtain spectral images in the 400 to 1000 nm range. PCA was used to remove unwanted information and ANN was used to develop a prediction map to determine the number of *E. coli* in the sample. The results of the study proved that hyperspectral imaging could be used to detect *E. coli* contamination in fresh spinach. Yang et al. (2010) examined hyperspectral fluorescence imaging to determine fecal contamination in leafy vegetables such as spinach and romaine lettuce. The imaging system consisted of an electron-multiplying charge-coupled device (EMCCD) camera, a spectrograph, lenses, and two ultraviolet lights (320–400 nm) for illumination. The results of the study showed that wavelengths of 666 nm and 680 nm provided better detection of fecal contamination and the authors concluded that this technique could be successfully used for detection of fecal contamination on romaine lettuce and spinach.

Sugar-end defect, also known as translucent ends or jelly ends, is a defect of potatoes (*Solanum tuberosum* L.). French fry processors rate this as one of the major defects because it deteriorates the quality of the final product. The affected potatoes show a difference in fructose, glucose, sucrose, and starch concentration between proximal and distal ends. It is caused by plant stress during the growing season, which results in accumulation of excess sugar during storage. Groinig et al. (2011) studied the hyperspectral imaging for in-line quality control of potatoes affected by sugar-end defect. The imaging system was the HELIOS-EC3 NIR system working in the wavelength range of 900 to 1700 nm. The system classified the affected and sound potatoes, and the classification accuracies were 91.7%, 94.4%, 8.3%, and 5.6% for true positive, true negative, false positive and false negative, respectively. Groinig et al. concluded that this technology has a potential for inline quality control of potatoes.

Mushroom (*Agaricus bisporus* [J.E. Lange]) is a commonly consumed edible fungus around the world. Due to the presence of a high amount of water content, storage at temperatures below 0°C results in freeze damage, and water lost after thawing results in enzymatic browning. Gowen et al. (2009b) investigated the potential of hyperspectral imaging to identify mushrooms subjected to freeze damage. Experiments were conducted at three time periods: May, August, and September 2008 with a total sample size of 144 mushrooms (48 for each test). Data from May and August were combined to create a calibration set (96 mushrooms), and September data were treated as an independent set to evaluate the performance of the model. Samples were maintained overnight at 4°C and the next day, 24 undamaged mushrooms were separated in 3 groups of 8 mushrooms. The undamaged samples were tested after 24 h and 48 h storage. The other 24 mushrooms were split into 3 groups of 8 mushrooms and kept in a freezer at –30°C ± 3°C for 24 h. After removal from the freezer, samples were tested after thawing for 45 min and again tested after 24 h while were stored at 4°C ± 1°C. The imaging unit was comprised of a CCD camera, a spectrograph (Specim V10E) covering a spectral range of 400 to 1000 nm, zoom lens, light source, and a computer system. PCA and LDA were used to classify sample spectra into freeze-damaged and undamaged samples. The classification accuracy was 100% for undamaged mushrooms and 97.9% for freeze-damaged mushrooms. Gowen et al. concluded that hyperspectral imaging could be used for detection and monitoring of freeze-damaged mushrooms even before visible damage is evident.

Many research studies have been conducted for quality monitoring of food and agricultural products using hyperspectral imaging, but not much research has been conducted on dairy products. However, Gowen et al. (2009a) has stated that a broad range of quality control and safety testing on dairy products could be implemented using hyperspectral imaging. During homogenization, the size distribution of fat globules in milk could be assessed using hyperspectral imaging, because fat concentration in milk varies spatially. Hyperspectral imaging by means of spatial characterization of the spectral response could provide improved coagulation characterization and curd formation processes. During spray drying, moisture distribution profile maps could be generated using hyperspectral imaging, which could be used to determine the effects of different drying parameters on the quality of the final product. Any problem occurring during the drying process, such as equipment malfunction, could be determined by nonuniform moisture profiles in a product. Hyperspectral imaging could also be used to calculate the particle size distribution and monitor the blending homogeneity, thereby increasing the quality of the final product.

5.3.4.2 Nuts and beans

Black walnut shell is hazardous and in the walnut processing plant, it sometimes gets mixed with the pulp. Walnut cracking machines are currently used to remove the majority of the shell, but it still requires human intervention to completely remove the shell fragments. In the walnut processing plant, manual pickup of shell is the most labor-demanding work because walnut shell looks very similar to walnut pulp in both size and color. Hence Jiang et al. (2007) developed an alternate technique to remove walnut shell from pulp based on hyperspectral imaging. A hyperspectral imaging system was developed by the Instrumentation and Sensing Lab at U.S. Department of Agriculture (USDA), which consists of a CCD camera, a spectrograph (ImSpector V9), a C-mount lens, two halogen lamps, and an image acquisition and processing unit. Walnuts were cracked using a nut cracker and four sample groups were considered for the study: dark pulp, light pulp, outside shell, and inside shell. A support vector machine (SVM) method based on Gaussian kernel was utilized to differentiate the walnut pulp and shell, and the results of SVM are compared to the PCA and Fischer's discriminant analysis (FDS) methods. Using the SVM method, an accuracy of 90.3% was achieved for walnut shell and pulp classification, which was better than PCA and FDS methods.

Mung bean (*Vigna radiata* L.) is a pulse crop widely grown in India and is greatly infested by cowpea weevil (*Callosobruchus maculates* F.), which deteriorates the quality of the mung bean kernel during the storage period. Commonly used detection methods such as Berlese funnel, visual inspection, whole grain flotation, carbon dioxide production, and acoustic have one or more limitations, for example, time consuming, destruction of sample, subjective, reduced accuracy and unable to detect life stages of infestation of the grain. Kaliramesh et al. (2013) studied the detection of cowpea weevil using hyperspectral imaging. The imaging systems consisted of an InGaAs camera (SU640-1.7RT-D) with liquid crystal tunable filter, a lens, and an illumination source. Twelve percent moisture content mung beans were mixed with 150 cowpea weevils. After 24 h kernels with single eggs were collected and incubated at 30°C and 70% relative humidity to obtain various life stages of the weevil. Using LDA and QDA methods, classification models were developed. The classification accuracy for detecting uninfested and infested kernels was 85% and 82%, respectively. The classification accuracies were higher for kernels with pupal and adult stages compared to kernels with eggs and larval stages.

Soybean is a famous crop in East Asia and Japan, and the taste is attributed mainly to the sweetness and presence of amino acid content. A nondestructive method for appropriate estimation of fructose, glucose, sucrose, and nitrogen content would furnish useful information for the farming community to facilitate appropriate harvest time. Monteiro et al. (2007) examined the ability of hyperspectral imaging in the NIR and visible region to determine the sweetness and amino acid content of soybean. Thirteen varieties of soybean

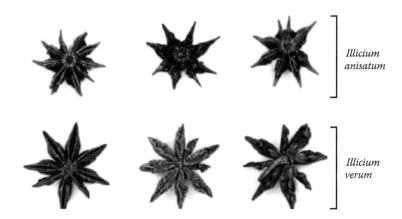

Illicium anisatum

Illicium verum

Figure 5.5 Images of *Illicium anisatum* and *Illicium verum*. (From Vermaak, I. et al., *Journal of Pharmaceutical and Biomedical Analysis*, 75, 207, 2013. With permission.)

grown in experimental plots at Yamagata University were used for the study. Images were obtained using a hyperspectral sensor ImSpector and images were acquired between 400 and 1000 nm with a resolution of 5 nm. An artificial neural network method was used and a performance analysis of regression models was conducted. The nonlinear regression model of the second derivative resulted in excellent predictions for fructose, sucrose, glucose, and nitrogen concentrations. The regression models from the hyperspectral data set reduced by PCA provided the worst correlation. Monteiro et al. concluded that hyperspectral imaging could be used to determine the amino acid content and sweetness in soybean crops.

Chinese star anise (*Illicium verum* Hook. f), native to Southern China and Vietnam, is mainly used as a traditional medicine and as a spice in China and India. Japanese star anise (*Illicium anisatum* L.) looks very similar to *I. verum* (Figure 5.5). Since Japanese star anise contains compounds that are neurotoxic, adulteration or mistaken identity has resulted in undesirable side effects in many infants and adults. Vermaak et al. (2013) assessed the ability of hyperspectral imaging to differentiate between Chinese and Japanese star anise. Authentic specimens of *I. anisatum* and *I. verum* were purchased from American Herbal Pharmacopoeia (California). The sisuChema shortwave infrared (SWIR) hyperspectral pushbroom imaging unit with a spectrograph coupled with a HgCdTe detector and halogen lamps was used to acquire images. PCA and PLS-DA methods were applied for data analysis. The results of the study showed that classification accuracy of 98.42% was obtained for *I. anisatum* and 97.85% was obtained for *I. verum*. Vermaak et al. concluded that SWIR hyperspectral imaging is a nondestructive technique that could be used to detect whole dried fruit of *I. anisatum* and *I. verum*.

5.3.4.3 Meat

The meat industry has stringent quality control regulations to maintain the quality and to improve safety for consumers. During cold storage of meat, unfavorable conditions or temperature fluctuations cause unwanted growth of microorganisms, which deteriorate the quality and safety of the product. Also, when the total viable count (TVC) of bacteria in meat grows above a stipulated limit, it becomes unsafe and when consumed results in serious health issues. A conventional plating method is widely used to calculate the number of viable microorganisms and a similar method to determine psychrotrophic plate count (PPC) is implemented by detection of colonies plated on solid medium and maintained at refrigeration temperatures. Although economical and providing good results, it is laborious, tedious, and destructive. Barbin et al. (2013) examined the capability of NIR hyperspectral imaging for determination of TVC and PPC in pork samples. Fresh pork meat from the *longissimus dorsi* muscle (loin) were obtained from an industrial plant and cut into chops of 1.5 cm thickness and stored at refrigerated temperatures (0°C and 4°C) for 21 days before images were acquired. The imaging system consisted of a spectrograph, CCD camera, lens, and a computer. LDA models were constructed to categorize samples based on hyperspectral data and a PLS approach was used to fit the spectral data obtained from the sample to the logarithmic values of TVC and PPC. The best regressions with R^2 of 0.86 and 0.89 for log (TVC) and log (PPC), respectively, were obtained. Barbin et al. concluded that the results are very promising and hyperspectral imaging has a great potential for determining spoilage due to bacteria in pork samples.

Minced meat constitutes a major portion of processed products like hamburgers, patties, and sausages, and contains varied levels of fat. Current techniques used to analyze chemical composition of meat are time consuming and subjective to errors. Hence a fast technique to determine fat content in minced meat is required. Barbin et al. (2012a) studied the ability of NIR hyperspectral imaging for fat quantification in minced meat. The pork samples from four different muscles—*longissimus dorsi* (LD), *semimembranosus* (SM), *semitendinosus* (ST), and *biceps femoris* (BF)—were obtained from a meat supplier (Rosderra Irish Meats Group, Roscrea, Co. Tipperary, Ireland). Hyperspectral images were obtained using pushbroom NIR hyperspectral system in the reflectance mode and the fat content was also measured using standard methods (AOAC Official Method, 2008). The imaging system comprised of a spectrograph (ImSpector N17E), a camera with C-mount lens (Xeva 992, Xenics Infrared Solutions, Belgium), two tungsten halogen lamps, a translation stage, data acquisition software, and a computer. Partial least square regression (PLSR) was used to determine the amount of fat using spectral information. The coefficient of determination obtained by PLSR model was 0.95, showing that NIR has good potential to predict fat content in minced meat.

Pork quality attributes result from a combination of various characteristics of fresh meat including color, softness, and water holding capacity, which are the basic lean quality traits. Pork quality is classified into different grades: RFN, DFD, and PSE. Reddish-pink, firm, and nonexudative (RFN) is the highest quality meat. Dark purplish-red, firm, and dry (DFD) has a hard and sticky surface with high water-holding capacity and pH resulting from long-term stress due to improper handling. Pale or pinkish gray, soft, and exudative (PSE) meat is the least favorable meat with undesirable appearance and excessive shrinkage. Traditional methods depend on average measurement of smaller areas of pork samples and hence are not ideal for monitoring the entire product in a commercial production facility. Barbin et al. (2012b) explored hyperspectral imaging in the NIR range from 900 to 1700 nm for classification and grading of pork. Seventy-five fresh samples from various grades of quality obtained from *longissimus dorsi* muscle were used for the experiment. Pushbroom hyperspectral imaging systems used in Barbin et al. (2012a) was used to obtain spectral images. PCA was applied to extract important features from the images. The results showed that there was significant variation among the three quality grades (RFN, DFD, PSE) at wavelengths of 960, 1074, 1124, 1147, 1207, and 1341 nm. Pork could be classified into different grades with an overall accuracy of 96%. The authors concluded that hyperspectral imaging could be useful for classification of pork samples but the major limitation is the high magnitude of data and correct selection of the representative region of interest (ROI). The first limitation could be overcome by selection of one or more critical wavelengths and the selection of region of interest should be established by utilizing various image processing regimes on the chosen wavelengths.

Pork quality varies depending on texture (firmness), color, and exudation (drip loss). In addition to the three grades of pork (RFN, DFD, PSE), two more classes have been named: RSE (reddish, soft, and exudative) and PFN (pale, firm, and non-exudative) and these are recognized as important quality defects in Canada. Another quality parameter of pork is the marbling, which is the mixing of fat with lean in the muscle. The marbling scores are based on size, number, and distribution of fat particles, which is usually assessed subjectively by human inspection. Qiao et al. (2007) determined the possibility of utilizing hyperspectral imaging for pork quality and marbling assessment. Fresh pork samples were commercially obtained and cut into 1 cm thick loin samples. A total of 40 samples including 10 samples of RFN, PSE, RSE, and PFN each were used for imaging. The imaging system consisted of a spectrograph (ImSpectorV10E), a CMOS camera, illuminator, conveyor, data acquisition software, and a computer. The spectral analyses were performed using PCA and ANN for classification. The results showed that classification accuracy of RFN samples was perfect and it was easier to classify RSE samples, but PFN samples were confused with PSE and RSE samples. The RFN and RSE samples were classified accurately and the total corrected ratio was 75% to 80%. They concluded that hyperspectral imaging could be used to assess pork quality and there is also a potential to use textural features to detect marbling scores of pork.

The main quality characteristics used to select the meat products are visible fat, uniformity in color, and maximum water-holding capacity. Of these, the quality of fresh meat greatly depends on the water-holding capability of the meat, which is important both technologically and economically for processors and consumers. Conventional techniques used to determine water-holding ability, such as drip loss, filter paper wetness, and centrifuge force, are elaborate and destructive. ElMasry et al. (2011a) explored the potential of hyperspectral imaging to determine the water-holding capacity of beef. Three types of muscles—*M. longissimus dorsi* (LD), *M. semitendinosus* (ST), and *psoas major* (PM)—were selected for the study. The pushbroom imaging unit consisted of a spectrograph (ImSpector, N17E), CCD camera and lens, and a computer. The spectral range was between 890 and 1750 nm, but due to low and noisy response in the 850 to 910 and 1700 to 1750 nm ranges, only the 910 to 1700 nm range was used to build calibration models. PCA and PLSR models were developed, and the PLSR model provided a coefficient of determination $\left(R_{CV}^2\right)$ of 0.89 and standard error from cross-validation (SECV) of 0.26%. Six wavelengths—940, 997, 1144, 1214, 1342, and 1443 nm—were selected as critical to construct prediction models, which resulted in R_{CV}^2 of 0.87 and SECV of 0.28. ElMasry et al. concluded that the hyperspectral technique has potential to determine water-holding capacity of beef samples with reasonable accuracy. ElMasry et al. (2011b) explored NIR hyperspectral imaging for quality grading of cooked, sliced turkey hams, because ham grading is monitored by human inspection based on standards. Four ham samples were prepared from turkey breast using various levels of brine injection: premium (B1), medium-high (B2), medium-low (B3), and low (B4) quality hams. The ham blocks were cooked to a core temperature of 74°C and refrigerated at 4°C before slicing. Spectral information was examined using PCA and data from the 910 to 1710 nm range were used for model development. The results showed that from the 241 wavelengths only eight (980, 1061, 1141, 1174, 1215, 1325, 1436, and 1641 nm) were chosen as optimum wavelength for turkey ham classification. The results showed that NIR spectral imaging has the potential to be developed into a robust and nondestructive method to classify turkey ham slices.

Tenderness of beef is an important quality characteristic to satisfy consumer needs. For steaks with guaranteed tenderness, consumers are ready to pay a higher price. But the current USDA grading standard is mainly dependent on degree of marbling and does not always classify based on tenderness. Naganathan et al. (2008) evaluated the capability of visible/NIR hyperspectral imaging for prediction of tenderness in beef. Hyperspectral imaging showing the spectrum for lean and fat pixel of beefsteak is shown in Figure 5.6. Beefsteaks (*longissimus dorsi* muscle) were obtained from four packing plants and the samples were aged 14 days and kept in vacuum packages. Images were obtained using a hyperspectral imaging unit that consisted of a spectrograph (ImSpector V10E), a CCD camera, linear motorized slide, and six tungsten halogen lamps for illumination. The spectral range was between 400 and 1000 nm with 2.8 nm spectral band resolution. During imaging, steaks were taken out from vacuum packages, oxygenated for 30 min, and images were obtained. After image acquisition, steak samples were cooked and slice shear force (SSF) values were measured. Depending on SSF values, steaks were grouped into three tenderness classes: tender (SSF ≤ 205.80 N), intermediate (205.80 N < SSF > 254.80 N), and tough (SSF ≥ 254.80 N). PCA was carried out on the region of interest to decrease the dimensions along the spectral axis and canonical discriminant analysis (CDA) was performed to develop a canonical discriminant model. The model achieved an accuracy of 96.4% on three tenderness categories. Based on the results, it was stated that hyperspectral imaging could be used to classify beef based on tenderness, which would enhance the economic prospects of cattle producers and processors, and could also meet and satisfy consumer expectations.

Enterobacteriaceae is a group of bacteria containing many foodborne pathogens, including *Escherichia coli*, *Shigella*, and *Salmonella*. Detection of these pathogens is very crucial for food safety, and conventional methods used to monitor these bacteria consume more time and are destructive in nature. Feng et al. (2012) assessed the ability of hyperspectral imaging to monitor bacteriological contamination in chicken fillets. Sample chicken fillets packed in plastic trays were bought from stores, and samples of 10 g were taken and subjected to imaging after which traditional tests using the standard pour plate

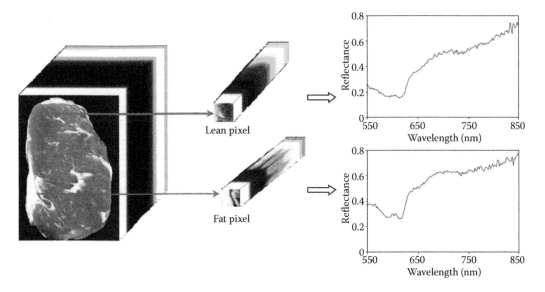

Figure 5.6 Hyperspectral image of beefsteak highlighting the spectral signatures of lean and fat pixel. (From Naganathan, G.K. et al., *Computers and Electronics in Agriculture*, 64, 225, 2008. With permission.)

technique were carried out. The image acquisition system described in Barbin et al. (2012a) was used for acquiring images. PCA and support vector regression (SVR) were used to construct models using spectral data. Using full wavelength, coefficient of determination (R^2) was 0.87 and when the model was simplified by using only eight wavelengths (930, 1034, 1021, 1158, 1195, 1268, 1398, 1658 nm), the resulting R^2 values were 0.94 and 0.92 for calibration and prediction models, respectively.

In the meat industry, detection of meat authenticity and adulteration has become very crucial and received significant attention in the recent past. Although food authenticity is increasing, incidences of food fraud or mislabeling is difficult to appraise. Identification of different meat species is performed manually which is time consuming, tedious, and subject to human error. Kamruzzaman et al. (2012a) investigated the categorization and authentication of red meat using hyperspectral imaging. Meat samples from *longissimus dorsi* muscles of beef, pork, and lamb were used for the study. The hyperspectral imaging system described in Barbin et al. (2012a) was used for the experiments. The spectral data were analyzed by PCA and PLS-DA methods. Six wavelengths (957, 1071, 1121, 1144, 1368, 1394 nm) were determined as important wavelengths and used in developing classification models. An overall classification accuracy of 98.67% was obtained in classifying lamb, pork, and beef. The results proved that hyperspectral imaging could be used to detect various red meats and the system could be installed in the meat industry with minimum modifications of the existing industrial setup. They also suggested that since this study was conducted in off-line mode, further research should be performed at an industrial scale in on-line applications.

Poultry meat with pathological issues should be identified and segregated from the processing line to ensure safety of the product supplied to the consumers. Traditional inspection is carried out by human inspectors who inspect on an average 30 to 35 samples per minute during an 8 h day. These conditions may result in repetitive motion injuries and fatigue problems resulting in human error. Especially in poultry, tumors are not easy to identify as other diseases during visual inspection because their spatial signature seems more of a distortion of shape rather than a discoloration. Hence, Kong et al. (2004) examined the ability of hyperspectral fluorescence imaging for detection of poultry skin tumors. For fluorescence measurement, two fluorescence lamps (Model XX-15A, Spectronics Corp, New York) provided a near uniform ultraviolet excitation on the sample area. The hyperspectral image contained 65 spectral bands of fluorescence at wavelengths ranging from 425 to 711 nm. Using PCA analysis, important features were extracted from two spectral peaks identified as spectral bands to detect tumors. Their study showed that hyperspectral fluorescence imaging has a potential to detect skin tumors in poultry.

Although bacterial contamination of chicken carcasses is influenced by many factors, the fecal contamination at the processing facility is an important cause. The important reason for fecal contamination is the bursting of the intestine during processing thus releasing the fecal material. Since there exists a zero tolerance for fecal material in poultry, development of a classification tool to identify contamination in poultry carcass has become very crucial for food safety audits. Park et al. (2007) examined the ability of hyperspectral imaging using a spectral angle mapper (SAM) algorithm to detect fecal contamination. After processing operations, carcasses containing fecal materials were sent to the USDA imaging lab for analysis. The clean samples were imaged first and then were contaminated with ingesta and feces of various types, spot size of contaminant, and location on carcass. A transportable imaging system (Figure 5.7) specifically designed and fabricated for mobile purposes consisted of a spectrograph (ImSpector V9), a CCD camera with

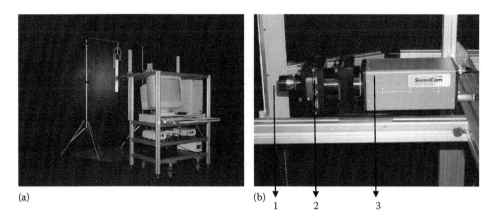

Figure 5.7 A portable hyperspectral imaging system. (a) Complete imaging arrangement and (b) motor driven line scan hyperspectral camera: (1) focusing lens, (2) spectrograph, and (3) CCD camera. (From Park, B. et al., *Biosystems Engineering*, 96, 323, 2007. With permission.)

C-mount lens, frame grabber, halogen lamp, and a computer. A spectral angle mapper (SAM) algorithm was chosen due to its better performance compared to other algorithms. To select the ideal classifier using a SAM algorithm, regions of interest were generated from an uncontaminated region (wing, thigh, and breast) and surface contaminated areas (caecum, colon, duodenum, and ingesta). The mean classification accuracy increased from 75.31 to 89.08 and then to 90.13 as the spectral angle (α) increased from 0.1 to 0.2 and then to 0.3. The kappa coefficient (κ), which represents the classification accuracy based on a confusion matrix, increased from 0.0614 ($\alpha = 0.05$) to 0.7169 ($\alpha = 0.1$). Park et al. concluded that hyperspectral imaging using a SAM classification method could identify various fecal contaminants in poultry carcass and hence could be used in food safety inspection.

Park et al. (2010) developed a hyperspectral imaging system for poultry fecal detection in real time. A pilot-scale test has demonstrated that the technique could be implemented on a large-scale poultry processing facility for detection of fecal and ingesta contamination at a speed of 140 samples per minute. The challenging aspect during the system development was to reduce false positives, since Park et al. (2006) showed a high accuracy of 96.4% for fecal detection, but false positives ranged from 147 to 443 for a total contaminant of 1066 spots. To reduce false positive errors due to the presence of feathers, cuticle, broken wings, and edge pixels, many solutions based on software and hardware had been created. For hardware, an additional optical trim filter was added. For software, various algorithms, including dynamic thresholding techniques such as kernel density estimation, fisher linear discriminant analysis, and textural analysis of hyperspectral images, were used. Their study showed that with real-time imaging algorithms combined with high-speed data acquisition, hyperspectral imaging could be a potential tool to detect fecal contamination by inspecting a minimum of 140 birds per minute.

5.3.4.4 Aquaculture

Salmon (*Salmon salar* L.) is an important species of fish with a production of about 1,400,000 t in 2009 which is worth over US$7 billion (FAO, 2011). The various products made from salmon are labeled as spoiled if quality changes such as emission of off-odors, discoloration, and formation of slime occurs to an unacceptable level. It is a great challenge for the salmon processing industry, because harmful microorganisms can grow rapidly and once consumed may create harmful effects for consumers. Current techniques for detection of deterioration in seafood are sensory based, chemical, microbiological, and biochemical methods. A major limiting factor for the sensory method is that considerably skilled and experienced panels are essential for reliable results and are very subjective. Other methods are laborious, consume more time, and are destructive in nature. Hence Wu and Sun (2013b) tested the time-series hyperspectral imaging for detection of spoilage in salmon. Two groups (22 fillets) were purchased from a supermarket and each fillet was cut into a 3 cm × 3 cm × 1 cm shape. The samples were left to spoil in a refrigerator at 4°C. Two hyperspectral imaging systems at 400 to 1000 nm and 880 to 1720 nm were used for the experiments. Hyperspectral data were acquired for 66 samples out of which 50 samples of data were used for calibration with the remaining data for prediction. After acquiring images, the standard plate count method was used to determine the total viable count (TVC) of each chop of the sample. Eight wavelengths—495, 535, 550, 585, 625, 660, 785, and 915 nm—were identified as critical for determining the total viable count of the salmon. Models were established using PLSR and least squares support vector machine (LS-SVM) methods. The coefficient of determination based on the model was 0.985 and hence the authors concluded that hyperspectral imaging could be used for fast and nondestructive detection of bacterial spoilage in salmon.

Texture is a critical quality factor that determines the overall quality of salmon, and soft flesh results in lower acceptability and quality downgrading of the salmon. Currently texture is measured based on two approaches: organoleptic assessment using taste panels and instrumental methods. Human inspection is laborious, subjective, and inconsistent, whereas instrumental techniques are destructive, time consuming, expensive, and require lengthy sample preparation. There is a lack of objective, noninvasive methods to assess the quality of salmon, which limits the ability of the salmon industry to supply quality products to the consumers. Wu et al. (2012b) performed textural analysis of salmon using hyperspectral imaging. Three groups (24 fillets) of fresh Atlantic salmon fillets—10 from Scotland, 8 from Norway and 6 from Ireland—were purchased. Images were acquired with a pushbroom line scanning hyperspectral imaging system (DV Optics Ltd., Padua, Italy) consisting of a spectrograph (Specim V10), a CCD camera, objective lens, halogen lamp for illumination, moving table, and computer. After image acquisition, the color value of each fillet was determined using a colorimeter. Texture profile analysis (TPA) parameters such as hardness, cohesiveness, and adhesiveness were measured using an Instron Universal testing instrument (Model 4411, Canton, Massachusetts). PLSR analysis was conducted to create quantitative models between spectral and TPA parameters. The results showed that a correlation coefficient (r_c) of 0.665, 0.555, and 0.606 and root mean square estimated by cross-validation (RMSECV) of 4.09, 0.067, and 0.504 were obtained for hardness, cohesiveness, and adhesiveness, respectively. The authors concluded that hyperspectral imaging could be used to determine the textural characteristics of salmon fillet in a consistent, fast, and noninvasive nature.

Nematode-infected fish was not regarded as a health risk but mainly considered a cosmetic problem. But as the popularity for undercooked seafood consumption increased, nematode infection has become a health risk. The two major types of nematode that infect Atlantic cod (*Gadus morhua* L.) are *Anisakis simplex* (Karl Rudolphi) and *Pseudoterranova decipiens*. Currently nematode removal is done manually, which is called trimming, and accounts for 50% of the production cost for Pacific cod. The fillet trimming is performed at room temperature, which increases the risk of bacterial infection and degradation due to enzymatic reactions. The efficiency for manual detection of *P. decipiens* is reported as around 68% in an ideal environment and only around 50% under a real-time industrial environment (Hafsteinsson and Rizvi, 1987). Hence there is a need for automatic nematode detection for the cod fillet industry. Sivertsen et al. (2012) conducted experiments based on hyperspectral imaging for automated detection of nematode in cod fillets. The inspection was carried out under industrial conditions, and during the testing, 127 fillet samples were collected prior to the trimming station and 20 fillets were collected after the trimming station. The nematode was grouped as pale or dark based on its white/yellow or red/brown color, respectively. The operating speed of the conveyor belt was 400 mm/s, which met the industrial speed requirement. The results of the study showed that a Gaussian maximum classifier detected around 60.3% and 70.8% of the pale and dark nematodes, respectively. These results were better than the results previously reported using higher resolution equipment with a slower conveyor speed and on par with the manual inspection results. Hence the authors concluded that hyperspectral imaging could be a potential technique to detect nematodes in cod fillets.

5.3.4.5   Sanitation in food industry

Increased foodborne illness and issues related to food contamination have resulted in development and implementation of strict sanitation measures in food processing industries. There is significant potential for imaging technologies to improve the sanitation protocols in the food processing facility. Lefcourt et al. (2013) developed a portable hyperspectral unit to monitor the effectiveness of sanitation procedures in food processing facilities. The imaging system consisted of a C-mount lens, liquid crystal tunable filter (VariSpec VIS, Caliper Life Science, United States), a CCD camera, back-correction optics, touchscreen monitor, and a laptop. The efficacy was tested with honeydew slices and cantaloupe melon pieces placed on a high-density polyethylene (HDPE) cutting board. The melon pieces were clearly identifiable at a wavelength of 675 nm and the juice trails made by melon were also evident at 675 nm. The juice trails were invisible to the naked eye and the ability to see the juice trails explains the sensitivity of the imaging system. The handheld hyperspectral imaging system could acquire spectra from 460 to 720 nm at 5 nm intervals in 11 s, and a fluorescence-based response to violet LED excitation can be identified under ambient fluorescent lighting at 475, 520, and 675 nm where the ambient lighting intensity is low. Lefcourt et al. showed that it was possible to detect any worn out HDPE surface as well as any residue of the sample. They concluded that a portable hyperspectral imaging instrument could be an important tool for regulating the efficiency of sanitation guidelines in food processing industries.

Escherichia coli O157:H7, *Staphylococcus aureus*, *Salmonella* spp., and *Listeria monocytogenes* are some of the most common bacteria that attach to food surfaces and other surfaces such as plastic, stainless steel, and glass. These bacteria form communities and are a major health concern for the food industry since the biofilm-associated microorganism can increase public health risks. Commonly used methods to detect bacterial contamination are polymerase chain reaction, colony counting methods, and immunology-based systems, which are time consuming and labor intensive. Jun et al. (2009) examined the possibility of the hyperspectral fluorescence imaging for evaluation of bacterial biofilm on stainless steel. Nonpathogenic *E. coli* O157:H7 strain 3704 and *Salmonella enterica* typhimurium ATCC 53648 were selected for the study. The imaging system was composed of an electron-multiplying charge-coupled device, spectrograph (VNIR Concentric Imaging Spectrograph, Headwall photonics, Massachusetts), and a lens. Images were obtained between 416 and 700 nm with a spectral interval of 4.79 nm. PCA was performed to analyze the images, and the results showed that maximum fluorescence emission were observed at a wavelength of 480 nm for both *Salmonella* and *E. coli* O157:H7 on stainless steel surfaces. Jun et al. concluded that the 480 nm wavelength band is best suited for developing portable imaging equipment for evaluating sanitary conditions of food processing machineries.

5.3.5 Engineering

The applications of hyperspectral imaging have spread across many sections of the engineering industry, including steel, plastic, pulp and paper, recycling, and object sorting applications. In the steel industry, many parameters are established by subjective evaluations, specifically in the slag characterization processes in the electrical arc furnace (EAF) and in the ladle furnace (LF). In EAF, chemical composition of slag cannot be monitored by visual inspection, and by having a greater understanding and knowledge of iron oxide content in slag, the production could be properly controlled and waste could be minimized. Gutierrez et al. (2010) assessed the potential of hyperspectral imaging for the steel foundry process. Their study showed that the technique provides an estimation of the element's chemical composition and enables optimization of the parameters to achieve the desired properties of steel. The results showed that better performance of slag characterization was achieved using a spectro-spatial model approach with 97% accuracy. They showed that hyperspectral imaging has promising potential to provide accurate real-time data for the slag samples coming from the refining and melting process.

Plastic packaging and other used plastic items could be a valuable resource in the manufacture of new plastic products and in the generation of energy. There is a global need to increase recycling to minimize environmental pollution and to make use of available resources. Recycling plastics and avoiding landfill use results in reduced CO_2 emission and saves lot of resources and protects our environment. There are around 50 kinds of plastics and there are many challenges in sorting and recycling. Existing techniques for separation depends on the variation in flotation properties in water, which separates lighter kind of plastics, such as polypropylene (PP), low density polyethylene (LDPE), and high-density polyethylene (HDPE), from heavier types of plastics, such as polyvinyl chloride (PVC) and polyethylene terephthalate (PET). Furthermore the lighter types—HDPE, PP, and LDPE—are difficult to separate among themselves. To produce high-quality recycled products, the waste plastic mixture must be sorted very accurately, which involves multiple separations and hence the process is very expensive. Serranti et al. (2010) developed a hyperspectral imaging technique for detecting impurities in secondary plastics. First they carried out investigations on three different wastes: bottom ashes, light fractions resulting from car dismantling (fluff), and waste glass fragments (cullets). Then they performed tests to assess the potential of the utilization of hyperspectral imaging in (1) secondary plastics feed characterization (different polymers and contaminants identification), (2) quality of different flow streams resulting from specific processing action, and (3) identification of PE and PP particles to set up new sorting strategies for their recovery. The sensing device consisted of an ImSpector V10E working in the VIS-NIR spectral range of 400 to 1000 nm with 2.8 nm spectral resolution. The results of the study showed that acquired spectra for particulate solid identified the different materials constituting the secondary plastic flow stream. Spectral plots clearly showed different materials present had different spectral signature. The different types of plastics (PVC, PET, PE, PP) could be identified as well as different contaminants, such as wood, foam, and aluminum. Through spectral analysis, it was possible to quantitatively identify undesirable particles and also their positions to implement automatic sorting strategies for their removal.

Sorting paper of different qualities is a tough task, and the significance of paper and cardboard sorting is increasing tremendously because improving the sorting efficiency can improve the price of secondary material and lower the requirement for chemicals in paper production. Tatzer et al. (2005) described an in-line material separating system using hyperspectral imaging for categorization of materials based on cellulose, such as paper, pulp, and cardboard. The system consisted of a camera with an InGaAs sensor, spectrograph (ImSpector N17, Specim Ltd., Finland) with a spectral range from 900 to 1000 nm and 13 nm spectral resolution, and halogen lamps for illumination. The spectral data were analyzed using PCA and LDA methods. The classification accuracy for the PCA model was 52%, 33%, 55%, and 70% for raw cardboard, color cardboard, newspaper, and printer paper, respectively. The classification accuracy of the PCA–LDA combined model was 93%, 81%, 95%, and 91% for raw cardboard, color cardboard, newspaper and printer paper, respectively. The results showed that a combined PCA–LDA model provided good classification accuracy and hence hyperspectral imaging could be used for in-line material classification of paper, pulp, and cardboard.

Development of an object sorting algorithm is a very challenging problem in pattern recognition. Paclík et al. (2006) studied the algorithm design for the real-world industrial sorting problems using hyperspectral imaging. They studied four groups of algorithms and the algorithms considered for the study operated in two steps: at the pixel and object level. They discussed not only the sorting accuracy of the algorithm but also estimated the computational complexity in executing the algorithm.

Picón et al. (2012) tested the hyperspectral imaging technique for the material classification process in the sorting of nonferrous objects present in the waste of electric and electronic equipment (WEEE) scrap. The WEEE scrap is sorted by mechanical, electrostatic, and densiometric sorting, after which the majority of the scrap contains nonferrous materials (copper, aluminum, stainless steel, lead, brass, and zinc) which is not possible to segregate by standard mechanical recycling process. The unsorted nonferrous objects are given away at a very low price compared to other nonferrous fractions. Hence, a technique to sort nonferrous material will significantly improve the profits of the WEEE recycling procedure. The system developed by Picón et al. (2012) consisted of a hyperspectral image acquisition unit, mechanical subcomponents that implement the WEEE vibratory delivery system, a conveyor, and pneumatic particle sorting mechanism. The material sorting algorithm consisted of hyperspectral data correlation, removal of background, labeling of nonferrous particle, data quantization, and material classification. The results of the study showed that the classification accuracy was around 96.87%, and the system was capable of processing scrap at the rate of 2.28 m/s. The authors concluded that the performance of the system has exceeded the economic threshold requirement for WEEE nonferrous material sorting.

5.3.6 *Medicine*

The type of information obtained with hyperspectral imaging technique may enable physicians to observe the features of different organs and tissues in good health and those affected by diseases. From the surgical perspective, the most important feature of hyperspectral imaging is that it captures and makes data available in real time. This is the major difference compared to other advanced imaging techniques such as PET scanning or MRI, which are performed before the actual treatment is determined or implemented. These are not interactive technologies or must be done preoperatively. Whereas hyperspectral imaging is a real-time technique and surgeons can assess surgical procedure in an ongoing manner and the presence of such feedback response in the operating room has resulted in more perfect performance of valve repair techniques (Freeman et al., 1997).

The inevitable presence of blood in surgical areas demands an effort to keep the areas as clean as possible. Monteiro et al. (2004) examined the potential of applying hyperspectral imagery as an intra-operative visual aid tool for surgical guidance. By processing and combining spectral reflectance information from different wavelengths of the spectrum, the possibility of revealing the images under the blood that is invisible to the naked eye was explored. An artificial neural network (ANN) approach to provide a nonlinear combination of pixel data from various wavelengths to reduce the effect of blood spilled over the area was proposed. Preliminary results were very promising and the use of hyperspectral imagery to serve as a visual aid during surgical procedures demands an online and automatic method. Research work has continued for generating RGB pseudocolor images, and developing an unsupervised version and further experiments need to be performed to define the limit of the thickness that blood can be seen through.

In traditional Chinese medicine (TCM), different parts of the body such as fingers, eyes, nose, and tongue are assessed. TCM consist of four processes in diagnosis: inspection, listening to internal sounds and evaluating smell, inquiry, and pulse feeling and palpation. Li (2012) evaluated the use of the hyperspectral imaging technique for tongue diagnosis. The human tongue is a vital organ that carries important information regarding the health of the body and the information includes tongue color, fissures or cracks present in tongue, sublingual veins, and tongue coating. The author developed an acoustic optic tunable filter (AOTF) based hyperspectral imaging unit that captures images of the human tongue at various wavelengths. Since an AOFT-based imaging system provided more information than a CCD-based system, the author suggested that it was possible to find more successful application in computerized tongue examination such as color analysis, tongue crack extraction and classification, and sublingual vein analysis.

Harvey et al. (2002) examined the potential of hyperspectral imaging for detection of retinal diseases. Hyperspectral imaging could provide retinal blood perfusion mapping based on spectral signatures of deoxygenated and oxygenated hemoglobin through which various retinal diseases could be identified. In patients affected by peripheral vascular disease, clinical decision making is based on patient health history, physical examination, and invasive and noninvasive testing. Hyperspectral imaging could provide quantitative and vital facts about the spatial tissue oxygen saturation for people affected with peripheral vascular disease. Among the various applications of hyperspectral imaging in medicine, tissue viability detection after plastic surgery, determination of hemorrhagic shock, and burns are important applications. Tissues that are affected due to insufficient oxygen are clearly visible from oxygen saturation maps developed from NIR spectral images obtained after surgery (Kellicut et al., 2004). Vascular endothelial dysfunction is common in type I and II diabetes patients and is an important risk factor for cardiovascular disease. Zuzak et al. (2001) tested a novel, noninvasive hyperspectral imaging technique for quantifying the percentage of hemoglobin existing as oxyhemoglobin as an index of skin tissue perfusion. To stimulate a condition of vascular endothelial dysfunction, N^G-monomethyl-L-arginine (L-NMMA) was infused in the brachial arteries of nine healthy individual for 5 min to inhibit forearm nitric oxide (NO) synthesis with the subjects first breathing normal air and subsequently inhaling NO at 80 ppm for 1 h. Visible reflectance hyperspectral imaging showed a significant decrease in the percentage of oxyhemoglobin in skin tissue when blood flow was lowered after inhibition of forearm NO synthesis and restoration of oxyhemoglobin with increased blood flow during NO inhalation. The hyperspectral imaging technique could provide an effective approach for monitoring skin hemoglobin oxygen saturation and assessment of therapeutic interventions in patients affected by vascular disease.

Inadequate blood supply to the intestines results in a condition called intestinal ischemia, and the sooner the condition is diagnosed, the better the outcome of the treatment. Akbari et al. (2010) studied the intestinal segment of the pig to determine the intestinal ischemia condition using hyperspectral imaging in the visible to near-infrared region (400–1000 nm). The results showed that normal and ischemic intestine showed different spectra in the wavelength region of 765 to 830 nm. The spectral difference between normal and affected regions may be because of relative abundance of hemoglobin and oxyhemoglobin. Randeberg et al. (2010) examined the potential of hyperspectral imaging to visualize skin bruises and vascular structures using image analysis and diffusion theory. Bruises were made in a swine model, images were acquired, and statistical analysis was performed to classify bruised areas. The results of the study showed that hyperspectral images could provide information on depth and extent of bruising and could also visualize vascular structures.

5.3.6.1 Cancer

Siddiqi et al. (2008) tested the hypothesis that detection of cancerous cells can be enhanced by use of a hyperspectral imaging technique. Their study revealed that normal cervical cells were identified with an accuracy of 95.8%, while high- and low-grade precancerous cells were identified with an accuracy of 93.5% and 66.7%, respectively. They concluded that hyperspectral imaging could be used in prescreening Pap test slides to increase the efficiency in Pap test diagnoses to determine cancerous cells. Panasyuk et al. (2007) examined the utility of hyperspectral imaging to aid in the identification of residual tumors during the surgery. During breast tumor resection, more than 30% of tumors recur locally unless radiation treatment is applied to completely destroy the cells. They developed an algorithm to differentiate between tumor and normal tissues, and the fragments of residual tumors of about 0.5 to 1 mm in size left intentionally during surgery were identified by a hyperspectral imaging technique. Freeman et al. (2005) demonstrated the potential of medical hyperspectral imaging for assessment of breast cancer and residual tumors. Tumors were induced in female rats. Freeman et al. studied 98 tumors and performed partial resection of 41 tumors. Hyperspectral imaging and histopathology were performed. The results showed that hyperspectral imaging correctly identified tumors in all cases, whereas standard histopathology failed to detect tumors in two cases. Freeman et al. concluded that based on the results, medical hyperspectral imaging showed great potential for detection of residual tumors over current tissue sampling procedures.

Kong et al. (2005) presented a hyperspectral fluorescence imaging and support vector machine for detection of skin tumors. Skin tumors cannot be seen visually with the naked eye like other pathological diseases because appearance of skin tumors seems more as distortion of shape rather than discoloration. Fluorescence data acquired by hyperspectral imaging has a significant amount of spectral information and hence increases the possibility of detecting tumors. The imaging system acquired images in the wavelengths between 440 to 640 nm. Image processing methods such as image smoothing using local spatial filter with Gaussian kernel increased the accuracy of classification and reduced the false positives. Classification accuracy of 99% was achieved for tumor tissue and an overall accuracy of 86% was achieved and hence they concluded that hyperspectral fluorescence imaging could be used for detecting skin cancers.

Martin et al. (2006) developed an advanced hyperspectral imaging unit for detection of cancer. The advanced hyperspectral system uses liquid crystal tunable filters (LCTFs) with a potential to record images at any number of wavelengths (10–100), a fiber probe meant for signal collection, an endoscope, an endoscopic illuminator, a CCD color camera, and an intensified charge-coupled device (ICCD) for fluorescence detection. Five nude mice were injected with tracheal carcinoma cells to induce tumor formation. Experiments were conducted in vivo because more accurate simulation of cancerous conditions can be obtained in vivo compared to experiments with extracted tissues. The results of the study showed that the imaging system could successfully distinguish between healthy and malignant mouse skin, and the results of this experiment could lead to advanced development in cancer diagnosis in humans.

Among the different types of cancer, prostate cancer is the most common type of cancer in men. Current diagnosis of prostate cancer depends on an ultrasound-guided biopsy, which requires tissue sample from the prostate for pathological examination, and it takes several days to obtain results. Akbari et al. (2012) examined the potential of hyperspectral imaging for detection of prostate cancer and proposed a support vector machine (SVM) for classification of tumor tissue. They conducted both in vitro and in vivo hyperspectral imaging studies to identify spectral signatures of both cancerous and normal tissues in animals. The analysis of images showed that spectral information from cancer tissues were distinct from those of healthy tissues and the cancer tissues displayed a relatively low intensity in the 450 and 950 nm wavelength range. Based on the preliminary study, they concluded that hyperspectral imaging has demonstrated the feasibility to determine prostate cancer. The major advantage of hyperspectral imaging is its ability to spectrally and spatially verify the spectral variation of various tissue types. Hyperspectral imaging could be useful not only for diagnosis but also to detect tumor margin and assess the tumor base following resection to be certain that tumor resection is complete, which lowers the complications and side effects and reduces operative mortality and morbidity.

Tongue cancer is a malignant tumor and if untreated may extend to the entire gums and tongue. Z. Liu et al. (2012) evaluated the capability of hyperspectral imaging for detection of tongue tumors. Due to the instinctive wriggling of the human tongue and the sound caused due to saliva, it is difficult to detect the tumor accurately, hence a hyperspectral imaging system based on an acousto-optic tunable filter (AOTF) was used. Since there was no medical hyperspectral database available, the authors constructed a database that included 65 different tumors and conducted partial resection of 34 tumors (Figure 5.8). For performance evaluation, the hyperspectral results were compared with histopathology results. The accuracy of the detection of tumors in the study was 96.5% and it was concluded that hyperspectral imaging has a great potential in detection of tumors.

5.3.6.2 *Diabetes*

Diabetic food ulceration (DFU) is a complication that may arise due to diabetes. Khaodhiar et al. (2007) examined the hyperspectral imaging as a new diagnosis tool to quantify tissue oxygenation, and detect systemic and microcirculatory changes associated with diabetes. The study was conducted on three types of subjects: healthy, type I diabetic patients having no ulcer, and type I diabetic patients with an ulcer on at least one foot. Type I diabetic patients were observed at the beginning, 6 weeks, 3 months, and 6 months, whereas healthy subjects were consulted only at the beginning and at 6 months. Data were collected using the HyperMedCombiVu-R system (HyperMed, Waltham, Massachusetts). The results of the study showed that tissue oxygen measurement using hyperspectral imaging could successfully detect and differentiate ulcers that started to heal and ulcers that do not heal. Also, differences were observed from healthy and normal nonulcerated skin tissue and

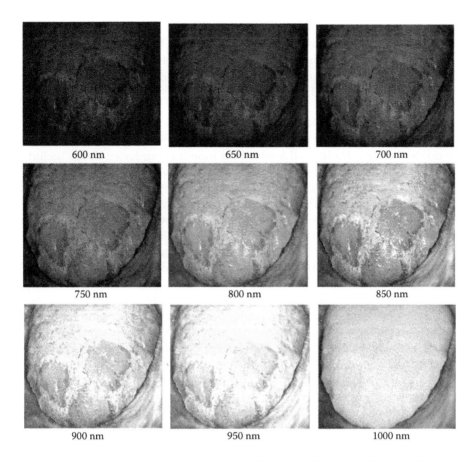

Figure 5.8 Examples of tongue tumor hyperspectral images. (From Liu, Z. et al., *Sensors*, 12, 162, 2012. Open access.)

skin tissue around the healing or nonhealing ulcers. They concluded that hyperspectral imaging has the ability to assist in the treatment of DFU by improving diagnosis and implementation of early interventions.

5.3.6.3   Blood vessel detection

During surgeries, detection of blood vessels is a critical and difficult task, and injury to blood vessels may result in serious complications. Akbari et al. (2010) examined the ability of hyperspectral imaging for detection of blood vessels. Differentiating between arteries and veins are helpful in many diseases, such as coronary artery disease, pulmonary embolism, pulmonary hypertension, renal hypertension, portal vein thrombosis, hepatic cirrhosis, lower extremity occlusive disease and deep venous thrombosis. In this study, two hyperspectral cameras (400–1000 nm and 900–1700 nm) were used, and a database was created for spectral signatures for various vein, artery, and abdominal organs. The hyperspectral data were acquired during a surgery on a swine and a support vector machine (SVM) was used for classification. The performance criteria for the procedure were analyzed by calculating a false positive rate (FPR) and false negative rate (FNR) for every blood vessel. The spectral reflectance of organ or tissue is dependent on its spectral characteristics, and the highest spectral difference between veins and arteries were at 650 to 700 nm wavelengths because of hemoglobin and oxyhemoglobin. Akbari et al. concluded that hyperspectral imaging is a noninvasive tool of great significance for surgeons to evaluate a large area during surgery and hence extension of surgeon's vision is a major achievement in the medical field.

5.3.6.4 Counterfeit drug detection

Counterfeit drugs are an important global issue and they are very difficult to differentiate from the original drugs. Traditional methods to monitor counterfeit drugs include visual monitoring, disintegration, and color reaction tests that reveal only rough fraudulent activities. Rodionova et al. (2005) studied the NIR spectrometry and hyperspectral imaging for counterfeit drug detection. Two types of drugs were tested but due to confidentiality, the chemical composition of the samples was not disclosed. Hyperspectral images were obtained for the two drugs using a Spectral Dimensions MatrixNIR camera in the wavelength range of 900 to 1700 nm. Three data sets were produced for three types of drugs: antimicrobial drugs with film-coated tablets, antispasmodic drugs with uncoated tablets, and antimicrobial drugs (crushed tablets without coating). PCA and soft independent modeling of class analogy (SIMCA) methods were used for analysis. The results of the first type of drug showed that two types of capsules had significantly varying composition and the differences in NIR spectra were so distinct requiring no mathematical data processing. For the second type of drug, two clusters were seen in the PCA plot and the object variance of fraudulent drugs was significantly higher than the variance between objects in genuine drugs. Multivariate image analysis performed on the third data set showed two distinct clusters that represented two tablet ingredients: genuine and counterfeit. The authors concluded that the difference between original and counterfeit drugs could be observed in the NIR spectra, and hence hyperspectral imaging has good potential to distinguish genuine and counterfeit drugs and may even substitute wet chemistry.

5.4 Advantages, limitations, and future of hyperspectral imaging

5.4.1 Advantages

The major advantage of hyperspectral imaging is that an entire spectrum of information is acquired at every pixel of the product being examined. It is a nondestructive and non-invasive method, and hence could be used for on-line quality inspection and monitoring. Hyperspectral imaging does not require any special sample preparation. Compared to conventional physical and chemical analytical methods, hyperspectral imaging requires less time, less sample preparation, no chemicals, and can be used to compute more than one feature at the same time (Lammertyn et al., 1998). Since hyperspectral imaging does not involve usage of any chemicals as in other chemical or biochemical methods, it is an environmentally friendly method.

Hyperspectral imaging could determine several constituents in a given sample without a need for doing multiple tests. For a given sample studied, hyperspectral imaging provides flexibility to obtain certain regions of interest within the acquired image of a specific sample. The main advantage of hyperspectral imaging is that it is possible to visualize the various biochemical components present in a sample based on spectral signature in a region of specific chemical composition where spectral properties may be similar (ElMasry and Sun, 2010). When the spectral data are analyzed and calibration models are developed and validated, hyperspectral imaging analysis becomes a very simple, easy, and time-saving method.

5.4.2 Limitations

Hyperspectral imaging is complex because of the huge amount of data gathered, and it requires large storage capacity and fast computers to process and analyze the huge amount of data acquired. A major drawback in hyperspectral imaging is the information overlap in adjacent slices, which makes the process of information extraction very challenging. The hyperspectral imaging requires a relatively long time for image acquisition and processing, which makes it difficult to be implemented in real-time on-line applications. Hyperspectral imaging is a time-consuming method, because after data collection it needs to be analyzed using a chemometric technique, which is a combined statistical and mathematical method to extract and interpret chemical information from the data and synthesize the results for the specific study. Hence modeling and data processing requires more time than data acquisition. Hyperspectral imaging is not suitable for liquid or other homogeneous samples such as suspension because continuous uniform motion of the sample averages the spatial information unless and until it is monitored at a very high detection speed such as fluorescence correlation microspectroscopy or fluorescence lifetime imaging microscopy (FLIM) (ElMasry and Sun, 2010).

5.4.3 Future

Application of hyperspectral imaging started with remote sensing and today it has extended to many fields, including agriculture, aquaculture, food, pharmacy, medicine, and engineering. Hyperspectral imaging applications in remote sensing cover areas such as mapping of water, vegetation, rocks, and geology. The application of hyperspectral imaging in agriculture includes determination of soil salinity, nutrient enrichment in soil, and detection of plants and weeds in the field. In the food industry, hyperspectral imaging has found many potential applications, including detection of bruises, physical and mechanical damage in the fruit, internal quality characteristics of fruits and vegetables, detection of pathogens and bacterial contamination in vegetables and fresh leaves, kernel hardness, germination potential, insect and fungal damage, and classification of cereal grains. Hyperspectral imaging for classification and grading of pork and beef, determination of fat content and water-holding capacity in meat, and detection of fecal contamination in meat has been studied and proved. Although the potential of hyperspectral imaging seems unlimited, there are certain limitations, such as high cost of the equipment, the large quantity of data acquisition, and complicated data processing, has resulted in dragging the technology away from the actual installation in real-time applications in the commercial world. If the technical difficulties are overcome by very high-speed computers and readily available algorithms for spectral data processing, the usage of hyperspectral imaging will become the most exploited and common technology in the near future.

chapter six

Thermal imaging

6.1 Introduction

The origin of thermal imaging dates to 1800 when astronomer Sir William Herschel was trying to reduce the brightness of the sun's image in a telescope using optical filter materials. He found that when using a red filter, a lot of heat was produced. He discovered infrared radiation in sunlight by passing it through a prism and measuring the temperature by holding a thermometer beyond the red end of the visible spectrum. He concluded that an invisible form of light is present beyond the visible spectrum and referred to this portion of the electromagnetic spectrum as calorific rays. In 1880, a major breakthrough was made by American astronomer Samuel Pierpont Langley, who invented the bolometer, which was used to measure infrared or heat radiation. In 1929, Kálmán Tihanyi, a Hungarian physicist, was the first to invent an infrared-sensitive electronic television camera for anti-aircraft defense in Britain. In the 1950s to 1960s, a single element detector to scan scenes and produce line images was developed by Texas Instruments, Hughes Aircraft, and Honeywell. This basic detector resulted in the development of modern thermal imaging. In 1978, a Raytheon R&D group patented ferroelectric infrared detectors, and FLIR Systems Inc. was founded as a provider of infrared imaging systems installed on vehicles for conducting energy audits and fire detection applications. In 1980, the microbolometer was developed, and in 1994, Honeywell was awarded a patent for microbolometer detector array. Thermal imaging technology, which was initially developed for military applications, has now expanded for use in firefighting, law enforcement, security, transportation, industrial, food and agriculture, and other industries (FLIR, 2011a).

6.2 Principle and components of thermal imaging

6.2.1 Principle

All bodies whose temperature is above zero Kelvin (–273.15°C) emit infrared radiation. The infrared radiation lies between visible light and microwaves in the electromagnetic spectrum. The infrared radiation has a wavelength in the range of 0.70 to 1000 μm and the infrared radiation could be classified as near-, middle-, and far-infrared radiation based on their wavelengths. The total amount of radiation emitted by any object depends on the temperature, surface condition, and thermal properties of the object. A black body absorbs all the radiant energy and emits a hundred percent of its energy, which is called an ideal body and does not exist in reality.

The radiant energy striking a material could be dissipated in three ways: absorption, transmission, and reflection. The total quantities of radiant energy that are linked with each mode of dissipation are termed absorptivity, transmittivity, and reflectivity of the object. The emissivity of an object is defined as the ratio of radiant energy emitted by an object to the amount of radiation emitted by a black body at the same temperature:

$$e = W_O/W_b$$

where W_O is the total radiant energy of an object at a temperature T and W_b is the total radiant energy emitted by the black body at the temperature T.

For a black body, at a steady state temperature, all the energy absorbed is emitted, so the emissivity of a black body is equal to 1, that is, Absorptivity = Emissivity = 1.

But for all objects that are not black bodies: Absorptivity + Transmittivity + Emissivity = 1. Energy radiated from the black body is described by Planck's law as

$$W_\lambda = C_1/\lambda^5 (e^{C_2/\lambda T} - 1)$$

where W_λ is the spectral radiant emittance per unit wavelength and unit area (W/m²µm); λ is the wavelength (µm); C_1 and C_2 are the first and second radiation constant, respectively; and T is the absolute temperature (K).

According to the Stefan-Boltzman law, the amount of radiation emitted by an object per unit area is directly related to the emissivity of the object and its temperature:

$$E = \sigma \varepsilon T^4$$

where E is the amount of radiation emitted by an object per unit area (W/m²), σ is the Stefan-Boltzman constant (5.67×10^{-8} W/m²K⁻⁴), ε is the emissivity of the object, and T is the temperature of the object (K).

Thermal imaging is a nondestructive technique that estimates the amount of infrared energy emitted from the surface of an object. A thermal camera converts the infrared energy into a thermal map referred to as a thermogram. Thermography is a technique of acquisition and analysis of temperature data using noncontact thermal imaging devices. Thermography can be classified as passive or active based on whether a heating source is used. When a thermal camera observes a scene and detects the thermal radiation emitted by the object without imposing an additional heat flow to the object, the method is called passive thermography and is widely used in various applications such as civil, mechanical, electrical, metallurgical, and process engineering. In situations where no natural temperature differences are present or if envelopes of objects are too thick for identification of structural elements beneath the surface, active thermography methods are used by applying heating (or sometimes cooling) to the surface of the object and monitoring the change in temperature through time. One application of active thermography is defect detection, such as delamination, cracks, and subsurface defect detection. The most popular methods of active thermography for nondestructive testing are pulsed thermography and lock-in thermography (Skala et al., 2011). The choice of the method is dependent on the proposed application, material thermal properties, defect location, and its thickness. In pulsed thermography, using a short duration high peak power pulse, the sample is warmed and the thermal response of the surface is recorded. The thermal camera acquires images of the sample at a predefined time interval thereby monitoring the thermal decay within the sample, and the resultant time series images could be analyzed. The requirement of a high power source (e.g., laser beam, flash lamp) is the limitation of pulsed thermography. Lock-in thermography is based on thermal waves produced inside the object and the excitation frequency is chosen based on samples of thermal characteristics and geometrical dimensions (Mulaveesala et al., 2012). Lock-in thermography is also referred to as modulated thermography in which sinusoidally varying thermal energy is applied to a target to produce thermal waves and hence to excite flow of heat within the material. The thermal camera observes the sample at the time of modulated excitation and measures the resultant oscillating temperature field (Gowen et al., 2010). The thermal imaging system normally operates in two wavelength ranges: 3 to 5 μm in the middle wavelength infrared region (MWIR) and 8 to 14 μm in the long wavelength infrared region (LWIR).

6.2.2 Components

The components of thermal imaging are not complicated and are composed of a target, infrared lens, detector, signal processing unit, and image processing and display unit (Figure 6.1). The target is the object of interest that emits infrared radiation. The radiation from the target passes through the Earth's atmosphere and is then received by the infrared lens.

6.2.2.1 Infrared lens

The lens of an infrared camera focuses the incoming radiation to the detector element. The most commonly used materials for lenses are silicon (Si), germanium (Ge), zinc selenide (ZnSe), and zinc sulfide (ZnS) (Brock, 2012). These materials are transparent to infrared radiation and allow the infrared radiation to pass through. Long-range infrared cameras require large lenses that are heavy and significant support for stability.

6.2.2.2 Detector

The detectors convert the energy into an electrical signal. The detector or detector array in a thermal camera is responsible for the thermal and spatial resolution of the camera. The infrared detectors are of two types: thermal and photon. In the photon detector, radiation is absorbed inside the object by interacting with electrons bound to lattice or to impurity atoms. Photon detectors display excellent signal-to-noise performance along with a quick response, but in order to accomplish this they need cryogenic cooling. The need for cooling is the major drawback for widespread use of photon detectors because they become heavy, bulky, inconvenient to use, and costly. Based on the type of interaction, photon detectors are further classified into intrinsic, extrinsic, free carrier, and quantum well detector. In a thermal detector, as the incident radiation is absorbed, the material temperature changes, which results in certain physical property change that is used to produce an electrical output. Thermal detectors can work at room temperature, have limited sensitivity, and slower response but are easy to handle and inexpensive (Ciupa and Rogalski, 1997).

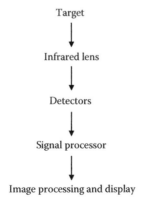

Figure 6.1 Components of a thermal imaging system.

6.2.2.3   Video signal processing

The detector element provides electronic output that is processed to produce a thermal image or temperature measurement. Signal processing is very essential to remove any background noise present along with the necessary signal.

6.2.2.4   Display

The image generated by the signal processing element is viewed on a computer monitor or separate external display, such as a small direct view display located in the infrared camera itself.

6.2.2.5   Important factors to be considered in selection of camera

There are certain key requirements to be considered when selecting a thermal camera for specific purposes. The factors include camera resolution or image quality, accuracy, thermal sensitivity, camera functions, and software requirements of the camera (FLIR, 2011b).

6.2.2.5.1   Spatial resolution.   The spatial resolution is the camera's ability to differentiate between two different materials within the field of view. The spatial resolution or image quality is a crucial factor and the most basic models have a resolution of 60 × 60 pixels, whereas more advanced models have a resolution of 640 × 480 pixels. Most thermal imaging cameras have a resolution of 320 × 240 pixels, which deliver good image quality. The spatial resolution of a camera basically depends on various factors such as distance between the object and camera, lens system, and detector size (Bagavathiappan et al., 2013).

6.2.2.5.2   Thermal sensitivity.   Thermal sensitivity of a camera describes the smallest temperature difference a camera can detect. A camera with high thermal sensitivity can detect very small temperature differences between the object of interest and the surroundings. The thermal sensitivity is usually denoted in Celsius (°C) or millikelvins (mK). The advanced cameras used in industrial applications have a thermal sensitivity of 0.03°C (30 mK). The common parameters used to measure the temperature resolution are noise equivalent temperature difference (NETD), minimum detectable temperature difference, and minimum resolvable temperature difference.

6.2.2.5.3   Accuracy.   All temperature measurements are prone to error and thermal cameras are no exceptions. Accuracy is expressed both in percentage and degree Celsius. The industry standard for accuracy of temperature measurement is ±2% or ±2°C. The measured temperature may deviate from the actual temperature within the mentioned percentage or absolute temperature.

6.2.2.5.4   Temperature range.   The temperature range of an infrared thermal camera implies the maximum and minimum temperatures that can be determined using an infrared camera. Typical temperature values for infrared cameras available in the market range from –20°C to 500°C, and the range can be extended by using various filters.

6.2.2.5.5   Camera functions and software.   The emissivity of the object is a parameter of significant importance, and thermal cameras should permit operators to set the emissivity and reflection. Another critical feature is the option to set the span and level of displayed thermal image, because without this option the camera would detect temperature of the whole scene, which may not be necessary in many instances. Most thermal imaging cameras come with the basic software package that allows a basic temperature measurement analysis to be performed.

6.3   Applications of thermal imaging

6.3.1   Agriculture

Agriculture is the oldest known industry and started as soon as humans inhabited the Earth. The adoption of newer technology in agriculture has become very important to feed the world. With the growing population and associated growth in the agricultural industry, modern technologies are adopted in agriculture in every possible way. Thermal imaging is one such technology that has been experimented, tested, and adopted in various fields of agriculture. The knowledge of soil water status; canopy temperature; respiration rate of plants; identification of plant stress; monitoring various diseases and infections of plants, leaves, and fruits; and yield estimation are essential in successful practice of agriculture. The applications of thermal imaging in all these agricultural areas have played a role and are described in this section. Table 6.1 lists thermal camera models; specifications; and applications of thermal imaging related to agriculture, grain, and soil water status.

6.3.1.1   Soil water status

Traditional methods to measure soil moisture content of agricultural land are spot measuring techniques, such as soil sampling and time domain reflectometry. Sugiura et al. (2007) developed a system based on thermal imaging to monitor soil water status. The system consisted of an unmanned helicopter equipped with a global positioning system (GPS) and a navigation sensor along with a thermal camera. The experiments were conducted in a paddy field near Hokkaido, Japan, and the soil moisture content was calculated by the oven-drying method. Images were acquired at 10:00 a.m. and 3:00 p.m. on the same day. The images captured by the camera included errors due to atmospheric effects, which were corrected for atmospheric transmissivity and a model was developed for estimating soil water content. When the initial images were used, the determination coefficient between temperature and water content was 0.64 and 0.62 at 10:00 a.m. and 3:00 p.m., respectively. Whereas when the image correction was applied, the determination coefficient increased to 0.69 and 0.67, respectively, at 10:00 a.m. and 3:00 p.m. The results showed that a correlation exists between water content and surface temperature and hence thermal imaging could be a potential technique for monitoring soil water conditions in an agricultural field.

6.3.1.2   Estimate canopy temperature and identify plant stress

Better crop management and irrigation management could be provided by monitoring the stomatal closure and rate of transpiration from the plants. The canopy or leaf temperature is based on the rate of evapotranspiration from the surface of the canopy. Thermal imaging could be a potential technique to estimate plant temperature, which acts as an indicator of stomatal closure and stress due to lack of water. Leinonen and Jones (2004) studied the thermal and visual imaging for estimating the temperature of canopy and plant stress both in greenhouse and field conditions. In the greenhouse condition, broad beans (*Vicia faba* L.) were studied by exposing one group of plants to drought stress and a control group that was watered every day. In the field conditions, mature grapevine (*Vitis vinifera* L.) was studied. Thermal images were acquired with an Infrared Solutions SnapShot 22 camera. After acquiring visible and thermal images, stomatal conductance of *V. faba* was determined using an AP4 porometer. Thermal indices calculated based on the thermal imaging were more accurate and could be utilized to measure the stomatal conductance in the plant canopy. Also, in the field conditions, thermal imaging provided an accurate estimation of distribution of temperature of shaded and sunlight exposed areas of canopy, thus making

Table 6.1 Thermal Camera Model, Specifications, and Applications Related to Agriculture and Soil Conditions

Thermal camera model	Company	Camera specifications: wavelength, geometric, and thermal resolution	Emissivity	Application	Reference
TH7102 MX	NEC, Tokyo, Japan	8–14 μm; 320 × 240 pixels; 0.06°C	0.95	Pathogen detection in grapevines	Stoll et al., 2008
Varioscan 3201 ST	Jenoptik, Jena, Germany	8–12 μm; 240 × 360 pixels; 0.03 K	1.0	Measurement of canopy temperature	Lenthe et al., 2007
ThermaCAM SC2000	FLIR Systems, Oregon	7.5–13 μm; 320 × 420 pixels		To estimate crop water stress in cotton	Sela et al., 2007
Infrared Solutions SnapShot 525	Alpine Components, East Sussex, UK	8–12 μm; 120 × 120 pixels	0.95	To monitor plant stress in grapevines	Stoll and Jones, 2007
NA	NA	8–14 μm; 320 × 240 pixels	1.0	To estimate soil water status	Sugiura et al., 2007
VARIOSCAN 3201 ST	Jenoptik Laser, Jena, Germany	8–12 μm; 240 × 360 pixels; 0.03 K	NA	To monitor downy mildew in cucumber leaves	Oerke et al., 2006
Infrared Solutions SnapShot 225	Alpine Components, East Sussex, UK	8–12 μm; 120 × 120 pixels	0.95	To estimate canopy temperature	Leinonen and Jones, 2004
Inframetrics 760 E	FLIR Systems	8–12 μm	NA	To measure leaf temperature during thermal weed treatment	Rahkonen and Jokela, 2003
FLIR-AGEMA THV 1000	NA	8–12 μm	NA	To measure temperature anomalies in greenhouse	Ljungberg, and Jönsson, 2002
ThermaCAM PM250	FLIR Systems, Massachusetts	3.4–5 Mm; 256 × 256; 0.1°C	1.0	For screening of defective stomatal regulation	Merlot et al., 2002
Inframetrics 760	FLIR Systems, Massachusetts	NA	NA	To characterize freezing of barley plant and leaves	Pearce and Fuller, 2001
ThermaCAM SC500	FLIR Systems, Burlington, Ontario	7.5–13 μm; 320 × 240 pixels; 0.07°C at 30°C	0.98	To detect fungal infection in wheat	Chelladurai et al., 2010
ThermaCAM SC500	FLIR Systems, Burlington, Ontario	7.5–13 μm; 320 × 240 pixels; 0.07°C at 30°C	0.98	To detect wheat insect infestation; to identify wheat class	Manickavasagan et al., 2008c, 2010

it a possibility to study temperature differences as a potential indicator of stomatal conductance and plant stress.

Stoll and Jones (2007) examined the potential of thermal imaging to monitor plant stress. The study was performed on mature grapevines (*Vitis vinifera* L.) and the two conditions were no irrigation and complete irrigation. Thermal images were acquired with an Infrared Solutions SnapShot 525 thermal camera. The study showed that temperature difference could be related to the water status of the grapevine, because nonirrigated vines showed higher temperatures compared to the fully irrigated vines and also temperature difference existed between sunlit and shaded sides of the canopy. There was no significant temperature difference between the berries of two treatments except on one day (July 25, 2006) when solar radiation was high and wind speed was low. The difference of temperature between water stressed and nonstressed plants provides a basis to identify the onset of plant stress due to changes in stomatal aperture. Stoll and Jones concluded that thermal imaging could provide leaf temperature variation, which could be used to identify plant stress and thereby schedule irrigation based on the requirements.

Grapevine (*Vitis vinifera* L.) is widely affected by *Plasmopara viticola*, a pathogen that causes downy mildew in grapevine. The pathogen penetration occurs through stomata, indicating that a relationship may exist between *P. viticola* and transpiration. Stoll et al. (2008) studied the variability of leaf temperature of grapevines of both infected and noninfected plants in well-irrigated and nonirrigated greenhouse conditions. Thermal images were acquired using a uncooled focal plane array TH7102MX infrared camera. The different treatments were (a) control that was completely irrigated and noninoculated vines, (b) fully irrigated and inoculated vines, (c) not irrigated and noninoculated vines, and (d) not irrigated and inoculated vines. The results of the study showed contrasting temperature effects due to the pathogen infection on fully irrigated and water deficient plants. The pathogen growth resulted in a higher temperature of leaf at the infected region in irrigated vines. In water stressed plants, pathogen-infected vines displayed a reduced temperature at inoculation regions compared to other portions of the leaf. Irrespective of plant water status, analysis of temporal and spatial sensitivity of temperature profile could distinguish between normal and pathogen-infected portions of the leaf. The authors concluded that they were not able to explain the mechanism that causes the contrast effect on leaf temperature, however, infrared thermography is a potential technique for temporal and spatial analysis of the effect of *P. viticola* under various plant water conditions.

Leaf water potential (LWP) is the commonly accepted parameter to monitor and determine the water status and crop water stress in plants. But LWP measurements are time consuming and laborious and since measurements are made at only certain points in the field, they are not representative of the entire field. Sela et al. (2007) examined the potential of thermal imaging to estimate and map the crop water stress in cotton plants. Experimental plots were planted with cotton, *Gossypium barbadense* (L.) and hybrid of *Gossypium hirsutum* × *Gossypium barbadense* with different irrigation treatments ranging from overirrigation to nonirrigation. Thermal images of fields were acquired with an uncooled ThermaCAM SC2000 camera with a microbolometer sensor with a spectral range of 7.5 to 13 μm. Digital images were obtained with a digital camera (DSC-F717, Sony Inc., Tokyo, Japan) that was connected to the thermal camera. The empirical crop water stress index (E_{CWSI}) was plotted against leaf water potential (LWP) and they both showed a linear fit with a good correlation ($R^2 = 0.76$) and standard error of prediction (SEP) of 0.24 MPa. The regression coefficient (R^2) of the flowering stage model decreased to 0.58, whereas the boll filling stage increased to 0.87 with an improved SEP of 0.20 MPa. The result of the study has shown that measurement of LWP could be performed under a range of climatic conditions, water stress levels, and for different phenological stages. LWP maps using thermal imaging can support decision making in scheduling irrigation and can help to determine the defects of the irrigation system and highlight the patches of problematic soil within agricultural fields.

In management of crop protection, computer-aided diagnosis has been used especially for detection of infection rate. In disease epidemiology of plants, leaf wetness and temperature are important parameters. Lenthe et al. (2007) studied the potential of thermography to monitor surface temperatures to differentiate microclimate in wheat by considering leaf wetness as the critical parameter for occurrence of leaf diseases. Infection levels of *Puccinia triticina* (fungal pathogen causing leaf rust), and *Septoria tritici* (causing leaf blotch of wheat) were monitored at the time of thermal imaging. The thermal images were acquired with a Varioscan 3021 ST camera. Based on the study Lenthe et al. concluded that they could not differentiate between disease-affected leaf areas by temperature of canopy or to distinguish plots with *Septoria* from a healthy canopy. These results led to the assumption that other abiotic factors have a significant effect on the local canopy temperature compared to the extent of diseased leaf area.

6.3.1.3   *Measurement of leaf temperature*

Weed control using thermal treatments involves various physical methods such as low or high temperatures or electrical fields. Plant temperatures measured using contact sensors such as thermocouples or thermistors are laborious and have many error sources. Rahkonen and Jokela (2003) conducted experiments with infrared imaging to measure the spatial and temporal difference of leaf temperature while performing thermal weed control. To determine the temperature of leaf, one leaf was flamed at a time with an LPG burner on one side while the temperature was measured on the other side of the leaf using an infrared radiometer. The plants tested were rape seed (*Brassica rapa* L.), Benjamin tree (*Ficus benjamina* L.), and so-thistle (*Sonchus arvensis* L.). Thermal images were acquired using an Inframetrics 760E camera with an HgCdTe detector. Images acquired at maximum temperature showed a significant spatial variability on the surface temperature of leaves. The average leaf temperature at the time of image acquisition was 64°C with maximum and minimum temperatures being 97.0°C and 24.6°C, respectively. They concluded that spatial and temporal variation of the leaves could be measured using infrared radiometer imaging and hence the technique could be used during thermal weed control treatment.

Abscisic acid (ABA) has a crucial role in the growth of plants and seeds, and it promotes the acquisition of nutritive reserves, dormancy, and tolerance to desiccation. The stomatal closure induced due to ABA is very important for plants when conserving water by lowering the water loss due to transpiration. Merlot et al. (2002) conducted experiments to determine the ability of thermal imaging to separate Arabidopsis mutants that exhibit defects in stomatal regulation. Thermal images were acquired using a ThermaCAM PM250 infrared camera. The thermal images acquired 3 days after drought stress showed that the temperature of the leaf was high and homogeneous showing the homogeneity in stomatal closing response. The temperature of ABA-insensitive plant leaves were around 1°C lower because ABA-insensitive mutant failed to close its stomata and the same type of results were observed with ABA-deficient mutants. The result of the study has shown that thermal imaging could be used to isolate ABA-deficient or mutant plants.

The survival of wild grass and other species of crop depends to a certain degree on the tolerance of freezing. To control and to avoid freezing damage, knowledge of spread of freezing within a plant helps to explain the susceptibility of various parts of the plant. Pearce and Fuller (2001) conducted experiments to study the freezing of barley leaves

(*Hordeum vulgare* L.), and grass species (*Hordeum murinum* L. and *Holcus lanatus* L.) using infrared thermal imaging. Freezing of *H. vulgare* and *H. murinum* was performed in an environment chamber providing a constant cooling rate of 2°C per h, whereas freezing of *H. lanatus* was observed in situ at the time of mild natural frost in February 2000. An infrared camera, Inframetrics 760 with a HgCdTe detector, was used to monitor the freezing of the samples. The video images were analyzed from the beginning to the finishing of freezing events, frame by frame, and the dimensions of leaves and plants used in the study were measured. Based on this data, rate and time for spread of freezing between the regions was determined. In the tests conducted in the laboratory, 0.4% of leaf water froze distributed in alternative strips of high and low freezing intensity. Similar results were observed for *H. lanatus* in the field. The parts of uprooted barley froze in the following sequence: nucleated leaf, roots, older leaves, young leaves, and secondary tillers. When the freezing event occurred from one leaf to the other, crown delayed the spread to other leaves and roots and the delay was longer at less than –2°C, thereby protecting the leaves from freezing during mild frosts. The infrared thermal imaging study provided better understanding of the process of freezing that occurs in plants during frost.

Cost reduction from energy resources is a key issue in greenhouse production. Ljungberg and Jönsson (2002) studied the potential of infrared thermography to map the temperature inconsistencies of plants grown in a greenhouse where temperature was maintained using gas-fired infrared heaters. The study consisted of one greenhouse heated with a small gas infrared heater and another greenhouse with a traditional water heating system. Both the greenhouses were fitted with a computer controllable climate curtain roof and wall system. The computerized system controlled the humidity and temperature in the greenhouse by optimization of various parameters. The thermogram of plants indicated that the gas infrared heating unit failed to provide a homogeneous energy distribution, but it resulted in a very aggressive distribution of heat compared to the water heating system. The results of the study indicated that infrared thermography is a potential technique to calibrate greenhouse heating systems, determine temperature inconsistencies of heat sources and heat distribution systems in greenhouses, and to indicate the irregularities in the growth of plants.

6.3.1.4 Insect and fungal damage in grain

The fungi growth in stored grain deteriorates the various quality characteristics such as germination, appearance, free fatty acid value, produces off-odors, and also results in the production of mycotoxins. Fungal growth that affects grain could be classified as two types: field fungi and storage fungi. Field fungi results in lesser damage and could be controlled by standard drying procedures, whereas storage fungi could cause significant loss. Chelladurai et al. (2010) examined the possibility of infrared imaging to detect fungal infection in stored wheat. Canada Western Red Spring (CWRS) wheat was selected for the study and wheat was infected with *Aspergillus glaucus*, *Aspergilus niger*, and *Pencillium* species. Images were acquired using an uncooled focal plane array type ThermaCAM™ SC500 infrared thermal camera (Figure 6.2). For the classification of normal and fungal infected samples, quadratic discriminant analysis (QDA) and linear discriminant analysis (LDA) models were used. Classification accuracy of 100% for sound samples, and 97% and 96% for infected samples were achieved using pair-wise (healthy versus fungal infected sample from each species) LDA and QDA models, respectively. Four-way (one healthy and three fungal infected samples) LDA and QDA models resulted in relatively lower accuracies for fungal infected samples because of nonsignificant variation in the temperature features of various fungal infected samples.

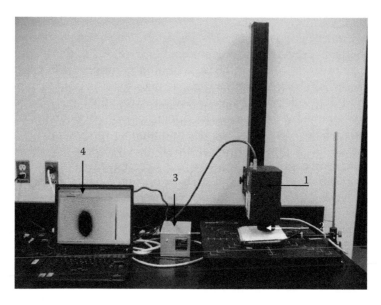

Figure 6.2 Thermal imaging experimental setup for fungal detection, sprout damage detection, insect detection, and wheat class identification of grains: (1) thermal camera, (2) close-up lens, (3) PID controller, and (4) data acquisition system. (Courtesy of University of Manitoba, Winnipeg, Canada.)

Preharvest sprouting of grain results in increased harvest losses, decreased test weight, and reduced seed viability, and the products made from sprout-damaged kernels are of poor quality. Visual inspection is mostly used to monitor sprout damage, but it is subjective and unreliable because most of the damage occurs even before germination is visible. Vadivambal et al. (2010a) examined the possibility of thermal imaging to determine preharvest sprouting of wheat. Thermal images were acquired for 1000 healthy and 1000 sprout-damaged kernels using a ThermaCAM™ SC500 (Figure 6.2). LDA, QDA, and artificial neural network (ANN) were used to classify healthy and sprout damaged kernels. The results of the study showed that classification accuracies were 88.2% and 98.1% for LDA, 88.7% and 95.1% for QDA, and 99.4% and 91.7% for ANN for healthy and sprout-damaged kernels, respectively. The determination of sprout damage in barley was studied by Vadivambal et al. (2010b) using the similar experimental setup, and the classification accuracies were 78.7% and 87.0% for LDA, 78.9% and 87.5% for QDA, and 88.5% and 87% for a NN, respectively for healthy and sprouted kernels. The results of the study have shown that thermal imaging technique has a potential to determine sprout-damaged kernels.

Insect infestation is a major problem in stored grain, and it affects the quality and quantity of grain. The Berlese funnel method is the widely used procedure to detect insects in Canadian grain handling facilities, but it requires time and provides less accurate results for detecting early life stages of insects. Manickavasagan et al. (2008a) studied the capability of thermal imaging to detect insect infestation in wheat kernels. CWRS wheat kernels infested with rusty grain beetle (*Cryptolestes ferrugineus* [Stephens]) were used for the study. Images were acquired using an uncooled focal plane array ThermaCAM™ SC500 camera (Figure 6.2). Algorithms were developed and classification was performed using LDA and QDA. The classification accuracy using QDA was 83.5% and 77.7% for infested and healthy kernels, respectively. Using linear function, the accuracy was 77.6% and 83.0% for infested and healthy kernels, respectively. The authors concluded that thermal imaging has the potential to detect infestation in wheat grain but could not identify the life stage of the insect present in the kernel.

Wheat classes are determined by hardness, color, and growing season, and since every class has various end uses, mixing of classes is not allowed in grain handling facilities. In grain handling facilities, visual inspection is performed, which is subjective and less accurate. A reliable and on-line method for testing of wheat classes is essential to classify wheat. Manickavasagan et al. (2010) evaluated the ability of thermal imaging to detect various wheat classes. Major wheat classes used for the study were Canada Western Amber Durum (CWAD), Canada Western Extra Strong (CWES), Canada Western Hard White Spring (CWHWS), Canada Prairie Spring White (CPSW), Canada Western Red Spring (CWRS), Canada Western Red Winter (CWRW), Canada Prairie Spring Red (CPSR), Canada Western Soft White Spring (CWSWS). Images were acquired using a ThermaCAM™ SC500 thermal camera. The authors conducted three different types of discriminant analyses using QDA models: (1) eight class model, (2) red wheat and white wheat classes separately (four class model), and (3) pairwise comparison in red and white classes (two class model). The classification accuracies using bootstrap technique were 76%, 87%, 79%, and 95% for eight class, red class (four class), white class (four class) and pairwise (two class), respectively. The results showed that misclassification occurred in the eight-class and four-class models, whereas two-class models provided higher classification accuracies. They concluded that although classification accuracy was lower for eight- and four-class models, thermal imaging has the ability to classify two classes of wheat that look similar and are difficult to differentiate by visual inspection.

6.3.2 Food

6.3.2.1 Quality of fruits and vegetables

The water content of fruits and vegetables influences their properties, and the loss of water due to transpiration depends on various factors, such as size and type of fruit, temperature and humidity of surrounding air, and air flow around and against the product. When heat is transmitted from the product, a temperature decrease on the surface could be observed and this temperature change could be monitored and measured by thermal imaging. Hellebrand et al. (2001) showed that thermal imaging could be useful for evaluation of climatic stress at postharvest stages of fruits, assessment of freshness of horticultural products, microbial infestation resulting in local temperature differences in fruits, ripeness, and mealiness of apples. Table 6.2 shows the details of the thermal camera model, specifications, and applications of thermal imaging related to fresh produce and food materials.

For long-term storage of fruits, the moisture from the surface of fruits must be dried off to prevent microbial activities. Gottschalk and Mèszáros (2012) explored the potential of infrared thermometry for heat and mass transfer analysis of surface drying of fruit. Thermal imaging was obtained for the temperature distribution along the surface of wet peach. The evaporation of surface moisture lowers the temperature and as soon as the surface was dried off, the temperature again increases to ambient air value, which could be seen by the temperature profile acquired by the infrared camera. The drying zone movement could be observed moving from the direction of airflow to the opposite direction. The temperature distribution on the surface was dependent on airflow direction and velocity, and was measured using thermal imaging. They developed a model to determine the heat and mass transfer from the surface of spherical fruit to the ambient air.

Watercore, a physiological disorder, results in translucent tissues due to the intercellular air spaces being filled with fluid. It is not possible to identify the disorder at the early

Table 6.2 Thermal Camera Model, Specifications, and Applications Related to Fresh Produce and Food Materials

Thermal camera model	Company	Camera specifications: wavelength, geometric, and thermal resolution	Emissivity	Application	Reference
FLIR PM545	FLIR Systems, Danderyd, Sweden	7.5–13 μm; 320 × 240 pixels; 0.1°C at 30°C	0.95	To monitor surface temperature during steam-disinfection of carrots	Gan-Mor et al., 2011
AGEMA 880 LWB	NA	8–13 μm; 0.007°C at 30°C	0.96	To detect watercore in apples	Baranowski et al., 2008
NA	NA	7.5–13 μm; 0.07 K at 30°C	NA	To monitor temperature during storage of potatoes	Geyer and Gottschalk, 2008
ThermaCAM P65HS	FLIR Systems, Massachusetts	7.5–13 μm; 320 × 240 pixels; 0.05°C	0.95	To detect citrus fruits for robotic harvesting	Bulanon et al., 2008
Varioscan 2011	Jenoptik, Jena, Germany		NA	To study water transpiration and quality monitoring of sweet peppers	Zsom et al., 2005
AGEMA 570	FLIR Systems	8–14 μm; 320 × 240 pixels; 0.1°C at 30°C	0.98	To estimate number and diameter of apples	Stajnko et al., 2004
ThermaCAM™ PM390	FLIR Systems, Portland, Oregon	3.4–5 μm; 0.07°C at 30°C	NA	Bruise detection in apples	Varith et al., 2003
ThermaCAM™ SC3000		8–9 μm; 20 mK at 30°C	NA	To evaluate the surface quality of apples	Veraverbeke et al., 2006
Varioscan 2011	Jenoptik Technologie GmbH	8–12 μm; 0.03 K at 300 K	NA	Evaluation of horticultural products	Hellebrand et al., 2001

(Continued)

Table 6.2 (Continued) Thermal Camera Model, Specifications, and Applications Related to Fresh Produce and Food Materials

Thermal camera model	Company	Camera specifications: wavelength, geometric, and thermal resolution	Emissivity	Application	Reference
AGEMA 880 LW	FLIR Systems	8–12 µm; 140 × 280 pixels	NA	To monitor maturity stages of apples and cherry tomatoes	Offermann et al., 1998
ThermaCAM E2	FLIR Systems	7.5–13 µm	0.98	To estimate the body temperature of pigs	Warriss et al., 2013
ThermaCAM P25	FLIR Systems, Italy	7.5–13 µm; 320 × 240 pixels; 0.08°C at 30°C	0.98	To assess the quality of pork and ham	Costa et al., 2007
ThermoVision A40M Researcher	FLIR Systems, Danderyd, Sweden	7.5–13 µm; 320 × 240 pixels; 0.08°C at 30°C	0.92	To monitor temperature during pelleting process	Salas-Bringas et al., 2007
Thermosensorik System CMT 384 M4	Thermosensorik GmbH, Erlangen, Germany	3.4–5.2 µm; 384 × 288	NA	Quality control of hazel nuts	Warmann and Märgner, 2005
Thermosensorik System CMT 384 M	Thermosensorik GmbH, Erlangen, Germany	3.4–5.2 µm; 384 × 288	NA	To detect foreign substances in food	Meinlschmidt and Märgner, 2002
ThermaCAM PM250	FLIR Systems	3.4–5.0 µm; 0.07°C at 30°C	NA	To measure internal temperature of cooked chicken	Ibarra et al., 2000
Agema model 782	AGA, Lidingo, Sweden	3.5–5.6 µm; 0.1°C at 30°C	NA	To detect skin surface temperature in pigs	Schaefer et al., 1989

stages because it becomes visible only when the injury is severe. Baranowski et al. (2008) examined the possibility of thermal imaging to detect watercore in apples. Gloster apples (*Malus domestica* Borkh) with the presence and absence of watercore were chosen, and thermal images were obtained with an AGEMA 880 LWB system. Apples stored at 1.5°C were taken to the measurement site maintained at an ambient temperature 20°C. When the surface temperature of the apples reached 7.5°C, thermal images were acquired. The apples were heated and the images were collected every 10 min during the heating process. After acquiring images, each fruit was cut longitudinally along the radial plane to check for the presence of watercore. The density, fruit firmness, and soluble solid concentrations were determined for the fruits using traditional methods. The change of temperature in the initial stages of heating (0 and 20 min of heating) plays an important role in assessment of watercore-affected and healthy fruit. The rates of increase of temperature per mass at the initial stages of heating for watercore-affected apples were significantly lower than the healthy apples. They stated that thermal imaging has the potential to determine watercore-affected apples by measuring temperature changes on the fruit surface during heating.

Postharvest treatment is very important in maintaining the quality of fresh fruits. Citrus surface drying (CSD) is an important processing operation. The common problem in citrus surface drying is the use of a very high air temperature or holding the product for a long period of time, which results in reduced sensory qualities in the fruit. Fito et al. (2004) examined the suitability of infrared imaging to develop a system for controlling industrial citrus surface drying by determining the final point in citrus surface drying. Fresh unwashed, uncoated oranges (*Citrus sinensis* L.) were bought from local orchards. A pilot drying plant was used to conduct drying experiments, and an AGEMA Thermovision 470 thermal camera was connected to the dryer to monitor and record infrared emission from the fruit surface. Oranges were dried at 20°C, 25°C, and 35°C with 1, 1.5, and 2 m/s air velocities. The point where surface drying was finished and peel drying started to occur was determined by the control of surface temperature of the fruit. To correlate drying time with air velocities, an empirical model was developed. Based on the results of the study Fito et al. stated that infrared thermal imaging could be a potential tool to determine the drying time and assess the fruit quality during surface drying.

Bruises in apples are difficult to detect visually or using automated sorting techniques. X-ray imaging and magnetic resonance imaging are among the successful techniques for detecting bruises but the associated high costs for equipment and installation make these techniques less practical for on-line fruit grading applications. Varith et al. (2003) examined the ability of thermal imaging to identify bruises in apples. Forty-five Red Delicious, Fuji, and McIntosh apples each were obtained from an orchard and bruised by dropping them onto a smooth concrete floor from 0.46 m and maintained at 26°C and 50% RH (relative humidity), for 48 h for bruise development. Apples were imaged for 3 min by a ThermaCAM™ PM390 camera while exposed to any one of the following three treatments: (1) forced convection heating in ambient atmosphere at 50% RH, 26°C; (2) forced convection heating in the same air heated to 37°C; and (3) forced convection cooling in ambient air at 50% RH, 26°C after heating in 40°C water for 2 to 3 min. Bruises were not detected in thermal images when the fruits were maintained at thermal equilibrium, whereas significant variation in temperature between bruised and healthy tissue were obtained during heating or cooling. Bruise detection accuracies were 100%, 86.7%, and 86.7% for Fuji apples for the three treatments, respectively. For McIntosh, bruise detection accuracies were 100%, 100%, and 86.7%, whereas for Red Delicious apples these were 66.6%, 40.0%, and 60.0%, respectively, for the three treatments. The temperature of bruised tissues were 1°C to 2°C cooler than the healthy tissue, and heating of bruised tissue was slower than healthy tissue indicating that thermal diffusivity was higher in bruised than healthy tissues. Due to higher thermal diffusivity, heat transfer from exterior into the healthy interior tissue was quicker than the surrounding tissue, thereby causing reduced surface temperatures in bruised tissues. The authors concluded that although bruises could not be detected in steady-state conditions, thermal imaging could be used to detect bruises in apples in packaging operations like those at the wax drying tunnel where changes in temperature of fruit occur due to external cooling or heating.

The quality characteristics of sweet pepper (*Capsicum annum* L.) is significantly influenced by mass or water losses because of transpiration during postharvest storage. Surface temperature differences between different parts, such as fruit body or stalk, could be found due to different water transpiration rates, and this temperature difference could be determined by thermal imaging. Zsom et al. (2005) investigated the effects of various storage conditions (10°C and 20°C, and with and without sealing in low-density polyethylene [LDPE] bags) on the quality characteristics of sweet pepper (two varieties: red variety Kárpia and white Hó) using nondestructive surface thermal imaging. Every 5 min for 1 h time period, surface temperature distribution of peppers were determined using liquid nitrogen cooled Varioscan 2011 thermal imaging camera. The mean surface temperatures of stalk and fruit were monitored using imaging software, and the differences in fruit mass over the measuring time period was measured using an electronic balance. The results of the experiment showed that fruit transpiration was higher in variety Kárpia owing to their significantly reduced tissue resistance to water vapor transfer. The calculated transpiration rates of the whole fruit surface was four times that of stalks and the difference in temperature between stalk and fruit suggested that drying of stalks were observed in samples stored at higher temperature without packaging (Figure 6.3). The temperature decreased rapidly in nonpackaged samples during the first day of storage at both temperatures. Zsom et al. suggested that efficient packing prevented excessive mass loss, and concluded that thermal imaging could be useful for quality monitoring of fresh produce during postharvest storage.

Linden et al. (2003) developed a measurement setup and a procedure for bruise detection of tomatoes using three types of temperature treatment. Sixty-nine uniformly grown

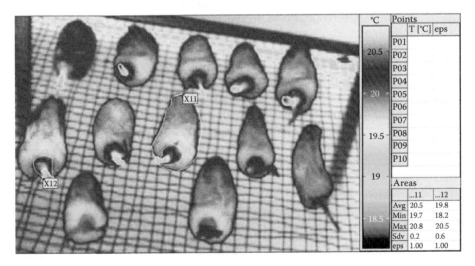

Figure 6.3 Surface thermal images of sweet pepper samples. (From Zsom, T. et al., *Journal of Thermal Analysis and Calorimetry*, 82, 239, 2005. With permission.)

tomatoes (*Lycopersicon esculentum* L.) were bruised by means of pendulum and stored at room temperature for 6 days. Thermal images were acquired on day 1, 2, 3, and 6 after bruising. The three treatments were: (1) cooling the fruit for 90 min at 1°C, (2) warming the tomatoes in the oven at 70°C for 1 or 2 min, and (3) warming the tomatoes in a microwave oven for 7 or 15 s. The images were acquired with the ThermaCAM™ SC3000 camera. A visual score from 0 to 4 was attributed for each image with 0 indicating a hardly visible or not detectable bruise and 4 indicating a clearly visible bruise. The results of the experiment showed that cooling the fruits were insufficient in revealing any bruised spots. Heating at 70°C for 1 or 2 min resulted in a decrease of 0.2°C or 0.3°C, respectively, at the impact location. A short microwave treatment for 7 or 15 s resulted in a temperature decrease of 0.3°C and 0.6°C, respectively, at the location of impact. The detected bruises showed some typical characteristics such as cold and regular circular shape, and hence based on the results it was concluded that thermal imaging could be a useful technique to detect bruise damage in tomatoes.

Offermann et al. (1998) studied the capability of pulsed infrared thermography (PIT) as a noncontact, nondestructive technique for inspection of apples (*Malus domestica* Borkh) and cherry tomatoes (*Solanum lycopersicum*) to characterize their varying stages of maturity. The samples were kept on a platform and energized by an intense light pulse by synchronously discharging four lamps. The resultant decay rate of temperature was measured by the AGEMA 880 LW infrared thermal camera with an HgCdTe detector. The experimental results showed that to a certain degree the samples can be differentiated by virtue of maximum skin temperature.

To maintain the quality of potatoes during storage, it is important to maintain a favorable environment inside the storage space, and a temperature of 4°C to 5°C should be maintained for long-term storage. In many storage facilities, potatoes are stored too cold in the lowest level and too warm in the top most level of the stack, which results in early sprouting in the upper level due to warm environment. Conventional temperature sensors only provide local temperature details, whereas thermal imaging could provide complete temperature profile of the storage room. Geyer and Gottschalk (2008) used an infrared camera working in the wavelength range of 7.5 to 13 μm and having a sensitivity of 0.07 K at 30°C. For comparison of thermal imaging and conventional techniques, two blackened metal sheets, serving as reference sheets, were fixed at a distance of 5 cm on the boxes with potatoes to ensure undisturbed aeration, and temperature changes were measured using contact thermometer. The results of the experiment proved that thermal imaging could be utilized for monitoring temperature or climatic changes in potato storage, and to measure temperature of potatoes and fluctuations in ambient air. The study showed that lowest temperature differences can be visualized by the infrared camera and desired storage temperatures could be maintained inside the box by installing additional cameras inside the store to get a better overview of temperature distribution in the room.

The use of insecticides and pesticides for pest control is being restricted to ensure the safety of consumers and protect the environment. To improve the appearance of carrots, they are hydrocooled before packing and there is a possibility of cooling water being infected with pathogens, hence surface disinfection is preferred after hydrocooling. Use of steam to disinfect agricultural produce was tested and preliminary studies in carrots by Afek et al. (1999) revealed the benefits of steam heat treatment over hot water treatment. However, accurate monitoring of the heat treatment chamber is essential to determine the surface temperature uniformity. Gan-Mor et al. (2011) studied the thermal imaging technology to develop steam disinfection for carrots and acquired images with a PM545 thermal camera. Thermal imaging accurately monitored the surface temperatures and provided appropriate guidelines for proper positioning of electric heaters to increase the uniformity of heating and reduce the overheating on the surface. The thermal images demonstrated that hydrocooling application before steam treatment prevented the tissue damage. The thermal images also showed that reduction of time duration after hydrocooling and before steam treatment also reduced the heat accumulation in the carrot tissue resulting in minimum tissue damage. Based on the study thermal imaging was considered as a potential technique to monitor surface temperatures of carrots and to optimize the heat and uniformity of temperature on the surface of carrots during steam disinfection.

6.3.2.2   Harvesting and yield estimation

Harvesting of citrus fruit is mostly performed by hand and the major challenge faced by citrus producers is the cost involved in the harvesting of fruit. Robotic harvesting is an alternative but the challenge in robotic harvesting is the fruit recognition. Bulanon et al. (2008) demonstrated the possibility of thermal imaging to separate the fruits from the canopy to assist in robotic fruit harvest. The study was conducted in an orchard located in Ocala, Florida. Images were obtained using the ThermaCAM P65HS camera with a focal plane array uncooled microbolometer. Images were captured for 24 h at every 15 min interval and other data such as surface fruit temperature, relative humidity, and ambient temperature were also recorded. The image processing steps involved histogram and segmentation procedures to determine the fruit from canopy. After thresholding, the images showed that fruit regions were easily detected from 4:15 p.m. until midnight, and other than this time period, canopy region was also detected as fruit region. The results showed that the higher true positive and lower false positive segmentation occurred during the time period when maximum temperature difference was observed between leaf and fruit. At this time, a mean true positive rate of 0.7 and false negative rate of 0.06 was achieved. Bulanon et al. stated that thermal imaging has the ability for fruit detection to support robotic harvesting of citrus fruits if implemented during the time period from late in the afternoon until midnight.

Estimation of yield of fruits is an important aspect, and predicting the number of fruits and size during harvesting are the basic aspects for prediction of future yield. At present, the "Prognosfruit" forecast model is the sole method for yield estimation accepted by European pear and apple producers. The major drawback of this method is that it is time consuming. Zhang et al. (1997, 1998) examined the potential of thermal imaging for counting fruits under natural conditions, and the results confirmed that the difference of temperature between apples and leaves was over 1°C. However, their experiment also showed that the temperature difference between branches and apples was much less when the weather was calm and clear, and no temperature difference existed between apples and leaves from midnight to early morning. Stajnko et al. (2003) evaluated the potential of thermal imaging to predict the number and size (diameter) of apples, which could be used for calculating the yield of the apple orchard. Apple (*Malus domestica* Borkh) trees were examined during four crucial stages of development of apple fruits: stage 1, after fruit drop (June 16, 2002); stage 2, 3 weeks later (July 7, 2002); stage 3, beginning of ripening (August 8, 2002); and stage 4, harvesting (September 2, 2002). Images were acquired using thermal camera AGEMA 570, and the images were digitized off-line using an image acquisition board with frame grabber. The algorithm involved global thresholding to separate background (grass, soil) and plant parts (branches, fruits, and leaves). After segmentation of leaves and fruits by thresholding, the images were filtered to remove the remaining noise. The results showed that a close correlation ($R^2 = 0.78$ to 0.81) was obtained between manually counted fruits and those estimated by imaging. For estimating of average yield per tree, the correlation coefficient ($R^2 = 0.69$ to 0.79) was obtained. The authors stated that thermal imaging has a great potential for estimating yield of fruits, but an algorithm needs to be improved to detect partially hidden spherical objects to increase the accuracy of detection.

6.3.2.3   Detection of foreign bodies in food

Presence of unwanted foreign objects in food materials is an important issue in the food industry. Foreign substances in food are mostly detected by various techniques such as mechanical, optical, and ultrasound methods. Imaging techniques such as X-ray imaging have been tested for detecting foreign substances in food but due to the higher cost involved, they are not commonly used. Meinlschmidt and Märgner (2002) evaluated the possibility of thermal imaging to identify foreign substances in food. The experimental setup consists of a conveyor belt that moves at a speed range of 1 and 50 m/min along a cooling or heating unit, and the samples move on top of the conveyor. A Thermosensorik System CMT 384 M camera with a HgCdTe detector was used for the study. The sample materials studied were cherries, berries, and chocolate contaminated with leaves, pedicel, stalks, and thorns. Further study was conducted on raisins and almonds with wooden sticks and stones mixed with them. The objects can be differentiated if the two substances have significantly varying heat conductivities. But a better parameter for detection of desirable food material and contaminant was the difference in the gray levels between the sample and the contaminants. The results of the study showed that it was possible to detect contaminants in the food materials using thermal imaging, but more work needs to be done to create algorithms that can detect even small and moving particles in the food materials.

Ginesu et al. (2004) evaluated the detection of undesirable foreign objects in food using thermal imaging. The two basic ways to differentiate between food material and unwanted materials is either by differing the emissivities or by using different heat conductivities or capacities of the material. But mostly the emissivity of food and foreign materials is not sufficient to get good contrast infrared images, so to obtain higher contrast images, the samples are either heated or cooled. They conducted study on almonds mixed with stones and pieces of cardboard and raisins mixed with wooden sticks. Thermal images were acquired using the Thermosensorik-System CMT 384 M. The results of the experiment showed that infrared imaging has the potential to be used for detection of foreign materials in food products (Figure 6.4).

6.3.2.4   Meat

With the increase in demand for ready-to-meat products, the major problem faced by processing industry is to achieve a right cooking of the meat product without under- or overcooking, because undercooking may result in food safety issues due to survival of bacteria, and overcooking may result in yield reduction due to loss of water content and juiciness. Since infrared thermal imaging needs no contact with the surface of the sample, Ibarra et al. (2000) evaluated this technique for noninvasive inspection of cooking processes of chicken. Sixty samples of chicken breast were cooked at constant oven temperatures (177°C) for varying periods of time between 5.8 and 7.6 min in an industrial oven (Model MPO-D2012, Heat and Control Inc.) to obtain various temperatures ranging from undercooked to overcooked conditions. Images were acquired using a ThermaCAM PM250. After cooking, the temperatures were measured every 30 s during the 10 min cooling time. Simultaneous internal and external temperatures were obtained using an artificial neural network. The neural network performed well and the internal temperature of

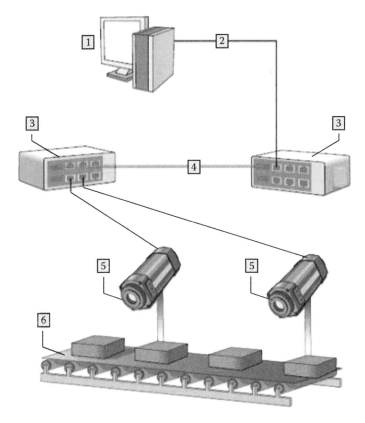

Figure 6.4 Typical food inspection system using thermal imaging camera: (1) computer, (2) Ethernet cable, (3) Ethernet switches, (4) fiber optic cable, (5) FLIR camera, and (6) food material on conveyor belt. (Image courtesy of FLIR Systems, 2013a, Thermal imaging cameras in the food industry, FLIR Commercial Systems, http://www.flir.com/cs/emea/en/view/?id=41781; accessed May 15, 2013. With permission.)

the sample was computed within a standard error of ±1.01°C for a time period between 0 and 540 s after cooking. The results of the study showed that combined thermography and neural network have the potential for noninvasive and high-speed monitoring of final temperatures in industrial cooking lines of meat products (Figure 6.5).

Costa et al. (2007) examined the capability of infrared thermography to evaluate the pork quality and suitability of ham to be processed into dry cured ham. The left and right hams of 40 pig carcasses were selected for the study. The left and right caudal and dorsal surface images were acquired using a ThermaCAM P25 thermal camera. The results exhibited an increase in temperature in hams with a reduced fat cover. The higher surface temperature of skin was owing to the thinner subcutaneous adipose tissue, which provided lower thermal insulation. Based on the study it was established that a relationship between fat content of ham and surface temperature exists, and hence infrared thermography is a valuable, fast, and noninvasive tool to compute the fat content of ham. It was concluded that thermography could be for assessment of ham and pork quality on the slaughter line.

Pale soft exudative (PSE) pork produces a significant economic loss to the swine industry and the ability to detect pigs prone to produce PSE pork is very valuable. Schaefer et al. (1989) investigated the potential of infrared thermography to predict the differences in

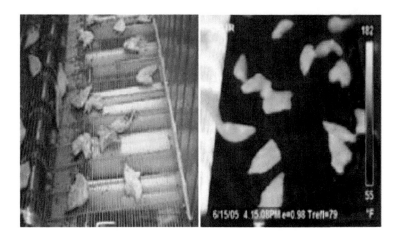

Figure 6.5 Infrared temperature measurements to check undercooked chicken fingers. (Image courtesy of FLIR Systems, 2013a, Thermal imaging cameras in the food industry, FLIR Commercial Systems, http://www.flir.com/cs/emea/en/view/?id=41781; accessed May 15, 2013. With permission.)

surface temperature of skin of three genotypes of pigs based on stress susceptibility. An AGEMA 782 thermal camera was used to obtain thermal images of external median and dorsal surfaces of all animal samples. The average mean temperature on the right exterior of carcass was 2°C more than the left side. This difference of temperature may be due to stunning procedure because all animals were stunned at the right side. High muscular contraction may occur due to high voltage stunning, which stimulates postmortem glycolysis and results in temperature increase on the stunned side. The analysis showed no significant temperature differences among the three genotypes of neither live animals nor the carcasses. However, swines with lower average side temperature showed a higher percentage drip loss and pale colored meat. They concluded that infrared thermography could be used to predict meat quality by determining the temperature differences within the meat sample.

6.3.2.4.1 Estimation of body temperature of pigs. Transportation of pigs at high temperature is stressful to pigs, which may lead to poorer quality of meat in terms of color, water holding capacity, and palatability. There are practical difficulties in measuring the temperature of pigs during transport and slaughter irrespective of the importance of the body temperature of the pigs. Warriss et al. (2013) estimated the body temperature of 384 pigs from 28 pigpens using thermal imaging. The pigs were killed and exsanguinated, and their core body temperature was considered to be the temperature of the blood lost from wound which was measured with an infrared thermometer (Raynger PM Plus, Raytec). Before the pigs were hoisted onto the dressing rail, an image of the side of the pig's head was recorded with a ThermaCAM E2 thermal camera. The serum samples were analyzed for cortisol and creatine kinase. The blood temperature of the pigs ranged from 35.6°C to 42.6°C (mean: 39.6°C ± 1.39°C) and the pig's ear temperature ranged from 27.3°C to 35.0°C (mean: 31.0°C ± 1.32°C). The ear temperature of pigs had significant correlation ($r = 0.71$) with the mean blood temperature. The serum creatine kinase had positive correlation with the mean ear temperature ($r = 0.55$) and the mean of serum cortisol had positive correlation with mean blood temperature ($r = 0.50$). The study showed that pigs with higher temperature were suffering from higher levels of stress, which affects the quality of meat.

6.3.2.4.2 Poultry feed.   In the manufacturing processes of food and feed materials, contact methods are used to measure temperatures that are not accurate in many cases because the materials easily agglomerate and it is hard to calculate moving object temperature using contact methods. Temperature is a crucial parameter during various stages of conditioning and pelleting process of animal feed, and an increase in temperature above the desired range affects the physical and chemical properties of end product. Salas-Bringas et al. (2007) explored the possibility of temperature monitoring during pelleting process of feed manufacturing using infrared thermal imaging. Images were acquired using a ThermoVision A40M thermal camera. The infrared camera was used for monitoring temperature of pellets at the die exit, the meal temperature at the conditioner outlet, and pellet temperature measured at the exit of the pellet press. The temperature was monitored throughout the process and it was shown that increase in temperature of the meal during pelleting was not just due to the die hole friction but also due to friction, stresses, and strains that occurred in the space between the die ring and the rollers. Salas-Bringas et al. concluded that infrared thermal imaging aids in the temperature monitoring of sticky and fast moving objects. The study of temperature distribution through infrared imaging requires improved instrumentation designed to perform in moist, dusty, and oily industrial environments.

6.3.3   Applications of thermal imaging in engineering

Thermal imaging has a wide range of application in the civil engineering and is most widely used in inspection of buildings and structures. The most commonly used applications of thermal imaging in building inspection are to visualize energy losses, source of air leaks, presence of moisture and mold, locate water infiltration in flat roofs, detect missing or defective insulation, determine faults in supply lines and electrical lines, and detect the presence of any construction failure (FLIR, 2011c). Infrared thermography could be used in aerospace engineering and the most common types of abnormalities such as delamination, water ingress, node failure, and core crushing could be detected efficiently using thermographic techniques (Ibarra-Castanedo et al., 2008). Table 6.3 provides the details of thermal camera models, specifications, and applications of thermal imaging in engineering.

Condition monitoring is one of the major uses of infrared thermography, that is, monitoring the condition of various machineries and processes, such as wear and tear of pipelines, leakage in valves and pressure vessels, inspection of electrical equipment, and monitoring deformation in plastics and engineering materials. Bagavathiappan et al. (2013) reviewed the application of infrared thermography for condition monitoring in various domains such as for assessment of structures such as buildings, bridges, sewer and water systems, monitoring of electronic and electrical components, monitoring of deformation that occurs during tensile or fatigue loading, inspection of machineries, corrosion monitoring, and application of infrared thermography in nuclear and aerospace industries. Figure 6.6 shows the application of infrared thermography in condition monitoring of machinery, level of liquids in industrial components, inspection of PCBs, motor shaft belt, transformer circuit breakers, and electrical panels.

Reinforced concrete is an important construction material widely used in many civil engineering practices due to its high strength, durability, and sustainability. The reinforced concrete may result in corrosion and loses its strength when exposed to undesired environmental conditions, which could result in catastrophic structural failure unless otherwise detected at an early stage. Mulaveesala et al. (2012) explored frequency modulated

Table 6.3 Model and Specifications of Infrared Thermal Cameras Used in Engineering Applications

Thermal camera model	Company	Camera specifications: wavelength, geometric, and thermal resolution	Application	Reference
SC6100	FLIR	3.0–5.0; 640 × 512 pixels	To monitor failure in aluminum alloys	Antoun and Song, 2012
T360	FLIR	7.5–13 µm; 320 × 240 pixels; 50 mK	To determined overall heat transfer coefficient in buildings	Fokaides and Kalogirou, 2011
FLIR S65	FLIR System	320 × 240; 0.08°C	To monitor subsurface deterioration in concrete bridges	Washer et al., 2010
Raytheon Radiance HS	Raytheon Co., Waltham, Massachusetts	3.0–5.0 µm; 256 × 256 pixels; 0.015°C	Mechanical fatigue testing of alloys	Wang et al., 2000

thermal wave imaging (FMTWI) for inspection of concrete structures to detect surface and subsurface features such as voids, corrosion, and cracks. Experiments were conducted on a 6.7 cm thick concrete specimen, which contains a 4 cm thick mild steel rebar 13.24 cm long. To examine the corrosion detection abilities, artificial corrosion was stimulated by introduction of four groove cuts of different widths with around 5 mm loss of material from the bar surface. The sample temperature distribution was monitored by an infrared thermal camera and the temperature rise for a given incident heat flux was recorded. The results of the study showed that the amount of corrosion in the concrete specimen was determined by frequency modulated thermal wave imaging and the technique has a great potential to detect hidden corrosion in concrete structures.

Infrared thermal imaging could be a potential tool to detect heat losses, damaged or defective insulation in walls and roofs, leakage of air, and moisture sources inside the building that could affect the building (Figures 6.7 through 6.9). Fokaides and Kalogirou (2011) studied the potential of infrared thermography to determine the overall heat transfer coefficient (U) in building envelopes. A FLIR T360 infrared thermal camera that performs in the range of 7.5 to 13 µm wavelength was used for the study. It was suggested in the study that infrared thermography of the building should be conducted either during night time or on a cloudy day to prevent the issue of temperature increase due to incident solar radiation on a sunny day. The study was conducted in Cyprus during the summer and winter seasons. The measured infrared thermography results were validated with results obtained from relevant European standards. The results showed that the percentage absolute deviation between the values from standards and measured heat transfer coefficient was at an acceptable range of 10% to 20%. The greater deviation in the building element was from the roofs followed by glassy surfaces mostly due to thermal inertia effects that could not be controlled.

The deterioration of concrete bridge components that occurs due to corrosion is a major challenge in maintaining the stability of bridge. Deterioration occurs at the embedded reinforcing steel due to expansion of corrosion products and resulting stresses in the concrete. Traditionally infrared thermography has been used to inspect concrete bridge

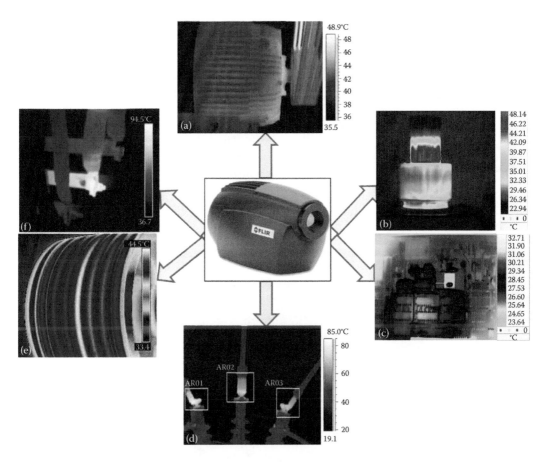

Figure 6.6 Condition monitoring applications of infrared thermography. (a) Monitoring of machineries where abnormal surface temperature distribution is an indication of a probable flaw. (b) Inspection of liquid levels in industrial components. (c) Inspection of printed circuit boards. (d) Typical thermal images of a transformer circuit breaker where the faulty regions can be clearly seen as hotspots. (e) Inspection of shaft belt where the thermal anomaly is due to overtightening of a belt. (f) Condition monitoring of three phase electrical panel where local hotspots are developed due to load imbalance. (From Bagavathiappan, S. et al., *Infrared Physics and Technology*, 60, 35, 2013. With permission.)

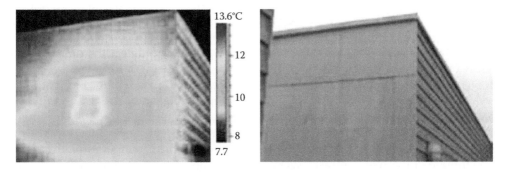

Figure 6.7 Building with concrete–insulation–concrete sandwich construction showing a missing insulation. (Image courtesy of FLIR Systems, 2011c, Thermal imaging guideline for building and renewable energy applications, FLIR Systems AB, Täby, Sweden. With permission.)

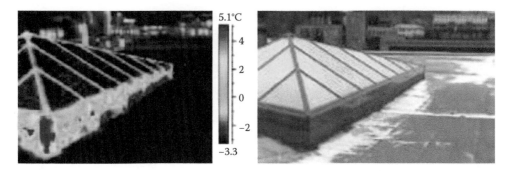

Figure 6.8 Glass roof above an atrium that is not air tight and warm air escape captured by thermal camera. (Image courtesy of FLIR Systems, 2011c, Thermal imaging guideline for building and renewable energy applications, FLIR Systems AB, Täby, Sweden. With permission.)

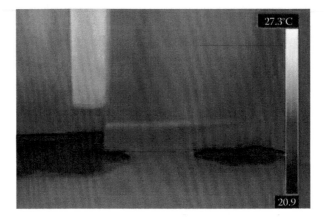

Figure 6.9 Moisture intrusions in floor detected with thermal camera. (Image courtesy of FLIR Systems, 2011c, Thermal imaging guideline for building and renewable energy applications, FLIR Systems AB, Täby, Sweden. With permission.)

decks because a bridge deck deteriorates more rapidly due to exposure to direct sunlight during the day and hence the damage is greater than for portions not exposed to sunlight. Washer et al. (2010) studied the subsurface deterioration in concrete bridges using thermography. They studied the daily temperature changes to detect the damage in the soffit area of the bridge, which is not typically accessible during a routine inspection. A FLIR S65 thermal camera was used to capture images of the surface of the block at 10 min interval for 24 h/day. Solar loading, wind speed, rainfall data, and relative humidity were recorded by an onsite weather station with the goal of determining the environmental conditions that were best suited for detection of subsurface features in concrete. The data were analyzed to determine the relationship between ambient temperature change and the magnitude of thermal contrast. Based on the results of the test block, a field test was conducted for assessment of the condition of the soffit area of a bridge. The results of the study showed that the technology could identify potentially problematic areas of concrete where the potential for spalling could occur and the concrete could fall onto the traffic.

Rao (2008) reviewed the applications of infrared thermography in civil engineering and stated that the technology has many applications in structural assessment, identifying the source of damage, evaluation of potential of damage in concrete and masonry, and in the identification of moisture ingress and flow through the pipes. The moisture penetration under the windows of the masonry structure could be identified by the temperature difference, because presence of moisture reduces the temperature at the location of moisture presence. The plumbing and the flow of sewage water through pipes could be monitored using thermal imaging. Similarly, thermal imaging could also be used to identify the state of fresh as well as hardened concrete and any obstruction to the flow of concrete could be monitored from the temperature patterns of the thermal image. Thermal imaging could be useful in testing the reinforcement bars for tensile strength. The thermal pattern of the bar could be obtained during tensile strength testing and the temperature of the bar increases with load and the temperature rise was uniform along the bar in the elastic region. However, the temperature of the bar starts increasing locally in the region of failure and the temperature was lower away from the critical section.

A major challenge in the packaging industry is to determine flaws such as cracks, voids, and delamination. Liu and Dias (2002) evaluated the ability of thermography to detect the defects in electronic packages. When an object is subjected to heating, a flaw in the material, such as a void or crack, alters the diffusion rate depending on the size and location which alters the temperature in the surrounding regions of flaw and ultimately changes the temperature profile on object surface. Inspection of thermal interface material (TIM) defect detection was performed by applying a heat pulse to the packaged surface. Four samples with different TIM defects were collected: (1) without TIM defect, (2) TIM delamination, (3) lack of TIM, and (4) no TIM. The samples were analyzed by a scanning acoustic microscope in reflective mode, and an infrared camera was used to monitor the change in thermal response on the surface. The temperature of regions with TIM delamination as in samples 2 and 3 was hotter than the adjacent regions. A well-defined cooler temperature was observed in sample 1 due to good TIM coverage, while there was no cooler region in sample 4 due to no TIM. The results of the study confirmed that infrared thermography could be a potential tool for TIM defect analysis in electronic packages.

In the development of engineering materials, such as alloys, knowledge of damage initiation and evolution at the microstructural level is essential for development of superior materials. Antoun and Song (2013) developed an infrared imaging method to visualize and monitor damage evolution in aluminum alloys. After heat treatment, polishing, and etching of 7075-T651 (aluminum alloy) are completed, a thermal camera (SC6100, FLIR) was used to acquire images of grain boundaries in the aluminum specimen. Images were also acquired while the specimen was subjected to quasistatic tensile loading to track changes. Preliminary results using thermal imaging showed that changes at the grain boundaries occur with increased loading, which could be used to improve the development of models to enable deformation and failure prediction in metallic alloys.

Mechanical properties of structural materials are tested by cyclic fatigue tests that determine the life span of a material under cyclic loading. During cyclic fatigue tests, based on the applied stress, the temperature of the specimen increases, and temperature measurement using single point contact thermocouple is not suitable because only limited information could be obtained. Wang et al. (2000) studied the potential of high-speed infrared imaging during mechanical fatigue tests. ULTIMET® alloy, which is a copper chromium based super alloy from Haynes International Inc., was used for the study. A Raytheon Radiance HS infrared camera was used for the image acquisition of the entire process, and an image was captured every 6 s until failure. The results of the study showed that infrared imaging is a potential tool to understand the fatigue studies and during the fatigue process, four stages were observed: the initial increase of temperature, equilibrium, the temperature increase before failure, and the decrease in temperature after the failure. The infrared imaging made it possible to study the initiation and propagation of fatal crack, and the thermoelastic plastic behavior was observed when plastic deformation was caused due to maximum stress in the material.

6.3.4 Applications of thermal imaging in bio-medicine

Since the 1970s thermography has been in use in the field of medicine, but due to low detector sensitivity and poor training in thermography there was low acceptance of this technique. The early breast cancer detection and demonstration project (BCDDP) performed between 1973 and 1981 clearly demonstrated the shortcoming of both mammography and thermography. It was explained that infrared imaging was able to determine the likelihood of a patient to have breast cancer but could not accurately determine the location of lesion. Hence, it was not accepted as a stand-alone technique; however, it could be used in a multimodality screening environment (Jiang et al., 2005). Modern thermal imaging systems comprised of advanced thermal cameras with very high detector sensitivity and sophisticated software solutions resulted in wider acceptance of the technique in medical diagnostics. Thermography can be used as a diagnostic tool in oncology, allergy diseases, angiology, plastic surgery, rheumatology, and many other diseases (Mikulska, 2006). Infrared imaging has numerous applications in medicine ranging from cutaneous blood flow modeling, monitoring the activity of the peripheral nervous system, angiopathies, and evaluation of postural disorders (Merla and Romani, 2006). Conci et al. (2011) examined the potential of thermal imaging for 3D modeling of the human body with special interest on breast geometry, identification of tumors, and early diagnosis of breast diseases.

The infrared camera used for medical imaging should have the following minimum requirements. The camera should have high spatial resolution of 340×240 pixels because high spatial resolution highlights the temperature difference between two spots. Medical CE (Conformité Européenne) certification is recommended, and a narrow calibration range for normal human temperature range (20°C–40°C) is recommended for a detailed temperature measurement. Medical examination software capable of exporting functions and properly designed tools for data analysis and image fusion is a requirement for medical imaging cameras (Hildebrandt et al., 2010).

6.3.4.1 Cancer/tumor

The use of infrared thermal imaging in medical oncology is dependent on the fact that tumors normally have a higher blood supply and a higher metabolic rate, which results in increased temperature gradient between tumor affected and healthy tissue. Infrared thermal imaging could be used to identify these hot spots and thereby determine and diagnose tumors. Research has been carried out to explore the potential of infrared thermal imaging for breast cancer diagnosis. Keyserlingk et al. (1998) studied the infrared imaging of breast in 100 patients with stage I and stage II cancer, and stated that sensitivity of mammography was 85% while that of combined techniques of infrared thermography along with mammography was 95%. Parisky et al. (2003) examined the efficiency of infrared imaging to examine the suspicious lesions from mammography and showed that infrared imaging had a high sensitivity of 97% to 99% and could differentiate benign from malignant lesions. Wang et al. (2010) evaluated the diagnostic potential of infrared imaging and established an interpretive age-adjusted multivariate model for infrared imaging of breasts. In 1982, the U.S. Food and Drug Administration (FDA) approved infrared thermography as an added tool for effective breast cancer diagnosis. Arora et al. (2008) examined the effectiveness of digital infrared thermal imaging (DITI) for detection of breast cancer. Ninety-two patients, who had been advised for breast biopsy due to suspicious ultrasound or mammogram, were assessed using a DITI system, the Sentinel BreastScan (SBS, Infrared Sciences Corp., Bohemia, New York). The results of the study showed that DITI detected 58 of 60 cancerous growths with 97% sensitivity and 44% specificity. The low rate of specificity in the pilot study was because of the selective patient population with suspicious findings on previous radiological tests. To assess the true specificity, an independent population with nonsuspicious breast pathology will be required. Digital infrared thermography is noninvasive, painless, and has no harmful radiation associated in the process. However, the limitation of DITI is that it is only a thermal recording of physiological measure and must be used as a secondary tool to another method such as ultrasound or mammography. The limitation of DITI is that infection of inflammation could also result in temperature variation, which may result in false positives; hence infrared thermography could be used along with other procedures to detect breast cancer. Ng (2009) reviewed the potential of thermography as a noninvasive method for detection of breast tumor. It was suggested that thermal imaging should be performed in a stable environment with minimum interference because skin surface temperature is dependent on the skin blood perfusion and surrounding environmental conditions. With the stringent standardized protocols for thermogram interpretation, an average sensitivity and specificity of 90% was achieved for breast thermography. To recognize thermal imaging as a potential technique to detect breast cancer, the major recommendations include: thermal radiation theory, patient preparation, standardization of imaging system, examination environment, protocol for image acquisition, protocol for image analysis, reporting, archiving, and storing. Figure 6.10 shows the abnormal temperature differences between the breasts indicating cancer in the left breast.

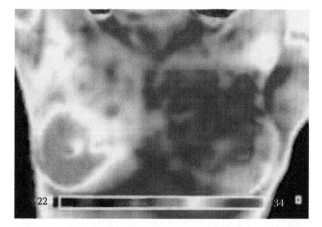

Figure 6.10 Abnormal temperature differences between breast indicating breast cancer in the left breast. (Image courtesy of FLIR Systems, 2013b, FLIR thermal imaging cameras help determine the functionality of anti-allergy medicine, http://www.flir.com/cs/emea/en/view/?id=41183; accessed May 15, 2013. With permission.)

6.3.4.2 Diabetes

Diabetes is a chronic disease, and the International Diabetes Federation has determined that around 61.3 million people in India were affected in 2011 and may increase to 101.2 million by the year 2030. Sivanandam et al. (2012) explored the potential of thermography in diagnosis and prognosis of diabetes from a study group. According to the American Diabetes Association, the diabetes threshold was set as $HbA_{1c} \geq 6.5\%$ (7.7 mmolL^{-1}). (HbA_{1c} occurs when hemoglobin joins with glucose in the blood. When glucose sticks to these molecules, a glycosylated hemoglobin molecule is formed, which is known as A1c and HbA_{1c}.) They studied a total of 62 subjects of which 32 were control and 30 were diabetic, and thermal images were acquired using a thermal camera (ThermaCAM FLIR T400, FLIR Systems, United States) with a thermal sensitivity of 0.05°C at 30°C. The results of the study showed that HbA_{1c} had a negative correlation with the carotid region and the average temperature of skin was lower than the control population at the forehead, knee, tibia, and palm. As HbA_{1c} increased, the temperature of skin decreased which enabled early detection of disease compared to HbA_{1c}. The reduction in skin temperature might be due to reduced basal metabolic rate, high insulin resistance, and poor blood perfusion. The results of the study showed better specificity, sensitivity, and accuracy in detecting diabetes as compared to HbA_{1c}. They concluded based on the study that infrared thermography could be a potential prediction and diagnostic tool for diabetes.

Barone et al. (2006) examined a noninvasive technology for early detection of inflammation using visible 3D imaging and a thermal imaging technique. The objective was to develop an optical system along with a 3D visual scanner and a thermal imaging system to focus on pathologies resulting in ulceration and laceration caused due to advanced diabetic conditions such as diabetic foot disease (DFD). The optical system consisted of a monochrome digital camera (1280 × 960 pixels), thermal camera (FLIR A40, 320 × 240 pixels) detecting radiation in the range of 7.5 to 13 μm with a thermal sensitivity of 0.1°C at 30°C and a multimedia video projector (1024 × 768 pixels). The results showed that temperature difference between healthy skin and regions where microcirculation problems occur could be detected. The experimental study has shown that the proposed methodology could be a potential technique for physicians to improve the quality of their diagnosis on diabetic patients affected by DFD. Figure 6.11 shows the thermal imaging of foot disease of a diabetic patient and control subject.

6.3.4.3 Pediatrics

Saxena and Willital (2008) evaluated the feasibility of infrared thermography for clinical applications in the pediatric population. Based on the study of 483 patients over a period of 10 years, it was found that infrared thermography was an excellent noninvasive technique useful in the follow-up of tumor, vascular deformity, and finger or toe amputations due to reimplantation, burns, and vascular growth. They suggested that infrared thermography is a valuable tool in the emergency room for faster diagnosis of extremity thrombosis, abscesses, varicoceles, gangrene, inflammation, and infection due to wound. Based on their wide experience over a significant period of time with the pediatric population, infrared thermography was considered a noninvasive technique that could be used without any undesirable side effects and that requires no anesthesia and can be performed repeatedly for follow-up treatments.

6.3.4.4 Arthritis and arteriosclerosis

Rheumatoid arthritis (RA), an inflammatory disease, results in swelling, pain, deteriorates the function of joints, and could not be easily detected at early stages. The severity of the

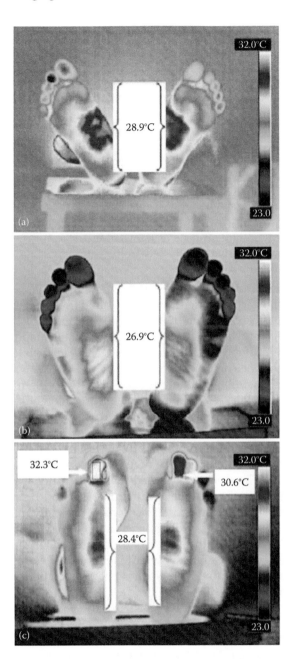

Figure 6.11 Thermal imaging of the foot. (a) Control subject, (b) diabetic patient, and (c) diabetic patient with early signs of ulceration. (From Sivanandam, S. et al., *Endocrine*, 42, 343, 2012. With permission.)

disease could be delayed if the disease is diagnosed at an early stage. Frize et al. (2011) examined the potential of infrared imaging to detect RA. The study was conducted in 18 healthy subjects and 13 patients affected by RA. The IR camera used to acquire images consists of an uncooled microbolometer focal plane array of 320×420 pixels operating in the range of 7.5 to 13 μm wavelengths. The thermal images were obtained from joints of hands, palms, wrists, and knees, and then analyzed. The results of the study showed that

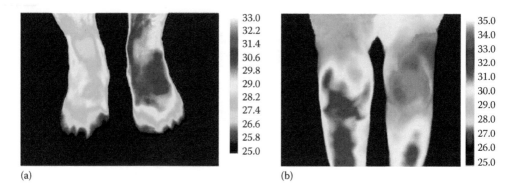

Figure 6.12 (a) Chronic inflammation of left forefoot due to sports injury. (b) Rheumatoid arthritis of right knee. (From Ring, E.F.J., and K. Ammer, *Physiological Measurement*, 33, 33–46, 2012. Reproduced by permission of IOP Publishing.)

the metacarpal phalangeal joint of the index and middle fingers and the knees are the best for diagnosis of the presence or absence of rheumatoid arthritis when compared to the palm, wrist, thumb, and proximal and distal interphalangeal joints. Frize et al. concluded that the presence of RA could be detected by infrared thermal imaging. Figure 6.12a shows the inflammation of a left foot due to sports injury and Figure 6.12b shows the thermal image of RA in the right knee of the patient.

Arteriosclerosis is an inflammatory disease, and the inflammation could initiate plaque development as well as result in complicated conditions like intra-arterial thrombosis. A method to identify the inflammation in coronary arteries may improve the prediction of acute coronary syndromes. Schmermund et al. (2003) examined the ability of thermography to determine the symptoms of arteriosclerosis. The result of the study has shown that an increase in temperature occurs at the region of inflammatory cellular macrophage infiltration. The study has proved that intracornonary thermography could provide insight into the location, extent of inflammation, and prognostic consequences. The preliminary results have shown that intracoronary thermography is safe and feasible, and could be performed on patients undergoing coronary angiography. Bhatia et al. (2003) studied the imaging of plaque with new techniques and stated that thermography is a promising technology to predict atherosclerotic plaques that are prone to rupture, and differentiate between stable and vulnerable plaques because temperature increase occurs at the site of inflammatory plaques.

6.3.4.5 Sports medicine

Hildebrandt et al. (2010) provided a summary of applications of medical infrared thermography (MIT) related to sports with a special attention on overuse and traumatic knee injuries. Research studies have shown that thermal images of both sides of the body are normally symmetrical and any temperature difference higher than 0.7°C could be considered as abnormal. They conducted a study on 35 female and 52 male Alpine skiers, because in alpine skiing a usual problem is the occurrence of injuries, such as patellae tendinopathy, which results in pain, tenderness, and swelling above tibial tuberosity. The result of the study showed that seven athletes showed symptoms with an average side temperature difference of 1.4°C, out of which four athletes complained of pain while others showed no symptoms at that time. Detection at an early stage and subsequent treatment could lower the severity of the symptoms. Figure 6.13a shows the image of a knee 6 weeks

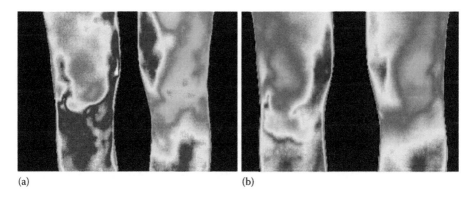

(a)   (b)

Figure 6.13 Infrared image of the anterior aspect of ACL rupture in right knee (a) and after 6 months of rehabilitation (b). (From Hildebrandt, C. et al., *Sensors*, 10, 4700, 2010. With permission.)

after an isolated anterior cruciate ligament (ACL) rupture and Figure 6.13b shows the same knee after extensive rehabilitation for 6 months.

Thermographic techniques have been used in neurosurgery, and the technique shows a qualitative relationship between cerebral blood flow and cortical surface temperature. Okada et al. (2007) examined the potential of thermal imaging in extracranial-intracranial (EC-IC) bypass surgery. Based on neurological examinations, 10 patients were recommended for EC-IC bypass surgery. A portable infrared camera (Tversus 100ME model, Nippon Avionics Inc., Tokyo, Japan) was used during intraoperative thermographic examinations. The cortical surface temperature was measured using thermography and the regional cerebral blood flow (rCBF) was calculated using a laser Doppler flow meter. A heterogeneous rise in cortical surface temperature due to blood flow via EC-IC bypass was observed during thermographic examination and the temperature increase was related to rCBF. Based on the study they concluded that thermal imaging is not only useful to monitor the blood flow distribution through the EC-IC bypass but also to assess the variation in the rCBF during the surgery. Ecker et al. (2002) studied high-resolution dynamic infrared imaging in various neurosurgical procedures and showed that infrared imaging could be a valuable supplementary intraoperative diagnostic tool during the examinations. Real-time evaluation of cerebral perfusion and cerebral vessel patency are the major applications of infrared imaging, and provides real-time intraoperative anatomical and physiological information.

6.3.4.6   Ophthalmology

Graves ophthalmopathy (GO), an autoimmune disease, results in inflammation of eyes and if it is in an active state, immunosuppressive agents are prescribed for patients affected with the disease. Chang et al. (2008) examined the feasibility of digital infrared thermal imaging (DITI) to monitor the inflammatory state and the effect of methylprednisolone pulse therapy administered in patients with GO. The temperature of the lateral orbit (the reference point), caruncle, upper eyelid, lateral and medial conjunctiva, cornea, and lower eyelid were measured using the Spectrum 9000 MB series (United Integrated Service, Taipei Hsien, Taiwan) thermal camera, and the room temperature was maintained at 23°C. The difference of temperature between each region and the lateral orbit was determined. The result of the study indicated that based on the heat produced in the inflammation of GO, DITI could be used to monitor the result of methylprednisolone pulse therapy in patients with GO.

Phacoemulsification is the most widely used surgical technique for cataracts. Immediately after the introduction of the technique, serious surgical complications such as burns on the cornea were observed due to a rise in the heat around the phacoemulsification probe tip. To assess the heating, utilization of a thermocouple was tested, but it was not widely accepted because a thermocouple provides only local temperature, and inserting a thermocouple during an invasive procedure may result in problems for both the patient and surgeon. Corvi et al. (2006) examined the potential of thermography to examine and compare three cataract procedures: (1) the Sovereign phacoemulsification system with conventional technique, (2) the Sovereign WhiteStar phacoemulsification system with a conventional technique, and the (3) Sovereign WhiteStar Phacoemulsification with a bimanual technique. The thermal camera used for the testing was AGEMA Thermovision (880 LWB, AGEMA Infrared Systems) with a temperature sensitivity of 0.05°C at 30°C. The maximum temperature obtained for each procedure at the time of surgery was 44.9°C, 41°C, and 39.5°C, respectively. The results showed that the Sovereign WhiteStar phacoemulsification with bimanual technique had the least thermal effect on the eye with minimal amount of heat transmission. The authors concluded that thermography could be a potential noninvasive temperature monitoring technique during cataract procedures without the need for any change in surgical procedure and without any discomfort to the patient and the surgeon.

6.3.4.7 *Other medical and pharmaceutical applications*

People with serious motor impairments who cannot communicate through speech or gestures need an alternate method to communicate. In rehabilitation engineering, the alternative ways to communicate are referred to as access pathways. Some of the physiological signals that have been explored are electrical, hemodynamic activity of the brain, and electrodermal response of the skin. Memarian and Chau (2009) explored the potential of infrared thermography-based technology as a means for people with motor impairment to communicate. Ten participants were cued to open their mouths and keep it open for one second before closing. After closing the mouth every time, a 3 s rest was provided before the next opening. A THERMAL-EYE 2000B video camera was used to record the videos, which were processed offline in MATLAB®. The detection of mouth opening was achieved with high sensitivity (average sensitivity: 88.5% ± 11.3) and specificity (average specificity: 99.4% ± 0.7). The advantages of the proposed thermography method over other access technology such as sip and puff and EMG-based switches are noninvasive, requires no contact, and does not need any sensors attached externally to the user, independent of lighting and color, and hence can be used any time indoors or outdoors.

Food allergy is a major issue in developed countries and the diagnostic procedures vary in their efficiency. Infrared thermography could detect small increases in temperature during the positive skin prick test (Larbig et al., 2006). Clark et al. (2007) investigated the possibility of infrared thermography for assessing food challenge outcomes by investigating the facial temperature changes that occur during the testing. Twenty-four children with a history of egg allergy were given an incremental dosage of egg, either cooked or uncooked, at 10 min intervals. The subjects were grouped as positive when undesirable symptoms occurred and grouped negative when no symptoms were noticed after consuming all the dosage of egg. Symptoms were recorded and images were acquired using a thermal camera (ThermaCAM 500, FLIR Systems, West Malling, UK) with 0.07°C sensitivity, and the test was stopped when either all the dosage had been consumed or an objective reaction had happened. The analysis of thermal images showed that average nasal temperatures of participants from the positive group were higher than the baseline temperature at every point of time, whereas average nasal temperatures of participants from the negative group were below the baseline temperature at any point. Based on the results, the authors concluded that facial thermography detects an increase in nasal temperature for the positive challenge group before any objective symptom occurs. Therefore, thermography could be used to determine food challenges, and more studies need to be conducted to validate these finding in bigger populations with different food allergens.

Varicocele is considered a major cause of male infertility and is characterized by retrograde flow in the internal spermatic vein. Gat et al. (2004) evaluated three noninvasive procedures to detect left and right varicocele: physical examination, ultrasound Doppler, and scrotal contact thermography. Based on the study, scrotal contact thermography was established as the accurate method with sensitivity, specificity, accuracy, and positive predictive value of 98.9%, 66.6%, 98.5%, and 100%, respectively, for the left varicocele, and 95.6%, 91.6%, 94.9%, and 98%, respectively, for the right varicocele. Doppler sonography resulted in the highest number of false positives and it was concluded that for the detection of varicocele, thermography is more sensitive and accurate and can be used as an independent method for screening.

Infrared thermography has the potential to determine the temperature of pharmaceutical materials during compaction. During compaction of pharmaceutical materials, localized high temperature regions are created by interparticle friction, which could sometimes attain the melting point of the materials. Bechard and Down (1992) explored the infrared thermography technique to investigate the heat released during compaction of pharmaceutical powders and granules. An infrared thermal camera (Model 470, AGEMA Infrared Systems, Ontario, Canada) with high sensitivity (0.1°C at 30°C) and compaction was carried out with a rotary tablet press (Korsch PH106, Korsch Tableting, New Jersey). The model granulation used was a blend of microcrystalline cellulose and spray-dried lactose, and magnesium stearate was used as the lubricant. The results of the study showed that hot spots were seen at tablet edges where the die-wall friction occurs and the cross-sectional thermal profile revealed a 3°C to 4°C temperature gradient across the tablet. The experiment showed that infrared thermal imaging could be used as a unique tool for evaluation of heat released during compaction of pharmaceutical materials.

The accuracy of determining the absolute temperatures depends on the features of the infrared camera, the heat-producing characteristics of the object, and the temperature of the room, which are very important for use of thermal imaging in physiology and medicine. Ivanitsky et al. (2006) performed a study to compare two infrared cameras in the wavelength ranges of 3 to 5 μm and 8 to 12 μm for the diagnosis of different vascular pathologies. The study was conducted on more than 100 patients, and the air temperature in the room was maintained constant, and all measurements were performed at the same distance between the patient and camera. The resulting human thermal portraits obtained from both cameras differed insignificantly. However, the cameras operating in the 3 to 5 μm range showed higher sensitivity to reflexes of skin exposed to external sources of heat radiation.

6.4   Advantages, limitations, and future of thermal imaging

6.4.1   Advantages

Most imaging systems require an illumination source to acquire images, whereas no illumination source is essential for thermal imaging. Moreover thermal imaging cameras can acquire images even in fog, rain, mist, and smoke, and are not affected by weather conditions making them useful for many applications in various fields. Infrared thermal imaging is a noncontact and nondestructive method. In engineering applications, it does not obstruct or restrict the use of structure during examination. The image can be instantly obtained, and can be stored, retrieved, and processed later as per convenience. Thermal imaging is useful in assessing historical structures without disturbing or damaging the structures, and large concrete and masonry structures such as chimneys, towers, bridges, and buildings (Rao, 2008).

In medicine, thermal imaging is a painless, noninvasive procedure and does not emit harmful radiation, hence no risk is involved to the patient and provides immediate results. The real-time information provided by thermal imaging can be used as an instant feedback. Thermal imaging is inexpensive compared to MRI because MRI may cost around $2000 to conduct each examination and $2 million for the equipment, whereas digital infrared thermal imaging costs around $200 for each examination and approximately $25,000 for the equipment (Arora et al., 2008). Other than medicine, even in other areas of application, the cost of infrared thermal cameras is relatively low compared to other imaging devices due to the volume production and suitability of their application in many fields. In the food and processing industries, obtaining real-time accurate temperature measurement without any contact with the object is the most significant advantage of thermal imaging.

6.4.2   Limitations

In medicine, as opposed to X-ray and MRI that examine the anatomy, thermography is used to test physiology and is normally not an independent method. The biggest challenge in thermal imaging is to combine and analyze the physiological and anatomical information provided by the thermal pattern of the skin surface (Hildebrandt et al., 2010). Another drawback is that if determining tissue temperature underneath the skin, the skin temperature may exhibit different correlations with the body temperature and may not be unique (Jiang et al., 2005). In medical thermal imaging, accurate temperature measurement is sometimes difficult to perform due to existence of different emissivities and the presence of casts and bandages (Vardasca and Simoes, 2013). Thermal imaging could see only through the surface and surface defects could be monitored by surface thermal fluctuations, but it cannot see through the solid object as in X-ray imaging. Thermal cameras cannot see through walls and glass, water, or any reflective surface as the infrared image is reflected the same as is image in a mirror.

6.4.3   Future

Thermal imaging is widely adopted in various industries, including engineering, medical, food, agriculture, military, security, and surveillance applications. The thermal imaging was initially developed for military applications but later spread across every industry. The power to see through darkness has provided an irreplaceable position in security, surveillance, firefighting, search and rescue operations in various emergencies, airplanes, ships, and even the latest model cars. Noncontact accurate temperature measurement has made thermal imaging a necessary component in the food and processing industry, agriculture, and various engineering industries such as civil, electrical, mechanical, and aerospace. In medical industry, the importance of noncontact temperature measurement by thermal imaging has been experimented, tested, and verified, and is currently used in various diagnostic and treatment procedures. The real-time temperature measurement of thermal imaging is a very important characteristic of thermal imaging for its adoption in the medical, food, and processing industries. With increased application of thermal imaging in many industries, the manufacturing of thermal cameras has dramatically increased, which has ultimately decreased the cost of production. Many portable and hand-held thermal cameras are available in the market a very economic price range, which has resulted in affordability of thermal cameras even by very small businesses. With its many advantages and affordable prices, thermal imaging will be the most affordable technology of the future.

chapter seven

X-ray imaging

7.1 Introduction

X-ray was discovered by Wilhelm C. Roentgen in 1895. X-rays are electromagnetic radiation that lies between ultraviolet rays and gamma rays (Figure 7.1). The wavelength of X-rays lies in the range of 0.01 to 10 nm, corresponding to frequencies in the range of 3×10^{16} to 3×10^{19} Hz and energies in the range of 100 eV to 100 keV. X-rays are produced by a vacuum tube that contains a cathode and anode, and the vacuum tube is enclosed in a glass or metal envelope. Electrons are released from the cathode and are accelerated by high voltage in the vacuum tube. When these electrons with high velocity collide on a metal target (anode), X-rays are produced.

The important properties of X-rays are that they are invisible rays and travel in straight lines. X-rays are ionizing radiation that have enough energy to remove tightly bound electrons from atoms thus creating ions and they travel at the speed of light. X-rays cannot be deflected by magnetic or electric fields. X-rays can be classified into soft and hard X-rays depending on their penetrating ability. Soft X-rays range from 0.1 to 10 nm wavelength and corresponding energies from 0.12 to 12 keV. Soft X-rays have longer wavelength, lower energy, and lower penetration power, whereas hard X-rays have shorter wavelength, higher energy (>10 keV), and hence higher penetrating power. Soft X-rays are suitable for agricultural and food products due to their lower penetration capacity and their ability to characterize the differences in density. Hard X-rays, owing to higher penetration power, are extensively used to image the interior of objects and hence are mostly used in medical imaging and airport security scanning applications. X-rays were originally used in medical diagnosis, but later on, applications of X-ray use in other fields, such as astronomy, agriculture, food, aquaculture, dairy, pharmaceutical, and security, were explored.

7.2 Components and principles of an X-ray imaging system

The important components of a biological X-ray imaging system are (1) X-ray source, which produces X-rays; (2) a detector and a camera that captures the real-time image of the object of interest; (3) an image digitizer that converts the captured video image into a digital image; and (4) an image processing system, including analog-to-digital (A/D) converter, frame grabber, and a computer to store and process the digital images. Basic components are shown schematically in Figure 7.2.

7.2.1 X-ray source

The important parts of an X-ray generator are the X-ray tube, high voltage generator, and the control console. The X-ray tube basically consists of cathode and anode, rotor and stator, tube casing, and tube cooling system. The various X-ray beam characteristics, namely, X-ray field uniformity, focal spot size, and X-ray energy spectrum, are determined by the design of the X-ray tube. These characteristics are important because they affect the spatial resolution and image contrast (Zink, 1997). The X-ray generator supplies the power

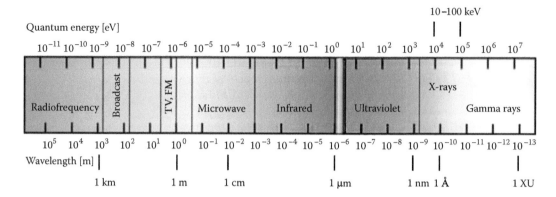

Figure 7.1 Electromagnetic spectrum. (From GE Measurement & Control.)

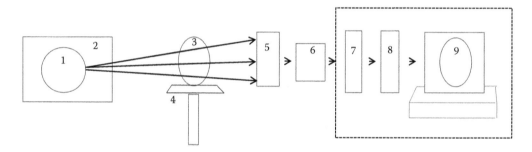

Figure 7.2 Basic components of an X-ray imaging system. (1) X-ray generator, (2) X-ray tube, (3) sample, (4) sample holder, (5) detector, (6) camera; image processor: (7) A/D converter, (8) frame grabber, and (9) image display.

required to produce X-rays, and X-rays are produced when electrons with high energy strike the target material, which is mostly tungsten or molybdenum. The focal spot is the origin of X-rays to produce radiograph and the focal spot size (or area) is the size of the target region over which X-rays are produced. The important characteristics of X-rays that determine the operating conditions are the voltage (or energy), current, and exposure time. The high voltage provided by the generator is selected according to the application and it determines the energy of the resulting X-rays. The peak voltage is called kilovoltage peak (kVp), and the current is based on the number of X-ray photons produced, which is represented in milliamperes (mA). Exposure time is the time during which high voltage is applied to produce X-rays. The amount of X-ray energy produced is controlled by the adjustment of voltage potential, X-ray tube current, and exposure time.

X-ray tubes and radioactive substances are two principal sources of X-rays. Radioactive substances produce monochromatic X-rays, whereas X-ray tubes produce polychromatic beams. X-ray tubes are most widely used for applications of X-ray radiography in the agriculture and food industry (Kotwaliwale et al., 2011).

7.2.2 Image intensifier

An image intensifier is a component that converts the low intensity X-rays into visible light and it amplifies the low level X-ray photons to visible image. The operating principle of an image intensifier is that X-ray photons penetrate the vacuum case where the X-ray photons are converted to optical photons, which are further converted to photoelectrons. Due to acceleration by the electric field, the photoelectrons are collected at the output phosphor and many optical photons are produced by each accelerated electron. Image intensifiers are specified by conversion factors, which represent how efficiently the image intensifier converts the X-rays to visible light (Wang and Blackburn, 2000).

7.2.3   Detectors and camera

The various types of detectors used for X-ray detection are gas detectors, solid state detectors, and charge-coupled device detectors. Conventionally, X-ray images are acquired either on photographic plates or films. X-ray films are most commonly used in medical applications because it provides a permanent record, and spatial resolution is typically in the range of 10 to 100 micron (Xradia, 2010). Photographic plates are similar to films in resolution and sensitivity, but they are reusable. But currently due to advancement in technology, X-ray images are acquired through digital methods. The major advantage of using digitized X-ray images is that they allow online quality monitoring of objects, such as food or agricultural produce or biological materials, along with the ease of storage and transmission and relatively lower time requirement for digital imaging. Haff and Slaughter (2004) reported that use of digital imaging saves time by a factor of four as compared to film radiographs. The various cameras used in X-ray imaging are CCD (charge-coupled device), line scan cameras, and flat panel sensors, because these cameras could be used in real-time imaging applications.

7.2.4   Image processing system (A/D converter, frame grabber, and computer)

The analog-to-digital converter is basically a device that converts the continuously varying analog signal to digital signal in binary form. The frame grabber captures video signals and converts them to digital form, which are displayed, transmitted, or stored. A computer attached to the imaging system serves as the software and hardware component to store and analyze the images using image processing algorithms.

7.2.5   Principle

The basic principle underlying X-ray imaging is that different objects absorb X-rays in different ways depending on the composition, density, and thickness. For instance, in the human body, bone absorbs X-rays much higher than soft tissues or cartilages, and hence they appear white in an X-ray image, whereas soft tissues such as muscles and cartilage appear gray and airspace looks black. The more the object absorbs the X-ray, the brighter it appears.

When any material is exposed to X-rays, the X-rays interact with the material and they lose their energy exponentially. This process by which X-rays lose their energy as it passes through objects is called attenuation. When passed through an object, photons present in a soft X-ray beam are transmitted, absorbed, or scattered, and the intensity of the photon is exponentially reduced, which is given by (Curry et al., 1990)

$$I = I_0 e^{-\mu z \rho}$$

where I represents the intensity of attenuated photons exiting through an object, I_0 is the intensity of incident photons, μ is the mass attenuation coefficient in square millimeters per gram (mm^2/g), ρ is the density of material in grams per cubic millimeter (g/mm^3), and z is the thickness in millimeters (mm). The ease of penetration of a material by a beam of sound, light, or other energy is described in terms of attenuation coefficient. A large attenuation coefficient denotes that the beam of light is easily weakened when it passes through the medium, whereas a smaller attenuation coefficient denotes that the intensity of the beam of light is not greatly reduced as it passes through the medium.

Intensity of X-rays depends on the number and energy of photons. The number of photons can be increased by increasing the tube current, and the energy of photons can be increased by increasing the peak voltage between the two electrodes (Kotwaliwale et al., 2003). There are many ways to attenuate X-rays, and it depends on how the photons interact with matter. There are three methods by which X-ray attenuation occurs: photoelectric absorption, Compton scattering, and pair production. When X-ray photons collide with an electron that is bound to an atom, photoelectric absorption occurs. Due to this collision, the electrons are knocked free from their orbit. When collision of X-ray photons occur with loosely held electrons, Compton scattering occurs. This kind of collision occurring between electrons and photons results in electrons being energized from photons, and the photons travel with less energy and in a different direction. Pair production does not occur at the energy levels typically used in the food industry (Peariso, 2008).

7.2.6 X-ray machine specification and type

Based on the application and the type of the product that needs to be monitored, there are basically three types of X-ray machines available for industrial applications: vertical beam system, horizontal beam system, or a combination of the two (Mettler Toledo, 2009).

7.2.6.1 Vertical beam X-ray system

The vertical beam system is the most common type of system used in which an X-ray generator is typically mounted on top of a cabinet and the X-ray beam passes downward through the object and strikes the detector. They are mostly used for objects that are smaller in depth compared to their length and width. In order to ensure that the entire object volume is inspected, the object should fit within the conical beam of the X-ray.

7.2.6.2 Horizontal beam X-ray system

Horizontal beam X-ray imaging units are used for objects that are higher in depth compared to the length and width dimensions. The X-ray generator is located at the sides of the product conveyor and scans the product through the sides. For low-density packaging such as cartons, plastic bottles, and plastic jars, a single horizontal X-ray beam system are used. A single horizontal beam system has one generator and a single X-ray beam scans the object as it passes along the conveyor (Figure 7.3a). For medium density packaging such as metal cans, a split dual beam arrangement can be used. From a single generator, the X-ray beam is funneled through a dual diverging collimator creating two separate angled beams, which helps in detecting small contaminants on the bottom or side walls of the container (Figure 7.3b). For high-density packages such as glass jars or bottles, dual X-ray generators are used, which produce two separate angled beams. For each product two images are obtained from different angles, which increase the efficiency of detection of contaminants (Figure 7.3c).

7.2.6.3 Combination beam system

In cases where even a dual beam system could not provide complete monitoring of the object, a combination of vertical and horizontal beam X-ray systems are used. These are

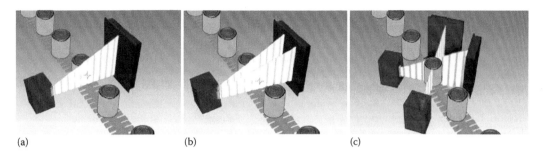

(a)   (b)   (c)

Figure 7.3 Schematics of different horizontal beam X-ray systems. (a) Single horizontal beam X-ray, (b) split dual beam X-ray, and (c) two beams of X-rays from two generators. (From Mettler Toledo, 2009, *Safeline X-ray inspection guide*. With permission.)

the most advanced X-ray systems available for the food industry for best possible detection and monitoring of products.

7.3   Present applications in bio-industries

The food and agriculture industry has started installing X-ray units for monitoring the quality of products to ensure that quality is not compromised during processing. Metal detectors in many industries are replaced by X-ray imaging due to their higher efficiency in performance. In the food and food processing industry, implementation of an X-ray imaging system as a part of an effective overall inspection system improves the product quality and to a great extent reduces the possibility of product recall, which would result in better brand name and greater business opportunity. The commercial applications of X-ray imaging in food industry are listed in Table 7.1.

7.3.1   Detection of contamination

Presence of physical contaminants in food products, such as broken pieces of glass, plastic, metal, or other unwanted materials, is a major concern in the food industry. It poses a serious health hazard to the consumer and compromised quality for the processor, which may even result in huge financial losses due to product recalls. Metal detectors are mostly employed to detect unwanted physical impurities. But the trend is changing in the food and processing industry to replace metal detectors with X-ray imaging units.

Bottled mushrooms are inspected by an X-ray inspection unit at Zhangzhou Gang Chang Can Food Company (China) to identify and reject jars with any contaminants such as glass, stone, metal, and plastic, and handles up to 600 jars/min. The unit also ensures that the closure is in place and checks the fill level. The system also has a variable speed detection capability, which enables smooth handling of various line speeds without interrupting the inspection. Pukka Pies, a well-known UK brand that produces 50 million pies and sausage per year, has installed a T10 X-ray machine that is capable of detecting metal, glass, stone, and plastic as small as 1 mm. Orval Kent (Mexico) produces 80 different kinds of salad that are packed in PET jars of 4 and 8 lb (1.8 and 3.6 kg), and 1, 3, and 5 lb (10.45, 1.36, and 2.27 kg) flexible pouches. Orval Kent installed a PowerChek X-ray unit to detect metal, glass, plastic, and other foreign materials. If a foreign object is detected in a package, it is removed from the production line and sent to the quality control lab for further inspection (Reynolds, 2011). The Really Cool Food Company, a manufacturer that produces more than

Table 7.1 Commercial Applications of X-Ray Imaging in Food Industry

Model/manufacturer	Industry	Material	Application
GlassChek (Mettler Toledo, Zurich, Switzerland)	Zhangzhou Gang Chang Can food company, Fujian China	Bottled mushroom	Detection of stone, glass, metal, plastics
T10 XP (Mettler Toledo, Leicester, UK)	Pukka Pies, Syston, Leicester, UK	Pies and sausage	Detection of metal, glass, stone and plastic
AdvanChek (Mettler Toledo, Columbus, Ohio)	Really Cool Food, Cambridge City, Indiana	Organic entrees, salads	Detection of contaminants
X^4 (Loma, Hannover, Germany)	Bäckerei Brinker, Germany	Bakery	Detection of contaminants
X^4 (Loma, Hampshire, UK)	J.B. Groothandel, Vlees, Vriezenveen, The Netherlands	Meat	Detection of contaminants
X^4 (Loma, Hampshire, UK)	Culi d'Or, Velp, Holland, The Netherlands	Dessert	Stainless steel, ferrous and nonferrous metals, plastic, rubber, glass, and stone
X^4 (Loma, Hampshire, UK)	Central Food Services, Birmingham, England	Frozen meat	Metallic and nonmetallic contaminants
IX-GA-2475 (Ishida, Birmingham, UK)	Rose Poultry, Skovsgaard, Denmark	Chicken	Contaminants like bone, glass, shell, grit, plastic, and rubber
PowerChek (Mettler Toledo Safeline Inc., Tampa, Florida)	Orval Kent, Linares, Mexico	Fruit salad	Metal, glass, plastic and other foreign bodies
EZx (ThermoFisher Scientific, Waltham, MA)	Golden Boy Foods Inc., Burnaby, BC	Pouches of nuts, dried fruit, trail mixes	Detection of glass, metal, and foreign materials

120 prepared food products, installed an AdvanChek X-ray system from Mettler Toledo. The AdvanChek X-ray system uses a single beam X-ray generator along with data and image analysis software to detect any contaminant that are of different densities than the product being inspected (Hartman, 2009).

Bäckerei Brinker, a famous company in Germany that sells fresh baked, deep frozen, and partially baked bread throughout Europe, has installed an X-ray imaging system to detect foreign bodies (Packaging Europe, 2009). Meat processing plant J.B. Groothandel, a modern pig slaughterhouse in Netherlands, has installed an X-ray (X^4) unit for meat inspection. It processes about 300 tonnes of pig's head every week (Connecting Industry, 2009). Culi d'Or, a major dessert producer in Europe, has installed the latest X-ray (X^4) machine, which has high-speed technology and enables determination of metal and non-metallic contaminants such as metals, stainless steel, plastic, rubber, glass, and stone. More than the detection of contamination, it could also detect various defects in the product such as mass measurement and shape conformity (Loma Systems/Cintex, 2007). Central Food Services (England), a frozen meat processor, has installed Loma X^4, an X-ray machine to detect metallic and nonmetallic contaminants in its products packed in tinfoil trays. There are 97 different specifications of products that were preprogrammed in the X-ray unit, which ensures switchover of product in about 30 s without any mechanical changes (Loma Systems, 2012).

Eagle has a range of X-ray imaging units (Eagle pack 240 XE, Eagle pack 240, Eagle pack 320, Eagle pack 400 HC, Eagle pack 720, Eagle pack 1000) capable of 240 to 400 mm detection coverage at the belt and a high imaging speed up to 62 m/min. These units are capable of inspecting 300 items per minute and are ideal for using in confectionary, bakery and snack, dairy, meat, and poultry plants. There are different ranges of X-ray units for usage in rigid container product inspection such as products packed in cans, bottles, or jars.

Theo Müller (Germany) developed the SC 4000 L and SC5000 X-ray scanner to detect foreign objects even with a diameter of less than 1 mm, and the system is incorporated in its HACCP program to monitor the product. The X-ray unit is also capable of monitoring the filling level of its dairy products (OCS Checkweighers, 2013).

Detecting contamination in multitextured food, such as a bag of salad leaves or mixed nuts, is a great challenge. Material discrimination X-ray (MDX) technology is able to discriminate materials based on their chemical composition. This technology was originally used in security checking but it has been adopted in the food industry. This technology allows detection and rejection of inorganic contaminants such as rubber, plastics, stones, and glass (Woolford, 2011b).

The presence of bones in boneless poultry meat is one of the most common problems faced by the poultry industry. The poultry industry faces huge insurance claims and lawsuits, and about two-thirds are due to the presence of bones in foods labeled as boneless meat (Smith, 1999). Rose Poultry, the largest producer of chicken products (around 290,000 chickens per day) in Denmark, has installed the Ishida (IX-GA-2475) X-ray inspection system that can detect fragments as small as 0.3 mm in diameter and a variety of contaminants such as glass, bone, plastic, shell, grit, and rubber. The X-ray inspection unit operates at a speed of 160 fillets per minute per line (Ishida, 2008).

Removal of bone from poultry is a major challenge for the meat processing plant. Marel has designed a SensorX bone detection system that automatically determines the bone and other contaminants such as metal, stone, and glass (Figure 7.4). An accuracy of more than 99% on detection of calcified bone larger than 2 mm can be achieved by this unit with a false positive less than 3% (Marel, 2013).

7.3.2 Shell removal from whelk

Whelk (various kinds of sea snails used as food) is largely consumed as a food in Korea. Cape Mariner Enterprises Limited (CME), a Newfoundland and Labrador Company, processes whelk in large scale and exports to Korea. Presence of shell in whelk is a food safety concern as well as it reduces the market value of whelk. X-ray imaging technology is considered a potential technology to monitor for complete removal of shell in cooked whelk. Initial tests were performed and based on satisfactory performance of X-ray machines, CME has installed an X-ray detection and rejection equipment for whelk processing plants to improve the quality of the product and efficiency of the process (Fisheries and Aquaculture, 2009).

7.3.3 Inspection of pumped products

Food products in semisolid state or slurries, and fluids such as jams, ice cream, yogurt, juice, smoothies, melted chocolates, and sauces are inspected by X-ray units to detect

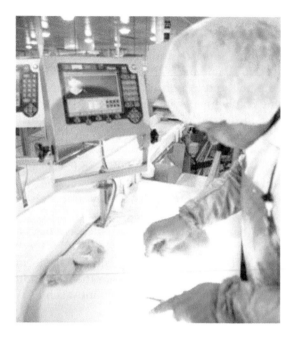

Figure 7.4 Poultry deboning with use of X-ray machine. (From Marel, 2013, X-ray bone detection, http://marel.com/Systems-And-Equipment/Poultry/Processes/Broilers/Deboning-and-skinning/1347/X-ray -Bone-Detection/1354/default.aspx; accessed November 30, 2012. With permission.)

contamination at an early stage of the production to minimize wastage and save costs. Due to the homogeneous nature of the product, detection of contamination is very high.

7.3.4 Determination of composition

Eagle has an X-ray unit for fat analysis using dual energy X-ray absorptiometry (DEXA) technology. This system measures chemical lean (CL) values with an accuracy of ±1CL. This X-ray unit determines not only the fat content of the meat but also inspects for metal, stone, glass, or bone contamination, and could check the mass of meat at a speed of around 145,000 kilogram of bulk meat per hour. Another new model of the Eagle X-ray unit (Eagle pack 400 HC) is especially designed for easy and efficient cleaning of packaged meat and poultry and dairy-based products to facilitate compliance with the food safety standards.

7.3.5 Detection of defects in products

X-ray inspection units could detect defects in food products to a great extent. The various examples in which food product integrity are monitored are undersize or oversize products, wrong boundary length such as short or big chocolate bar, cavity inside a block of butter, or cracks or splits in sausages (Ishida, 2009).

7.3.6 Monitoring packaging and sealing

Monitoring the proper sealing of food packages is as important as monitoring for contamination in the product. Improper sealing may result in contamination and rejection of the product. X-ray inspection units are used for monitoring the seal integrity of various packaged food products such as yogurt. A dual beam X-ray system identifies and rejects containers such as those dented, damaged, or upside down.

7.4   Agricultural and food product inspection and quality evaluation

Research studies are being conducted around the globe using X-ray imaging to improve the quality of agricultural and food products. The potential of X-ray imaging is not completely utilized in the agricultural and food industry sector and various researches are aimed at exploring the possibility of using X-ray imaging for various applications not currently available. Table 7.2 shows the various research studies on X-ray imaging in the agriculture and food industry.

7.4.1   X-ray quarantine for agricultural products

Globalization and the improvement in technology to import and export fresh agricultural products has strengthened countries' economies, but has also resulted in insect and pest invasion from one country to another causing serious damage. For instance, the Asian longhorned beetle arrived from China in wooden packing materials and got established in Chicago causing extensive damage to trees and the ecology (Poland et al., 1998). Chuang et al. (2011) developed an effective quarantine X-ray imaging system for detecting insect infestation in various fruits including apple, peach, and guava. The ability of the system was tested by introducing eggs of the pest inside the fruit and monitoring the development of the infestation stages. The system was able to detect the infestation in 2 to 3 days, even though there was no visible damage on the surface of the fruit. The results showed that the X-ray quarantine and pest infestation detector system could identify the infested sites at a success rate of 94% on the fourth day after the eggs were introduced into the fruit.

Jiang et al. (2008) developed an algorithm for quarantine inspection of fruits such as peach, guava, and citrus using X-rays. The basic aim of the study was to analyze the acquired X-ray images to detect pest infestation of fruits. The imaging setup consisted of an X-ray source (Hamamatsu L8601-01), a line-scan camera, a frame grabber, and a computer. The fruits were implanted with eggs of the Oriental fruit fly (*Bactrocera dorsalis* Hendel) and development of larvae was monitored by X-ray imaging and visual inspection. The acquired images were then processed using an image segmentation technique to determine the site of internal infestation. Then noise removal was performed by removal of background pixels and then adaptive thresholding was applied. The binary image obtained by adaptive thresholding contains cavities or tunnels made by pests, and hence, a hole-filling step was applied to fill these spots to create a temporary image followed by morphological filtering. Jiang et al. concluded that the developed algorithm could be used without significant modification for inspection and monitoring of various agricultural products with different densities and thickness.

7.4.2   Dynamic X-ray imaging

A novel X-ray imaging technology to identify moving objects in agricultural or packaged food was developed by Osváth and Szigeti (2012). This technology could be very useful for determination of pests in agricultural products or cargo that are shipped from other countries. Dynamic imaging provides two images at the same time, one is the conventional

Table 7.2 Research Studies on Potential Applications of X-Ray Imaging
in Food and Agricultural Industry

Model/manufacturer	Material	Application	Reference
Hamamatsu L8601-01, (Hamamatsu Photonics K.K., Tokyo, Japan)	Apple, peach, guava	Quarantine of agricultural products	Jiang et al., 2008; Chuang et al., 2011
NA	Agricultural or packaged food	Determination of pests	Osváth and Szigeti, 2012
NA	Agricultural products	Flow rate monitoring	Inanc, 2001
Faxitron X-ray cabinet (Faxitron Corp., Buffalo Grove, Illinois), LX-85708 (Lixi Inc., Downers. Grove, Illinois), Electonika 25 (ARI St. Petersburg, Russia)	Grain: wheat	Detection of insect infestation	Haff and Slaughter, 2004; Karunakaran et al., 2004a,b,c; Fornal et al., 2007; Haff and Pearson, 2007
Marel hf (Gardabaer, Iceland)	Fish	Pinbone detection	Andersen, 2003
XT60-60 (Matsusada Precision Co. Ltd., Kusatsu City, Shiga, Japan)	Apple, pear, peach	Internal quality evaluation	Ogawa et al., 2003
EaglePak (Smith-Heimann Systems Corp., Alcoa, Tennessee)	Onion	Internal quality evaluation	Tollner et al., 2005
43804N (Faxitron X-ray Corporation, Wheeling, Illinois)	Olives	Detection of infestation	Jackson and Haff, 2006
Faxitron X-ray cabinet (Faxitron Corp., Buffalo Grove, Illinois)	Pineapple	Detection of translucency	Haff et al., 2006
BJI-1U (Bo Jin Electronic Instrument Inc., Shanghai, China)	Apple	Internal quality evaluation	Yang et al., 2009
Philips Diagnost 97 (Philips Healthcare Inc., Andover, Massachusetts)	Tomato, orange, apple, pear, peach	Detection of fruit fly infestation	Yang et al., 2006
Faxitron cabinet film X-ray machine (Faxitron X-ray Corp., Wheeling, Illinois)	Almonds	Detection of pinholes	Kim and Schatzki, 2001
XTF™-5011 (Oxford Instruments X-Ray Technologies Inc., Abingdon, Oxfordshire, UK)	Pecans	Determination of defects and insect	Kotwaliwale et al., 2007
T80-1-60 (BMEI Co. Ltd., Beijing, China)	Chestnuts	Detection of internal defects	Lü et al., 2010

(Continued)

Table 7.2 (Continued) Research Studies on Potential Applications of X-Ray Imaging
in Food and Agricultural Industry

Model/manufacturer	Material	Application	Reference
Poskom XM-20BT (Poskom Co. Ltd., Goyang, Korea)	Fish	Bone detection	Mery et al., 2011
NA	Chicken	Bone detection	McFarlane et al., 2003
Pencil beam DXA scanner (Lunar DPX-L, Lunar Corp., Madison, Wisconsin)	Chicken	Determination of body composition	Swennen et al., 2004
Norland XR-26 Fan beam (Norland Cooper Surgical Inc., Fort Atkinson, Wisconsin)	Sheep	Carcass composition of live sheep	Pearce et al., 2009
F-scan X-ray unit (Xavis Co. Ltd., Gyeonggi-Do, Korea)	Apple	Watercore detection	Kim and Schatzki, 2000
Faxitron 43805 N (Hewlett Packard, Palo Alto, California) Inspector XR200 (Golden Engineering Inc., Indiana)	Wood	Evaluation of wood degradation by fungi and wood density	Roig et al., 2008; Tomazello et al., 2008; Moya and Tomazello-Filho, 2009; Lechner et al., 2013

image and the other will highlight the motion of the pest (or the object) by a different type of contrast. The static components fade away while the moving objects appear brighter. This dynamic X-ray imaging could be very useful for determination of insects and pests in agricultural products or packaged food.

7.4.3   Quantification and flow rate measurements

Inanc (2001) studied the possibility of using X-ray for yield and flow rate monitoring of agricultural products (corn, sugar cane) and chemicals (granular urea, monoammonium phosphate, diammonium phosphate, anhydrous ammonia, liquid fertilizer, muriate of potash). Insensitivity of X-rays to moisture variation and its noncontact nature has made X-ray a potential method for quantification and flow rate measurements. Inanc concluded that it is feasible to use X-ray for flow rate measurement of agricultural products in laboratories, but new detectors with dynamic range need to be developed for actual field measurements.

7.4.4   Detection of insect infestation

7.4.4.1   Grain

Haff and Slaughter (2004) developed a real time X-ray inspection system to determine the infestation of life stages of granary weevil (*Sitophilus granarius* L.). About 1500 kernels were X-rayed, and images were obtained in both film and digital method. The images were provided to human subjects for identification of infested kernels. Infested kernels were correctly identified 84.4% and 90.2% with digital and film images, respectively. However, when the insect life stage was higher than the third larval instar, the error in identification was less than 2% for both film and digital images or the accuracy in identification was more than 98%.

Haff and Pearson (2007) developed an algorithm for X-ray images for detection of granary weevil in wheat and Olive fly (*Bactrocera oleae* L.) in olives. They developed algorithm based on discriminant analysis using Bayesian classifiers, which was suitable for high-speed image analysis. The algorithm for detection of granary weevil had a 14.4% error comparable to that of human inspection, which had an overall error of 15.6%. Results on olives produced a 12% error for large infestation and 50% error for small infestation.

Fornal et al. (2007) developed a method for early identification of granary weevil life stages in wheat. Fifty kernels were glued to paper and placed in a petri dish along with adult *S. granarius* for 3, 5, 7, 10, 20, and 30 days. The adults were removed and the number of eggs laid were counted and marked based on plugs secreted on the kernel. X-ray images were obtained at 20 kV and 60 μA for 120 s. The algorithm for detecting insects was developed in three stages. First to adjust the visual quality, the "contrast enhancement" control was used. Next, filtration of the image was performed by a local equalization filter, which enhances the contrast near the edges making dark and light areas of the images clearly visible. Then thresholding of filtered images was performed. The results demonstrated that soft X-ray is suitable for early detection of granary weevil eggs in wheat at least 5 days after oviposition has occurred.

Vitreousness, which gives a glassy or translucent appearance that corresponds to high protein content, is the primary quality characteristic in classifying Durum wheat. The standards set by the Canadian market for Grade 1 Canada Western Amber Durum wheat is that the lot should contain more than 80% hard vitreous kernels (Canadian Grain Commission, 2005). Neethirajan et al. (2007a) studied the possibility of dual energy X-ray image analysis for identification of vitreous wheat kernels and determined the accuracy of classification of vitreous and nonvitreous kernels based on artificial neural networks and statistical classifiers. Their results showed that vitreous and nonvitreous kernels were classified with an accuracy of 93% for neural network classifiers and 89% for statistical classifiers. Neethirajan et al. concluded that dual energy X-ray image analysis technique has a high potential and could be used for classification of vitreous kernels in durum wheat.

Karunakaran et al. (2004a,b,c) conducted extensive research on detection of infestation by rusty grain beetle (*Cryptolestes ferrugineus* Stephens), red flour beetle (*Tribolium castaneum* Herbst), and lesser grain borer (*Rhyzopertha dominica* Fabricius) in wheat using soft X-ray imaging. The X-ray imaging system shown in Figure 7.5 consisted of a Lixi fluoroscope, a CCD black-and-white camera, a monitor to display the image, an image digitizer, and a personal computer to store and process the images. Infested kernels of wheat were prepared by implanting eggs into a hole made on the germ of the kernel with the help of a single hairbrush. The kernels were placed in a gelatin capsule and X-ray images were obtained at 15 kV and 65 μA for 3 to 5 s. The detection accuracy for the four stages of larvae of *T. castaneum* was 73% and 86% using statistical and neural network classifiers, respectively. The classification accuracy of *C. ferrugineus* was 75.3% and 95.7% by statistical and neural network classifiers, respectively. For *R. dominica*, the neural network classifier performed better and classified all uninfested kernels and 99% of infested kernels. Karunakaran et al. concluded that soft X-ray technique has a great potential to detect insect infestation in wheat.

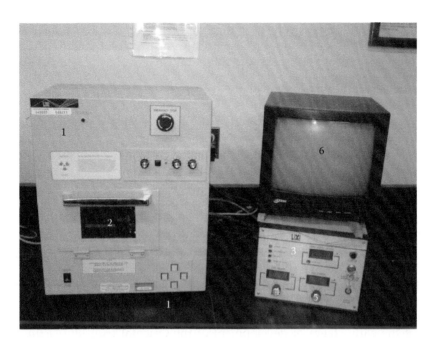

Figure 7.5 X-ray imaging system used for insect detection. (1) X-ray source, (2) sample, (3) Lixi fluoroscope, (4) voltage control, (5) current control, and (6) monitor. (Courtesy of University of Manitoba, Winnipeg, Canada.)

Nawrocka et al. (2012) studied the mass loss determination of kernels of wheat infested by granary weevil using an X-ray imaging method. Mass loss of kernels depends on the insect's life stage and hence finding the correlation between the developmental stage of the insect pest and the mass loss of the kernel could provide sufficient information to decide on pest management strategies and also could be helpful in determining the time of infestation. Initial mass of kernels were determined and placed along with adult granary weevils for 2 weeks and the infested kernels were then separated. X-ray images were taken 20 days after infestation and imaging was completed on the 66th day. The images were acquired on 20 fixed dates. The mass losses were calculated from X-ray images and the infested kernels were classified into six groups based on mass loss: sound, small larva (mass loss 0.5–3 mg), medium larva (mass loss 3.1–9.0 mg), large larva (mass loss 9.1–20.0 mg), pupae (loss of mass more than 20.1 mg), and adult emerged. They stated that it was more reliable to classify kernels based on mass loss and it could be used as an indicator of infestation time and location of infestation in grain.

Fungal growth affects the quality of grain and the major fungal species affecting cereals are *Aspergillus* spp., *Penicillium* spp., and *Fusarium* spp., which produce mycotoxins such as aflatoxin, Ochratoxin A, citrinin, and xanthoquinones. Mycotoxin affects the quality of grain and causes serious health issues to the consumers. Most of the methods currently used in the industry for determining fungal infection are time consuming and tedious, hence, Narvankar et al. (2009) examined the ability of soft X-ray imaging for detecting fungal infection in wheat. Sound kernels and kernels infected with fungi *Aspergillus niger*, *A. glaucus* group, and *Pencilliulm* spp. were selected for the study. Images were acquired for 300 kernels from each group using soft X-ray imaging system. The classification accuracy for a linear discriminant classifier and two-class Mahalanobis discriminant classifier were

82% and 92.2%–98.9%, respectively, for fungal infected kernels. The statistical classifier resulted in higher accuracy and lower false positive results compared to neural network classifiers. Narvankar et al.'s study showed that X-ray imaging has a potential for detecting fungal infection in wheat.

7.4.4.2 Produce

Infestation of mango by seed weevil (*Cryptorhynchus mangiferae* Fabricius) does not show any external indications, but it significantly affects the quality and results in a bigger loss for the mango processing industry and a greater restriction on the export of the fruit. A potential nondestructive technique to detect weevil infestation in mango was studied by P. Thomas et al. (1995) using X-ray imaging. Fruits of mango cultivar Neelam and Alphonso were brought to the laboratory in less than 3 days after harvest. X-ray radiographs of mango were obtained using a Polymat 501 X-ray machine operated at 40 kV and 800 mA. The fruits were then cut into halves to verify whether the fruits were healthy or weevil infested. X-ray radiographs showed darker gray areas of infested fruit corresponding to the disintegrated kernel tissue, whereas uniform and light gray areas were seen in radiographs of healthy fruits. The study suggested that X-ray imaging has a potential to monitor and detect seed-weevil-infested mango.

Yang et al. (2006) explored the possibility of determining the insect infestation of various fruits at the early stages of development of the Oriental fruit fly (*Bactrocera dorsalis* Hendel) using X-ray imaging. The various fruits selected for the study were orange (*Citrus sinensis* L.), apple (*Malus pumila* Auct.), pear (*Pyrus communis* L.), peach (*Prunus persica* L.), and berry tomato (*Lycopersivon esculentum*). Fruits were infested by artificially placing the eggs of the Oriental fruit fly inside the fruits. In every fruit, a pinhole was made, 12 eggs were implanted, and then instantly covered with surgical tape. For the control sample, the fruits were pierced and covered with surgical tape without implanting the eggs. Three replications were done for every fruit, and X-ray images were taken using the Philips Diagnost 97 X-ray system (40–50 kV and 12 mA). The earliest time to detect internal infestation in apples was 7 days, and a tunnel created by larvae was detected in X-ray images that matched the internal injury when the fruit was cut open. In pears and peaches, the internal injury was detected in 3 and 4 days, respectively, after implanting eggs, whereas the injury was serious at or after 6 days. It took 6 days to detect the infestation in cherry tomatoes and oranges. The study showed that the earliest time for detection of internal injuries by X-ray imaging for various fruits was different. The injuries caused by an insect's ovipositor may be too small to be detected by X-ray imaging, but the tunnel damage caused by larvae provided a good contrast on the X-ray images and was easily detectable.

7.4.4.3 Nuts

Aflatoxin, a mycotoxin produced by species of *Aspergillus flavus*, is considered a potential contaminant in many food products including nuts. Infestation of nuts by Navel orange worm (*Amyelois transitella* Walker) increases the probability of aflatoxin contamination. Grading and monitoring of pistachio nuts is conducted by manual inspectors by opening the nuts and visually inspecting for insect damage. Keagy et al. (1996) studied the possibility of X-ray image analysis as a nondestructive method for determination of Navel orange worm. Pistachio nuts were X-rayed (25 keV) with a Faxitron series X-ray system. They concluded that it is possible to determine insect infested nuts but 100% accuracy is not possible.

Navel orange worms bore small holes of less than 1 mm diameter (pinholes) in almonds and is the most common type of insect damage. It is very difficult to manually observe pinholes in almonds because the almond is still covered by a brown membrane, and hence an automated monitoring system to observe the interior of the nuts will be the most valuable detection method for the nuts processing industry. Kim and Schatzki (2001) studied the possibility of detecting pinhole damage found in almonds using X-ray imaging. X-ray images were obtained in two ways. First, almonds were imaged using a Faxitron cabinet film X-ray machine (60 s exposure, 32 keV, 3 mA), and digitization of images was performed using a Lumiscan film scanner. Next, line scan images of almonds were obtained using a line scanner (3 ms exposure, 35 keV, 30 mA). Scanned film images appeared sharper, had lesser noise, and higher resolution, but image acquisition time was longer. The algorithm was developed using image processing techniques, such as filtering and thresholding. The algorithm for line scanned images detected 74% of pinholes with 12% false positives, whereas with scanned film images 1% false positives were obtained. The algorithm provided better results on scanned film images compared to line scan images due to its limited horizontal and vertical resolution of 0.5 mm/pixel, which is insufficient to identify small pinholes.

Pecan nuts are infested by pecan weevil (*Curculio caryae* Horn) larvae. The nuts damaged by larvae could be easily detected by low specific gravity if the larvae have consumed the nut meat and exited the nut. But, it is difficult to determine if the larvae is present inside the nut. Kotwaliwale et al. (2007) explored the potential of X-ray imaging to determine the pecan nut quality. A soft X-ray imaging system (XTF™-5011) was used to obtain images at eight levels of X-ray tube voltage (15–50 keV in steps of 5 keV) and five current levels (0.1, 0.25, 0.5, 0.75, and 1.0 mA). Ten pecan nuts were fabricated with known defects and 30 nuts with unknown quality attributes were selected for the study. Preprocessing techniques were conducted to separate the region of interest from the background image. Manual segmentation was performed for each image with four distinct regions: (1) dark area, which represents the shell; (2) nutmeat, which is the area inside the shell portion; (3) central dark area, which represents the woody separator of pecan nuts; and (4) light area, which represents the gap between the nutmeat and shell. By applying contrast stretching, features of pecan nuts such as shell, air gap, nutmeat, defects, and presence of insects were clearly seen in X-ray images. Their study showed that defects and insects could be determined in pecan nuts by X-ray imaging.

Chestnut has a hard reddish brown shell that makes it very difficult to inspect using conventional techniques. Lü et al. (2010) studied the potential of X-ray imaging for nondestructive monitoring of chestnuts that are insect damaged, air-dried, or decayed. For the study, 475 nuts that were insect damaged, air-dried, decayed, or normal were obtained from cold storage. Chestnuts were imaged 20 at a time at 65 keV and 0.6 mA. After imaging, the shells were removed and the chestnuts were manually inspected. The irregular shape and size of chestnuts and the presence of many furrows on the surface of nutmeat made it difficult for segmentation to be performed. Hence to accurately evaluate the quality, a dynamic threshold segmentation algorithm was developed. The results showed that for healthy nuts, the classification accuracy was 87% with 13% false positives. For diseased nuts, classification accuracy was 93.5% with 6.5% false positives. The authors concluded that X-ray imaging has great potential to monitor the quality of chestnuts, and it took only 27 ms to inspect one nut, which is fast enough to be implemented on a real-time inspection unit.

7.4.5 Quality evaluation of agricultural products using X-ray imaging

With increased awareness on the quality characteristics of food, it becomes essential to monitor the internal quality characteristics of fruits and vegetables before they reach the consumer. Some conditions that occur on the inside of fruit, such as watercore damage in apples, split pits in peaches, and spongy tissue in mango, cannot be identified by inspecting the external surface. Conventional techniques fail to detect the internal damage due to the good appearance of the external features. Techniques like X-ray imaging can monitor the quality characteristics of fresh fruits and vegetables.

Kim and Schatzki (2000) developed an algorithm for detecting watercore in apples using X-ray imaging. It is very difficult to detect watercore in apples at the early stages based on visual inspection, because watercore does not affect the external appearance of the apple until it is very severe. Twenty boxes of Fuji and 20 boxes of Red Delicious apples were scanned with nine apples at a time using an X-ray unit at 49.9 to 50 keV and at 9.9 to 13 mA. After obtaining X-ray images, apples were cut into three slices and the watercore levels were evaluated based on a scale of 0 (good) to 4 (severe) indicating watercore-affected apples. The algorithm consists of two stages. The first stage was to extract features from the images and the second was to classify apples based on features extracted. A total of eight features was extracted and classified using an artificial neural network classifier. The classification gave a false positive of 5% and a false negative of 8%. The algorithm had the capability to sort apples irrespective of fruit orientation, but the stem-calyx axis should make a fixed angle with the X-ray beam and the speed of processing was on par with the current commercial processing lines.

Ogawa et al. (2003) studied the internal quality evaluation of apples, pears, and peaches using X-ray imaging. The soft X-ray generator used for the study was XT60-60 and the selected voltage and current was 60 keV and 3 mA, respectively. X-ray images were captured and analyzed and it was possible to detect split pits of apples and peaches.

Pineapple is an international crop and a common internal physiological disorder called translucency results in a water-soaked appearance of the flesh of the pineapple. A nondestructive determination technique for identifying translucency in pineapple is very limited. The size and skin toughness of pineapple poses a challenge for the use of near-infrared (NIR) spectroscopy, light transmission, or acoustic methods. Hence, X-ray imaging was explored by Haff et al. (2006) to determine translucency in pineapple. Pineapples of Gold cultivar with suspected translucency and healthy ones were used for the experiment. The pineapples were subjected to X-ray (30 keV, 3 min exposure) and then cut to determine the translucency on a scale of 1 to 5. The accuracy for determination of healthy pineapple and translucent pineapple using X-ray imaging was 95% and 86%, respectively.

Spongy tissue is an internal ripening disorder in mango, which results in damage to the mesocarp (flesh) and appears pale yellow and has an off-flavor (Subramanyam et al., 1971). Since the fruit appearance does not show any external symptoms during harvesting or at ripening, it is hard to determine the mangoes affected by spongy tissue. Thomas et al. (1993) studied the use of X-ray imaging of mangoes using 6R X-ray machine (36 kV, 10 mA) or Polymat 501 X-ray machine (40 kV, 12 mA), and 9 to 12 samples were placed in a single frame for X-ray photography. After imaging, the fruits were cut into halves for verification for the presence of spongy tissues. X-ray photographs showed indication of mesocarp damage by dark gray patches, whereas healthy fruits showed no dark regions. They concluded that X-ray imaging could be useful for quality monitoring and detection of spongy tissues in mangoes.

Deshpande et al. (2010) developed an X-ray imaging technique to determine the spongy tissue disorder in Alphonso mangoes. Initially, they used conventional X-ray imaging, and images were captured on X-ray film at 48 kV and 8 mA. The film was scanned using the scanner, but there was no significant information available from the image. Hence, further images were obtained using digital X-ray machines at 42 kV and 12 mA. The best contrast images were obtained when the X-ray source was set at 45 to 50 kV and 10 to 12 mA. The images were preprocessed and converted to gray scale images, and then morphological operations of region filling was performed. The image was segmented by thresholding and after the application of a linear filter, the area of interest was extracted and displayed. The images of affected mangoes showed dark areas, whereas there was no dark region present in the healthy fruits. They concluded that X-ray imaging could be used to determine spongy tissue disorder in mangoes and further study to optimize the parameters for reduced processing time will result in implementation of this technique for online quality evaluation of fruits.

Presence of voids in onions may be due to bacterial or fungal rots. Tollner et al. (2005) conducted a series of tests at the University of Georgia and Vidalia Onion Research Center to detect the quality of onion using X-ray machines. In 2001, two 100-onion batches were inspected using X-ray machines and visually inspected for internal quality. The accuracy of the test was greater than 93% and false positives were less than 6%. In 2002 and 2004, onions with mild to severe defects were passed through the X-ray machine multiple times without controlling the orientation of the onion. The X-ray detection unit was able to achieve 100% accuracy in onions with no or slight defects and 100% accuracy in rejecting onions with severe defects. Eighty percent of onions that passed visual inspection but identified as diseased by the X-ray unit showed the disease symptoms on cutting into halves and false positives were in the range of 10% to 15%. The normally accepted accuracy and false positive is 90% and 10%, respectively, and the experimental results are very close to the acceptable standards. Hence, they concluded that X-ray inspection is a commercially viable technology for detecting voids in onions.

7.4.5.1 Detection of body composition

Dual energy X-ray absorptiometry (DEXA) is a technique to determine the body composition of animals and poultry by using two X-ray beams of various energy levels. The DEXA is also used to accurately measure human body composition and fat content. Swennen et al. (2004) determined the in vivo body composition of a chickens using a pencil beam DEXA scanner. The measurements were based on attenuation of low (38 keV) and high (70 keV) energy X-rays. The whole body of a chicken was scanned and analyzed using total body scan software and the DEXA measurements estimated the fat and lean tissue mass (g), percentage (%) of fat, bone mineral content (g), and density (g/cm^3). These values were validated by means of chemical carcass analysis. The study showed that the most accurate results were obtained for lean tissue mass and body mass followed by mineral content and mineral density of bone. The accuracy was the lowest for fat tissue mass and percentage. The results obtained by DEXA were in good agreement with chemical carcass analysis for body and lean tissue mass, fat tissue mass, and percentage but not for ash weight.

Pearce et al. (2009) studied the potential of DEXA to predict carcass composition of live and dead sheep. A DEXA (Norland XR-26 Fan beam) scanner was used to measure the lean, fat, and bone content of both whole lamb carcass and live sheep, then compared with the results of chemical analysis. Their results showed that DEXA-measured carcass lean, fat, and bone content are all accurately measured with bone content being the most accurately predicted. They concluded that the potential to estimate live body composition would be a great advantage for researchers to have a better understanding of the interaction between genetics and environment and the influence on carcass composition.

7.4.5.2 Aquaculture (bone detection)

Pinbone removal in fish fillet is mostly done by manual labor commonly referred to as V cut, which results in approximately 7% to 8% of the valuable fish fillet weight removed during the process. Andersen (2003) developed an automatic pinbone removal and detection unit using X-ray technology. The fillets were manually fed and the pinbone removal units pulled the pinbones and were monitored by X-ray detectors indicating whether the fillet still contains pinbones. Fillets with remaining pinbones were retained at the station for further removal, while those without any bones were sent past the processing line. X-ray detectors could provide automatic and online detection of pinbones in individual fillet.

Mery et al. (2011) conducted experiments to identify bones in trout and salmon fillets using X-ray imaging. An X-ray system (Poskom XM-20 BT, 100 kV, 20 mA) powered by battery was used to acquire the images of fish fillet, and image processing techniques such as preprocessing, feature extraction, classification, and validation were performed to detect the bones. Cross-validation resulted in an accuracy of 100%, 98.5%, and 93.5% for large, medium, and small fish bones, respectively. When their methodology was validated for salmon and trout provided by the industry, higher detection accuracy of 99% was achieved.

Han and Shi (2007) proposed an image processing method to detect the bones in fish fillet using X-ray image analysis. The X-ray images were first subjected to image preprocessing, which involves morphological enhancement to highlight the region of interest (i.e., fish bone) and applying Gaussian and gray value distribution to reduce the amount of data. Then particle swarm clustering was applied to detect fish bones in the fillet and a detection rate of 85% was achieved.

7.4.5.3 Wood

Application of X-ray techniques in evaluation of wood quality has been assessed and studied by various researchers. The quality assessment of wood to be used in the construction and structural industry is very important because of the issue of biodegradation of wood by fungi. Fungi can decompose wood internally, which cannot be detected by external examination. Hence, nondestructive evaluation of the internal quality of wood is very essential. Tomazello et al. (2008) studied the nondestructive evaluation of Eucalypt (*Eucalyptus grandis*) wood using X-ray densitometry. Wood samples (20 mm × 10 mm) were placed on Faxitron X-ray film and X-rayed with 5 min exposure (16 kV, 3 mA). The radiographic films were digitized with a scanner (ScanJet 6100C/T). The results of the experiment showed that decay of eucalypt wood by white rot fungi could be detected by X-ray densitometry by a decrease in the mean, median, and maximum wood density. The biodegradation of cell wall components by mycelium of fungi resulted in reduction of wood density. The results of X-ray densitometry could also differentiate between sapwood and heartwood of eucalyptus due to differences in structural anatomy and chemical composition. The differences in sapwood and heartwood are reflected by the attenuation of X-rays due to variation in wood density.

Wood density variation within a tree may be due to genetic or physiological variation, and knowledge of wood density variation is essential to select sites and forestry practices and to predict end use of wood. Moya and Tomazello-Filho (2009) studied the wood density variation in Beechwood (*Gmelina arborea*) tree using X-ray densitometry. Thirty trees were selected and samples were prepared by cutting a slice 10 mm wide and 2 mm thick, and X-rayed on a film using a Faxitron 43805 N X-ray unit for an exposure time of 5 min (16 kV, 3 mA). Wood density values determined by X-ray radiograph showed that wood density was significantly affected by age of the tree, climatic conditions, and management practices. Trees from dry tropical conditions produced wood of greater density than those from dry conditions. The results showed that application of X-ray could establish tree ring demarcation and wood density variation from pith to bark of *Gmelina arborea*. Roig et al. (2008) studied the wood density of *Populus* trees from plantations in eastern Mendoza,

Argentina, using X-ray densitometry. Samples of 2 mm thickness were radiographed using the Faxitron 43805N unit for an exposure time of 5 min (16 kV, 3 mA). The anatomy of poplar growth ring showed a sustained increase of the intraring densities clearly showing a gradual transition from early to latewood density zones. The results showed a promising potential for evaluation of wood density properties.

In situ assessment of soundness and quality of structures are sometimes necessary in order to evaluate the quality of wooden structure in bridges, churches, or other such structures. To evaluate and analyze historical wooden structures, knowledge of strength and stiffness of timber is important. Lechner et al. (2013) evaluated the potential of assessment of timber density by X-ray technique. Fourteen different types of wooden specimen 64 × 94 × 30 mm were prepared and exposed to X-ray using a battery-powered portable X-ray source Inspector XR200. The results of the experiment provided accurate information on the density of the timber analyzed. The technique can also contribute to the detection of failure and deterioration of the wooden material in the early stages, which could increase the life and durability of the structure.

7.5   Medical applications of X-ray

The earlier application of X-ray was mainly focused on the medical field. The first X-ray image acquired by Wilhelm Roentgen was his wife's hand. But the real application of X-ray started with acquiring images of various body parts for diagnostic purposes. In spite of development of many newer technologies such as CT and MRI, plain X-ray radiography is used as an important diagnostic tool in many disorders. As X-rays pass through the object, they are absorbed in varying amounts depending on the density and composition of the material. Bones absorb X-rays well while soft tissues and muscles absorb lesser amounts of X-rays resulting in the contrast seen in X-ray images with bones representing white areas and gray areas represent the tissues. X-ray in the medical field is used for many types of examination. Some of the applications of X-ray are

- X-ray radiography to determine tumors, foreign objects, pneumonia, damages to bones and ligaments, etc.
- Mammography
- X-ray CT (computed tomography)
- Fluoroscopy
- Angiography
- Radiation therapy in treating cancer patients (U.S. Food and Drug Administration, 2012a)

Radiography is the science of acquiring images and visualization of internal organs of the human body for diagnostic and treatment purposes. Radiographic images can be obtained for vaious parts of the body such as the skull, teeth, chest, abdomen, pelvic area, spine, hands, leg, and any other specific area.

Mammography is the process in which low energy X-rays are used to obtain images of the human breast to screen for early detection of cancer or tumor growth. X-ray CT is a nondestructive imaging technique that captures and visualizes the internal features of solid objects. X-ray CT obtains cross-sectional images of the body in slices of 2D images, and by using reconstruction technique, produces 3D images of the area of interest.

Fluoroscopy is a medical imaging technique that uses X-rays to produce continuous real-time live images of internal organs of the patient using a fluoroscope. A fluoroscope is an instrument for observing the internal structure of opaque objects (living beings in medicine) consisting of an X-ray source and a fluorescent screen, and the subject is placed between X-ray source and screen. To perform minimally invasive procedures on ankles, knees, and joints, orthopedics depend on X-ray images for setting fractures or for replacement of metal works. Fluoroscopy is useful for assessment of the gastrointestinal tract, urinary tract, and musculoskeletal system (Dobranowski et al., 2013).

Angiography is a type of X-ray imaging technique used to visualize the blood vessels especially arteries, veins, and heart in human subjects by injecting a contrast agent into the blood vessel, which enhances the visibility of the structures. The contrast agent used is a radiopaque (high density) substance, and the blood vessels containing contrast show up dark on the image and areas without contrast show up bright.

X-rays are used in radiation therapy for treatment of cancer. The action of the X-ray is to break the bonds from cells by removing the electrons from atoms that results in treatment of cancer. The nucleus of cell contains DNA information and when the DNA bonds are broken, cell death occurs, and the destruction of tumor cells eventually results in destruction of tumor (Gerbi, 2011). External beam radiotherapy (EBRT) and brachytherapy are provided for treatment of various tumors. In external beam radiotherapy treatment, X-rays with high energy are directed toward the tumor from outside the body. Newer methods involve providing a higher dosage of radiation over a shorter period of time called accelerated irradiation. Brachytherapy involves placement of radioactive source (seeds or pellets) directly at the site of the cancerous tumor (American Cancer Society, 2012).

In spite of so many advanced techniques in radiology, chest X-ray is the most commonly performed examination and around 6.7 million chest X-rays are performed per year in the United Kingdom. In chest X-ray examination, the radiation dose is only equivalent to approximately 3 days of exposure to natural background radiation (National Radiological Protection Board, 2010). The lateral chest X-ray contains extensive information on the pleura, thoracic cage, lungs, heart, pericardium, mediastinum, and upper abdomen. Since many physicians could not read the lateral chest X-ray, they recommend higher dosage CT (Gaber et al., 2005). Feigin (2010) described the importance of lateral chest radiography and emphasized that the systematic approach of lateral chest X-ray radiograph could provide very valuable information. In modern chest imaging, if the frontal view shows any possibility of abnormality, CT is recommended by many radiologists, even though CT results in a much greater radiation dose than radiographs and may result in higher false positives that require further evaluation. Feigin has elaborated that lateral radiographs provide key findings that are not visible on the frontal view.

Brennan (2002) has stated that development of intra- and extraoral digital technology has made digital imaging a superior alternative to conventional X-ray film imaging. The advantages of digital imaging are image manipulation, which involves selecting the information of greatest value and suppressing the rest of the information; contrast enhancement; 3D reconstruction by which intra- and extraoral images could be reconstructed, easy image storage; and teleradiology, which means images can be sent to colleagues around the world for review.

7.6   *Applications of X-ray imaging in engineering industry*

New and advanced development in the field of X-ray detectors and micro to nano X-ray sources along with advanced imaging algorithms have resulted in new possibilities for application of X-ray in engineering industry. Due to advancement in X-ray imaging, it is now possible to observe and capture images of an object that was previously difficult because of low contrast, small dynamic range, low attenuation or small structural dimensions (Vavrik et al., 2011).

Shedlock et al. (2011) developed a mobile backscatter X-ray imaging system capable of imaging large areas, such as inspection of aircraft, in real time. The single sided imaging technique has made radiography an efficient method for inspection of aircrafts in highly congested areas and in areas backed by radiation attenuating structures. Backscatter X-ray imaging is a technique that allows images to be captured from one side of the object. In backscatter imaging, as the X-ray beam strikes the object, a portion of the incident radiation scatters back toward the source, which is measured by the radiation detectors that are placed adjacent to the radiation source. Backscatter X-ray imaging has many applications such as detection of corrosion, identification of foreign objects, detection of water intrusion, cracking, impact damage, and leaks in a variety of materials, and is also used for full body scanning in airport security.

Vavrik et al. (2011) has demonstrated that high dynamic range radiography has made it possible to detect fatigue crack in aircrafts by a high-contrast image. Such cracks otherwise will only be visible when the respective components are dismantled. Zschech et al. (2008) studied the potential of X-ray imaging techniques in the semiconductor industry. High-resolution X-ray imaging such as transmission X-ray microscopy and X-ray CT with a spatial resolution between 50 and 100 nm makes it possible to determine failure in micro- and nano electronic devices and to visualize voids and residuals in metal interconnects without any physical modification of the chip.

Vengrinovich et al. (2001) developed a new method of 2D and 3D X-ray image restoration of pipes in areas where access is restricted to monitor the pipelines. Accurate measurement of wall thickness of pipes is very important in the industrial environment. For the experiment, X-ray and gamma ray sources along with X-ray film or imaging plates were utilized for the data acquisition to reconstruct wall thickness profiles. The mean error for wall thickness estimation was around 200 µm, which corresponds to the spatial resolution of the data used for calculations.

X-ray has been used in many industrial applications to test the integrity of industrial products that are manufactured for various engineering purposes. In the automobile industry, a demand for light alloy castings has increased significantly over the last few years. To manufacture light alloy casting without compromising on the structural quality, automobile industries have installed an automatic X-ray inspection system to meet the growing market demands and to ensure the quality of the product. The use of X-ray to inspect castings at a high speed and in fully automatic mode is presented by Brant (2000). The inspection of materials is carried out by a collimated beam of X-rays that passes through the casting. As the beam passes through the casting, attenuation of X-ray occurs that is proportional to the thickness of the material as well as the presence of any voids or discontinuity in the casting. The X-rays then pass through the image intensifier and an image is produced based on the internal structure of the casting.

Most of the industrial radiographic applications are based on visual inspection of film-based X-ray images on the computer monitor. The range of applications of the Rolls-Royce imaging system includes measurement of crack length in welds, wall thickness in turbine blades, and movement of mechanical components in an aircraft engine during operational tests. Rogers (2000) replaced the current film-based imaging system with a digital electronic system. Laboratory tests have demonstrated the potential for improvement in the accuracy of measurement using digital electronic imaging compared to film-based imaging.

The application of radiography has been explored in the field of monitoring reinforced concrete facilities. The major advantage of using X-ray imaging in concrete testing is that the attenuation coefficient of steel, concrete, and air is 1, 0.3, and 0, respectively, which varies widely, thereby producing good X-ray images to test the concrete. X-ray imaging is both used in laboratory studies and in real-time applications to locate reinforcement, voids, and cracks as well as to determine the quality of grouting in prestressed concrete structures (Pla-Rucki and Eberhard, 1995).

7.7 Advantages and limitations of product inspection using X-rays

7.7.1 Advantages

X-ray is a nondestructive method to determine the internal quality characteristics of any product. Increased productivity can be obtained because X-ray units can be installed along the production lines to inspect different products, thereby increasing the efficiency and productivity of the entire process line. X-ray monitoring is ideal for high-speed monitoring and can handle 1500 products per minute or up to 10 tonnes per hour for bulk applications depending on the product (Mcrory, 2010). X-ray inspection of food products helps manufacturers and food processors to comply with global food safety standards such as Hazard Analysis Critical Control Points (HACCP), the Global Food Safety Initiative (GFSI), and Good Manufacturing Practices (GMP). X-ray is more convenient and relatively cheap compared to X-ray CT or MRI imaging equipment (Yacob et al., 2005). X-ray imaging does not require any sample preparation or very minimal preparation is needed. X-ray imaging has become very affordable, accurate, and easier to install and use in the industrial setup due to the technological advancement in the areas of high-voltage power supplies, solid state detectors, and computer speed and processing.

7.7.2 Limitations

One disadvantage of X-ray imaging is that it requires a high-voltage power supply to produce X-rays. X-ray imaging applications require a protective shielding and employees need to keep track of the radiation levels they are exposed to by use of a dosimeter.

Even though extensive research works have been conducted on detection of insect infestation in grain, still bulk grain could not be inspected by X-rays because the size and orientation of grain is such that it is difficult to determine insects, especially during developing stages such as larvae. The research studies conducted on detecting insect infestation have limited size samples (Haff and Slaughter, 2004; Karunakaran et al., 2004a,b,c; Fornal et al., 2007; Haff and Pearson, 2007) and hence it may not be effective in real-time bulk handling of samples in an elevator or a grain handling facility. The research needs to be extended to bulk samples, which will present challenges. The reason for the inability to use X-ray for bulk samples is that the size of the grain kernel requires monitoring speeds much higher than the speed of the existing computers and the lack of ability of X-ray machines to detect early life stages of insects (Haff and Toyofukku, 2008). Detection of early life stages of insects also becomes crucial depending on the end use of the grain. If the grain is for flour purposes and if it needs to be milled within a short period of time, presence of early life stages such as egg or first instar larvae does not pose a serious problem. On the other hand, if the grain is meant for storage for long term or for export, the presence of early life stages of insects is a serious concern because the insects may grow into complete adult and reproduce, which deteriorates the grain quality and affects the overall credibility of the system. The results of the laboratory research studies on insect identification are accurate under controlled conditions, but the practical feasibility of the technology in real time needs to be demonstrated. The real challenge lies in determining the infested kernel in large bins or rail cars. The performance of the X-ray imaging system needs to be assessed based on real-time conditions to make it a feasible technology in the near future.

The detection of split pits and normal pits in peaches using X-ray imaging was evaluated by Han et al. (1992) with 98% accuracy, but in order to achieve this, fruits needs to be placed in a specific orientation such that X-rays could penetrate from top to bottom or front to back during imaging. Hence, in a real-time situation, it becomes complicated to maintain a specific orientation of fruit to monitor the quality characteristics. X-ray imaging to detect watercore in apples explored by Kim and Schatzki (2000) showed that system could categorize sound and watercore-affected apples less than 5% to 8% false positive and negative ratio, independent of apple orientation. But the limitation was that the algorithm would work only when the stem-calyx axis makes a fixed angle with the X-ray beam. It was possible to detect glass contaminants in peat but they could not distinguish between stone and glass (Ayalew et al., 2004). X-ray imaging has certain limitations that hinder many applications to move forward from the research phase to the commercial phase. When solutions for these limitations are developed, X-ray imaging would be available for many commercial applications in the agriculture and food industry.

7.8   Cost comparison, safety, and future applications

7.8.1   Economics

The installation cost of an X-ray monitoring unit is seen as the most expensive part of incorporating imaging techniques in the agriculture and food industries. Installation cost is compensated by improved quality of the product, reduced wastage, and lower product recall due to effective monitoring by X-ray systems. Installation of X-ray units for quality monitoring increases the overall quality of the process and product, which eventually helps in increasing the credibility of the product brand name compared to the other products available in the market. Thus, break even for the initial cost of investment of X-ray units could occur in a short period of time, thereby eventually resulting in higher profits. Also, when consumers demand higher quality of food, it obviously increases the cost of production to ensure that the food meets all the safety standards. Hence, to ensure food free of contamination or other internal quality defects, a small premium in price for food could be justified. The total cost associated with installing and implementing an X-ray inspection system is definitely lower than the potential cost of failure, such as product recall or legal expenses, that may occur due to product contamination and health-related issues arising out of compromised product quality.

Mosqueda et al. (2010) studied the cost economics involved in the X-ray inspection technique in packaging of sweet onion based on simulation modeling. In a box of 50 to 70 onions, an average number of onions with internal defects could be around 10 to 22 per box in conventional methods, whereas using X-ray inspection, only 1 to 3 internally defective onions were found in a box. For the onions monitored by X-ray imaging, the estimated cost of producing an 18.14 kg box ranged from $9.00 to $12.00 for crop with low incidence of defects to $11.50 to $15.20 for high-defect incidence crop. The estimated selling price for each box of onions with 20%, 30%, and 40% profit margin was well within the historic price ranges. Mosqueda et al. study showed that it is economically viable to install X-ray machines for monitoring the quality of sweet onions and this could be extended for other products.

7.8.2   Safety

Although X-ray is an ionizing radiation, the exposure of food to X-ray is very limited and does not compromise the quality of the food. When an object is exposed to ionizing radiation, the energy absorbed by the object is called the radiation dose and the radiation dose can be described as the absorbed, equivalent, and effective dose. The total amount of energy absorbed by an object or substance is called absorbed dose and is expressed in grays (Gy). One gray is defined as the unit of energy (joule) deposited in a kilogram of a substance. When radiation is absorbed in a living substance, it may produce a biological effect, but an equally absorbed dose may not produce an equal biological effect because it depends on the kind of radiation. A radiation weighting factor equates various types of radiation with different biological effectiveness. This absorbed quantity is called equivalent dose and is expressed in sieverts (Sv). Radiation sensitivity of different tissues and organs are different and hence an effective dose is given by the equivalent dose multiplied by a factor related to the risk of a particular organ or tissue and is also expressed in sieverts (Canadian Nuclear Safety Commission, 2010). The maximum radiation dosage an X-ray machine operator in an airport receives is less than 1 mSv per year, whereas it requires 250 mSv for a person to result in nausea, vomiting, or diarrhea, and 2500 mSv to result in death (CATSA, 2010). The typical maximum dose for an X-ray system operator in a food industry would be less than 1 µSv (0.001 mSv) per hour. This radiation level would mean an operator working adjacent to an X-ray unit for 50 weeks a year and 40 h every week would receive 2000 µSv (2 mSv) per year, whereas the average natural background radiation every individual is exposed to corresponds to 2400 µSv (2.4 mSv) from the natural sources (Ansari, 2009). Hence an X-ray unit operator in a food industry is exposed to less radiation from his occupation than the exposure from the environment.

7.8.3   Shielding

X-ray units used in the food and agriculture industry come with a protective shielding to protect the operator, and the food passes through the X-ray units only for a fraction of a second. Hence, X-rays do not produce any undesired effect on the food materials. The most commonly used protective shielding for X-ray machine is lead. Proper shielding of an X-ray inspection unit is a mandatory requirement and certain units used for medical purposes are housed in a specially designed protective shielding room. But generally most industrial X-ray units have shields to protect the operators. Radiation protection plans involve monitoring the employee exposure to radiation levels and developing procedures for safe handling of equipment involving radiation exposure. Persons operating X-ray units and those involved in handling operations related to X-ray units are required to wear a dosimeter, a radiation measuring device that measures and records the amount of radiation the person is exposed to during the period of operation.

7.8.4   Future applications

The applications of X-ray imaging in the medical, engineering, and biological industries are continuously increasing compared to the previous decade. Many processing industries have incorporated X-ray imaging systems as a quality monitoring tool to provide complete product safety and to avoid costly product recalls and issues related to health claims. The design and implementation of X-ray installation in any food industry should be a strategic decision to be able to effectively implement the process at the critical points in order to achieve maximum benefits. The implementation of X-ray imaging should be proactive rather than reactive, that is, the technique needs to be used to prevent the occurrence of contamination rather than just detecting and eliminating the defects. High-speed industrial X-ray units and efficient image processing algorithms have resulted in X-ray imaging available for various applications for a wide range of industries. In the future, food and agriculture industries will continue to invest in X-ray imaging techniques to meet the demands of the food regulatory authorities and consumer on food safety initiatives, whereas X-ray imaging has become an irreplaceable technology in the medical field and it seems it will grow stronger in the coming decade.

chapter eight

X-ray computed tomography imaging

8.1 Introduction

X-ray computed tomography (CT) is an imaging technique that captures and visualizes the internal features of solid objects in a nondestructive manner. The objective of X-ray CT is to reproduce the internal structure of the desired object in 3D by using slices of 2D cross-sectional images and with the help of a technique called reconstruction.

With the development of modern computers and X-ray applications, X-ray CT became feasible in the 1960s. Godfrey N. Hounsfield, a British engineer, is the inventor of computed tomography with its successful practical implementation in 1972 at EMI Central Research Laboratory in the United Kingdom, although many people have contributed to the development of computed tomography. The medical community became very receptive for X-ray CT after the first medical images were obtained at Atkinson Morley Hospital in London in 1972 (Kalender, 2006). Hounsfield, an engineer, and Cornack, a physicist, were awarded the Nobel Prize for medicine in 1979 for their contribution to X-ray CT.

As with X-rays, X-ray CT was initially used in the medical field for obtaining images of patients, and computed tomography became a very important aspect in radiological diagnostics. But, later on, the applications of X-ray CT spread to various industries including engineering, agriculture, food, biomedical, electronics, and geological sciences. X-ray CT has the ability to show the internal characteristics, the difference in density, and atomic structure of the material, thereby enabling the study of the porosity, moisture movement, and the microstructure of the material.

8.2 Computed tomography

8.2.1 Principle of X-ray CT

An X-ray CT image is termed a slice because the image represents how an object would appear if it was cut or sliced along the plane. A CT image is made of voxels (volumetric picture elements), similar to pixels (picture elements) in digital images. In a CT slice image, the gray level corresponds to X-ray attenuation, which depends on the amount of X-rays dispersed or absorbed when they travel through each voxel. X-ray CT consists of exposing an object to X-rays from many orientations and calculating the reduction in intensity of X-rays along the linear path. The reduction of X-ray energy is explained by Beer's law, which describes the decrease in intensity as a function of X-ray energy, linear attenuation coefficient, and path length of the object being exposed to X-rays. Beer's law is expressed as

$$I = I_0 \exp(-\mu x)$$

where I and I_0 are the final and initial X-ray intensity, respectively, μ refers to the linear attenuation coefficient of the material, and x is the X-ray path length (Ketcham and Carlson, 2001).

The first-generation CT system is characterized by a pencil beam of X-ray that passes through an object and a single detector repeating the process at many angular orientations (Figure 8.1a). Second-generation CT is comprised of a fan beam of X-ray instead of the pencil beam and a single detector from the first generation is substituted by a set of detectors (Figure 8.1b). In third-generation CT, the fan beam and detector series surrounds the whole object and rotation of either the source-detector combination or the object is needed (Figure 8.1c and d). One variation in third-generation CT is that a part of the sample is outside the beam, but as the object revolves the entire object passes through the beam thereby permitting reconstruction of the whole object. Third-generation scanners allow

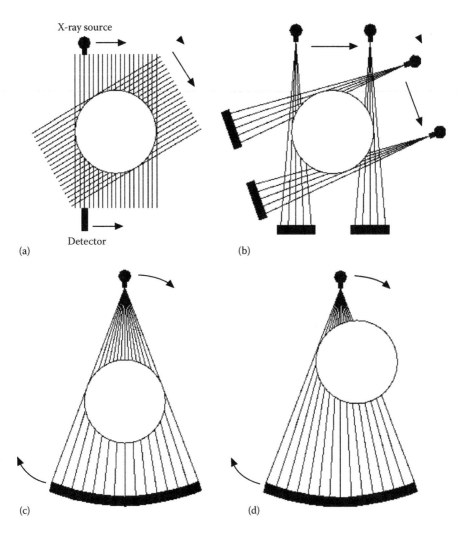

Figure 8.1 Different generations of CT scanners. (a) First-generation, translate-rotate pencil beam geometry, (b) second-generation, translate-rotate fan beam geometry, (c) third-generation, rotate-only geometry, and (d) third-generation offset-mode geometry. (From Ketcham, R.A., and W.D. Carlson, *Computers and Geosciences*, 27, 381, 2001. With permission.)

bigger objects to be imaged and the smaller objects move closer to the source thereby increasing the resolution of the image and are much faster than second-generation CT scanners. However, in third-generation scanners, the spatial resolution relies on the size and number of sensors present in the detector array and hence the speed is obtained by incorporating more sensors than the previous models. Fourth generation X-ray CT scanners comprise of fixed series of detectors and a single source of X-ray that moves around the object (Ketcham and Carlson, 2001). The fifth-generation CT scanner varies from the previous models because it does not involve mechanical motion and a circular array of X-ray sources are used that can be turned on or off electronically (Figure 8.2). The preliminary investigation and clinical testing of spiral CT was reported in 1989, and by 1992 CT manufacturers started making scanners incorporating slip ring technology and spiral CT capabilities with much higher scan speed and improved image quality (Kalender, 2006). In 2000, development in X-ray CT was growing with the addition of more rows to the detector arrays and simultaneous acquisition of many slices. In 2001, 16 slices were acquired simultaneously and it became 64 slices in 2006 with less than 10 s scan time.

CT scanners can be classified into two main categories: clinical CT and micro-CT. The field of view (FOV) of clinical CT scanners is about 40 to 50 cm, which is necessary to scan the whole human body. The spatial resolution of clinical CT scanners is only 2 to 3 cycles/mm, whereas micro-CT scanners provide a high spatial resolution of 100 cycles/mm with a field of view of a few centimeters (Arabi et al., 2010). Originally, X-ray CT was developed for medical applications and hence to maximize their effectiveness and minimize patient exposure, the medical CT system used low energy X-rays (< 125 keV) and large high-efficiency detectors to obtain as much information as possible. But later, as X-ray

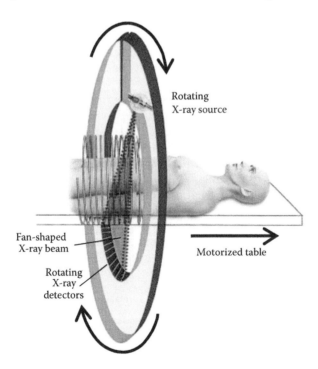

Rotating
X-ray source

Fan-shaped
X-ray beam

Rotating
X-ray
detectors

Motorized table

Figure 8.2 Spiral or helical CT scanner. (From Brenner, D.J., and M.A. Georgsson, *Gastroenterology*, 129, 328, 2005. With permission.)

CT was used in industrial applications, it demanded imaging of denser objects. Industrial application of CT does not have a limitation on radiation level or exposure time, and hence higher energy X-ray source and small detectors are used (Ketcham and Carlson, 2001).

8.2.2 Common configurations of X-ray CT

The most common configurations of X-ray CT are fan beam, cone beam, and parallel beam (Figure 8.3). In fan beam, collimators are used to reduce X-ray scattering thereby enabling additional X-rays to reach the detector. Thickness of slice is based on the aperture of the linear detector array. In cone beam configuration, instead of a linear detector array, a planar array is used and the beam is not collimated. In a single rotation,

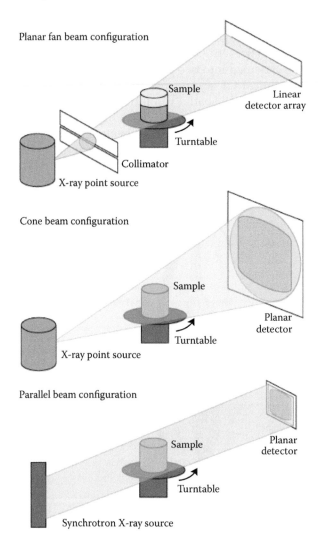

Figure 8.3 Configurations for CT scanners. (From Ketcham, R.A., 2012, X-ray computed tomography, Science Education Research Centre at Carleton College, Northfield, Minnesota, http://serc.carleton.edu/research_education/geochemsheets/techniques/CT.html; accessed February 10, 2013. With permission.)

the data for the whole object or a significant portion of the object can be obtained, and the data can be reconstructed depending on a cone-beam algorithm to obtain images. In parallel beam scanning, usually a synchrotron beam line is employed as the X-ray source. In parallel beam scanning, volumetric data are obtained without any distortion. The constraint is that the size of the object is limited based on the X-ray beam width (Ketcham, 2012).

8.2.3 Instrumentation or components of X-ray CT

The major components of X-ray CT are the X-ray source, the detector series that measures the intensity of X-ray attenuation, a rotational geometry along the material being scanned, and the image processor for image reconstruction and shielding. In medical CT, the scanning unit is called a gantry, which contains the X-ray tubes and detectors. The configuration of these components varies depending on the size, type, and composition of the object, and specific type of application. One set of X-ray intensity measurement for a given sample location and scanner geometry on all detectors is referred to as view. In X-ray CT, many sets of views of a sample for a range of angular orientation are obtained, which are used to create 2D images of the object that are called slices (Ketcham and Carlson, 2001).

8.2.3.1 X-ray source

Most CT systems use X-ray tubes while few of the systems use a gamma ray or synchrotron emitter as a monochromatic X-ray source. The effectiveness of the X-ray source for a particular application is dependent on focal spot size, intensity of X-ray, and the spectrum of X-ray energies generated. The focal spot is the area on the anode of an X-ray tube that is struck by electrons and from which X-rays are emitted. The resolution of image is dependent on the focal spot size. The spectrum of X-ray energy describes the penetrating ability of X-rays. High-energy X-rays have more penetrating ability than low-energy rays but they are less sensitive to variation in composition and density of the material. The X-ray intensity has a direct impact on the signal-to-noise ratio and hence the clarity of the image (Ketcham and Carlson, 2001).

8.2.3.2 X-ray detectors

A detector is either a crystal or ionizing gas, and when an X-ray photon strikes the detector, it produces light or electrical energy and a photodiode attached to the detector converts the light energy into electrical or analog energy. Two common types of detectors employed in X-ray CT are scintillation or solid state and Xenon gas. The image quality depends on the size and quantity of the detector and the efficiency of the detector in detecting the spectrum of energy produced by the source. The size and number of detectors are important, because the number of detectors determines the quantity of data that can be collected simultaneously. The quality of resolution for a single view and hence the overall image quality is dependent on the number of detectors. The X-ray energy determines the efficiency of scintillation detectors because the penetrating ability of higher energy X-rays is greater compared to lower energy X-rays and hence have higher ability to travel through materials without interactions (Ketcham and Carlson, 2001).

8.2.3.3 Image processor (digital acquisition system)

The analog signal produced by a detector is basically a weak signal that is amplified, and then the analog signal is converted to a digital signal by an A/D converter, which is part of a digital acquisition system. The digital signal is then passed on to an array processor, which performs the function of mathematical reconstruction of a CT image.

8.2.4 Microtomography

Microtomography is similar to computed tomography but the pixel sizes are in the range of micrometers. Microtomography and high-resolution X-ray tomography are similar terms and the machine is much smaller in size compared to the regular ones and are used to study smaller objects. X-ray microtomography has an ability to produce 3D images of an internal structure of an object at a spatial resolution less than 1 micrometer. Based on the spatial resolution, there are that three levels of micro computed tomography: mini-CT, micro-CT, and nano-CT; however micro-CT is the commonly used generic term (Ritman, 2011). The first X-ray microtomography was built by Jim Elliot in the early 1980s. The advantages of micro-CT are that the internal features of objects can be obtained with very high spatial resolution and the method is nondestructive (Landis and Keane, 2010). Another milestone in microtomography is the use of synchrotron radiation as a source of X-ray that could significantly enhance the image quality. Synchrotron radiation is the result of curving or bending of a beam of high-energy electrons in the presence of a magnetic field. The resultant light is much brighter than the light emitted by the conventional X-ray source. Higher brightness results in significant enhancement to the imaging and hence provides very subtle information and minute details about the sample. To maximize the efficiency of synchrotron X-ray source, size of the imaging object should be limited to 5 to 10 mm (Landis and Keane, 2010).

8.3 Applications of X-ray CT

The applications of X-ray CT in the agriculture and food industry are numerous, and Table 8.1 comprehends the various models of CT used in a variety of applications in the agri-food sector.

8.3.1 Forestry and agriculture

8.3.1.1 Knot detection in wood

The most important depreciation factors considered for estimating the price of timber are the frequency and size of the knots. Krähenbühl et al. (2012) studied knot detection in various softwood species and various moisture content woods using X-ray CT technology. The results of the study showed that X-ray CT could automatically detect and count all the knots in a given piece of wood. It took only a few seconds to detect the knots, whereas the commonly used method takes about an hour. Krähenbühl et al. concluded that X-ray CT is a robust nondestructive technique to determine knots in wood.

8.3.1.2 Assessment of wood decay

McGovern et al. (2010) evaluated the decay of wood using X-ray CT. The wood species Loblolly pine (*Pinus taeda* L.) was exposed to fungus Gloeophyllum (*Gloeophyllum trabeum* Pers.) for different time durations ranging from 1 to 12 weeks, and the decay was assessed using X-ray CT. From the acquired CT images, the specimen's volume and density were calculated. The results showed that wood samples exposed to 12 weeks of controlled decay resulted in 47% density reduction at the surface that was in contact with fungi, while the other surface lost only 28%. The wooden block exposed to controlled decay for a week

Table 8.1 Research Studies on Potential Application of X-Ray CT Imaging in the Food and Agricultural Industry

Model/ manufacturer	Parameters: slice thickness (mm); voltage (kV); current (mA)	Material	Application	Reference
Medical CT scanner	NA	Wood	Knot detection	Krähenbühl et al., 2012
X-ray CT (General Electric)	1.25 mm; 80 kV; 45 mA	Wood	Assessment of wood decay	McGovern et al., 2010
SMX-100CT-D (Shimadzu Corporation, Nakagyo-ku, Kyoyo, Japan)	1.8 mm, 43 kV, 90 mA	Wood	Tree ring measurement	Okochi et al., 2007
Somatom Plus medical scanner (Siemens, Germany)	1, 2, 5, and 10 mm; 120 kV; 165 mA	Loamy and silty soil	Assessment of soil structure	Rogasik et al., 2003
Somatom Plus	120 kV; 220 mA	Soil	Assessment of soil pores	Sander et al., 2008
Somatom Plus S Medical scanner (Siemens)	1–2 mm; 85–130 kV	Fine sand	Characterize phase distribution and pore geometry	Wildenschild et al., 2002
Cone beam scanner Oxford XTF5011 (Oxford Instruments, Bicester, Oxfordshire, UK)	50 kV; 0.5 mA	Wheat	Study the development of plant root in soil	Jenneson et al., 2003
Skyscan 1173 (Skyscan, Kontich, Belgium)	80 kV; 100 μA	Apple	Detect watercore in apple	Herremans et al., 2012
Skyscan 1072 micro-CT (Skyscan, Aartselaar, Belgium)	63 kV; 156 μA	Apple	Pore space quantification	Mendoza et al., 2007
TOSCANER-20000 (Toshiba Co., Japan)	150 kV; 3 mA	Mango; peach	Ripening assessment; quality evaluation	Barcelon et al., 1999, 2000
EMI 5005 scanner (Hayes, Middlesex, UK)	125 kV; 1881 mA			Brecht, 1991
CT Hilight Advantage (GE Medical Systems)	10 mm; 80 kV; 40 mA	Peach and nectarine	Evaluate the quality of fruits due to development of woolliness	Sonego et al., 1995

(Continued)

Table 8.1 (Continued) Research Studies on Potential Application of X-Ray CT Imaging
in the Food and Agricultural Industry

Model/ manufacturer	Parameters: slice thickness (mm); voltage (kV); current (mA)	Material	Application	Reference
Skyscan 1172	40 kV; 100 µA	Rice flour	Assessment of structure	Chanvrier et al., 2009
Skyscan 1072 (Bruker microCT, Kontich, Belgium)	50 kV; 100 µA	Cracker, soup inclusions	Visualization of internal structure	Dalen et al., 2007
Skyscan 1072 (Skyscan, Belgium)	100 kV; 96 µA	Chocolate, strawberry mousse, marshmallow		Lim and Barigou, 2004
Not available		Bread	Microstructure of bakery products	Miri and Fryer, 2006
Skyscan 1174 (Skyscan, Kontich, Belgium)	20 mm	Bakery products	Characterization of crust and crumb structure	Chevallier and Bail, 2012
Skyscan 1172 (Skyscan, Kontich, Belgium)	59 kV; 167 µA	Biscuits and breadsticks	Microstructural characteristics and sensory properties	Frisullo et al., 2010a
Skyscan 1072	60 kV; 100 mA	Bread	Evaluate internal crumb structure	Lape et al., 2008
Skyscan 1072 (Skyscan, Belgium)	100 kV; 96 µA	Potato	Evaluate microstructure during frying	Miri et al., 2006
Skyscan 1172 (Skyscan, Kontich, Belgium)	20 × 20 × 15 mm; 37 kV; 228 µA	Chocolate	Microstructural characterization	Frisullo et al., 2010b
Skyscan 1172 (Skyscan, Belgium)	50 kV and 200 µA; 100 and 100 µA	Bouillon	Microstructural characterization	Dalen et al., 2008
Skyscan 1172 (Skyscan, Belgium)	82 kV; 125 µA	Meat	Fat content determination	Frisullo et al., 2009
Skyscan 1072 (Skyscan, Belgium)	100 kV; 98 µA	Chicken nuggets	To determine porosity, pore size distribution, pore connectivity	Adedeji and Ngadi, 2009
Somatom AR (Siemens, Norway)	1 mm; 130 kV; 105 mA	Pork	Salt concentration in cured pork	Vestergaard et al., 2004
Somatom Emotion (Siemens AG, Germany)	80, 110, 130 kV; 106 mA	Salmon	Salt and fat distribution	Segtnan et al., 2009
Somatom 2CT body scanner (Siemens, Germany)	NA	Atlantic salmon	Slaughter yield and fillet yield	Einen et al., 1998

resulted in 5% density loss at the region in contact with fungi, while there was no loss of density at the opposite surface. The results suggested that X-ray CT could be used for assessment of decay in wood.

8.3.1.3   Tree ring measurement

Wooden cultural heritage objects are studied for measuring the age of the specimen, and tree ring measurement plays an important role in the age determination. When the surface is painted or deteriorated, it is difficult to clearly determine the tree rings and hence it becomes difficult for ring width measurement. Sampling or grinding a small portion of the object is performed but a nondestructive method to determine the age of wooden objects was not available until a decade ago, when X-ray CT was found to be useful to obtain images of the interior of the specimen. Development of small focal area X-ray tubes, image intensifiers with high sensitivity, and CCD cameras of very high resolution have made it possible to analyze the anatomical structure of various types of wood. Okochi et al. (2007) determined the possibility of tree ring measurements using microfocus X-ray CT for two wood varieties (Japanese beech and Japanese oak) and compared them with conventional soft X-ray radiographs. The microfocus unit is one in which the focal spot size is less than 100 μm. Advanced microfocus units have a focal size of 5 μm by focusing the electron beam on the target (TWI Ltd., 2012). Microfocus X-ray helps in obtaining minute details and a very high spatial resolution. The experiments were conducted using a microfocus X-ray CT (SMX-100CT-D) having a focal size of 5 μm, which is of great significance in obtaining high-resolution tomograms. The tube voltage and current was 43 kV and 90 μA, respectively, with a mean of 10 frames per view and 1800 views for one rotation of the specimen. The test specimens prepared for the study were 1.8 mm thick. The X-ray radiographs and micro-focus CT images of the thin specimens of Japanese oak and Japanese beech were compared and analyzed. The image quality of X-ray CT was lower than soft X-ray images due to grain noise, which is characteristic of CT images. They concluded that X-ray CT has the ability to determine the tree ring width by nondestructive means although limitations such as size of the specimen that could be handled and high cost of the device remains a constraint.

8.3.1.4   Assessment of soil structure

Soil has a complex morphological structure and most of the soil structure assessment methods are destructive in nature. X-ray CT could be used as a nondestructive technique to study soil structure with resolutions in millimeter scale. Rogasik et al. (2003) conducted a study to present the potential of X-ray CT for 3D visualization of macropores and calcu-lation of bulk density distribution within soil samples. Undisturbed loamy and silty soils were excavated for the experiment. The study was conducted using a Siemens Somatom plus CT scanner working at 120 kV and 165 mA. The scanning time was around 2 s per slice. The minimum slice thickness was 1 mm, while the slice thickness and spacing var-ied at 1, 2, 5, and 10 mm. With a slice thickness and spacing of 1 mm, soil samples were scanned horizontally. The soil was assessed immediately before and after compaction by a high-load sugar beet harvester. X-ray CT images revealed that before compaction, soil structure was characterized by high continuity and connectivity, and dry bulk density distribution was relatively homogeneous. Whereas after compaction, most of the macro-pores were destroyed and vertical continuity was destroyed. The results of the study thus enabled the visual assessment of soil structure conditions through X-ray CT imaging and revealed the relationship between soil tillage and soil structure of loamy and silty soils.

Sander et al. (2008) investigated the possibility of using X-ray CT to determine the size and arrangement of structural pores, aggregates, and distribution of bulk density of the topsoil and subsoil of two paddy fields that were 20 and 100 years old and referred to in the study as young (Y) and old (O), respectively. For the study, undisturbed soil (20 cm × 25 cm) samples were collected at a depth of 5 to 23 cm and 25 to 42 cm for field Y. For field O, samples were collected at depths of 0 to 18 cm and 19 to 38 cm. The soil samples were scanned using a medical CT (Siemens Somatom Plus, 120 kV, 220 mA) scanner. The CT images provided information on vertical bulk density and secondary pores were characterized by 3D plots of low density and air-filled regions. In the subsoil of both samples, aggregated structures were found and horizontal cracks were located. For the soil sample obtained from field O, the compacted horizon was larger and deeper compared to field Y. The bulk density for field O reduced suddenly compared to field Y where the bulk density gradually reduced with depth.

Macedo et al. (1999) examined soil samples using X-ray micro-CT with a spatial resolution of 100 μm. They investigated and presented the physical properties of undisturbed Latosol soil samples and minute details like pores, fractures, and mineral particles were observed. Macedo et al. concluded that microtomography could be used as a tool to study heterogeneous, opaque, and porous systems, such as soil and its characteristics, which could be used for better planning of agricultural activities.

8.3.1.5   Hydrology

Wildenschild et al. (2002) investigated the potential of X-ray CT in hydrology to study the phase distribution and the geometry of pores in porous media. The samples used for the study consisted of fine sand and slightly coarser material. In this study three types of CT systems—an industrial X-ray tube (400 μm resolution), a medical scanner (100–500 μm resolution), and a synchrotron based CT system (resolution of 5–20 μm)—were used. The soil samples were placed in concentric Lucite™ holders with various diameters ranging from 1.5 to 76 mm based on the type of CT. The images were studied, and the images with lower resolution provided macroscopic data regarding the variation in saturation for the bulk sample but hard-to-detect pore space features. The high-resolution images provided information regarding pore geometry but had lower phase contrast and hard-to-detect differences between drained and saturated images. They concluded that the choice of the CT system and specimen size is dependent on the objective of the study. If the objective is to study macropores and cracks, the best choice is an industrial or medical CT. To study the differences in saturation for a sample profile or to examine the effects of boundary, medical scanners are ideal because a large number of scans can be acquired in a short duration and images can be acquired for larger samples. If the purpose of the study is to investigate microscopic pores, a high-resolution synchrotron CT scanner is the best system.

8.3.1.6   Plant development study

Matsushima et al. (2009) studied the internal structure of peduncles from three rose cultivars using the Synchrotron X-ray CT to obtain high spatial resolution images to study complex tissues. "Bent neck" is a serious postharvest problem that occurs in roses, which results in upper peduncles bent prematurely thus lowering the flower quality. Bent neck may happen either due to lack of water conductivity and loss of water from the surface, but the objective was to investigate whether a link exists between bent neck and structural strength. Synchrotron studies were conducted at BESSY (Berlin, Germany), and roses were exposed to a monochromatic X-ray beam at 30 and 40 keV. The Synchrotron tomography clearly showed the structure of vascular bundles and parenchyma cells and no significant difference in the quality of image between 30 and 40 keV energy was observed. But due to irradiation, damage of cells was observed by chlorophyll fluorescence analysis and optical microscope images.

In plants, water balance maintenance is important and to transport water throughout the plant, xylem vessels must be refilled with water. But the process of refilling is not well understood due to inadequate methods. Lee and Kim (2008) investigated the synchrotron X-ray microimaging technique to study the refilling of xylem tissues of bamboo (*Phyllostachys bambusoides*) stem and leaves and to visualize the water entry in real time and in vivo. For every 0.5 s, the X-ray images were recorded at 10 ms exposure time. The water rise mechanism was evaluated by monitoring the water front in the successively acquired images. With this technique, it was feasible to study the water-rise kinetics and their association with xylem structure. This technique facilitated the study of both leaves and stem, and the study was conducted on 20 leaves and one stem to check the repeatability of the process. The authors concluded that Synchrotron X-ray CT imaging exhibited the xylem tissues of bamboo stem and leaves, and showed the meniscus movement in vessels refilling with water in vivo by noninvasive method and is a promising technique to examine the internal structure and water movement in plant tissues.

Soil constitutes a highly attenuating ferrous rich environment that makes MRI imaging not possible and X-ray tomography an ideal technique. Jenneson et al. (2003) designed a low dose X-ray microtomography unit suitable for sensitive living organisms. The system was used to obtain images during the initial period of plant growth immediately after germination of wheat (*Triticum aestivum* L.). The X-ray microtomography was a third-generation cone beam CT scanner with a minifocus X-ray source (Oxford XTF5011) with a focal diameter of 100 μm and working at 50 kV and 0.5 mA. The system could record 3D cylindrical samples of 25 mm in diameter and 25 mm height with a resolution of 100 μm in about 30 min. The radiation dose was determined to be 0.1 Gy, which was significantly below levels that could cause cellular damage. The projection data were then reconstructed and the length of root and volume were obtained from the data based on a 3D labeling routine. The results showed that the primary root grew 11 mm long on day 1 and 24 mm on the second day. The initial results showed that the X-ray CT designed for the purpose could be used to examine the growth of plant root in soil.

High-resolution CT uses a powerful X-ray source and sophisticated detector arrays, which offers higher penetration and density discrimination potential, thereby providing feasibility in imaging various types of new materials. Stuppy et al. (2003) examined various plant parts that have contrasting tissue density and varying X-ray attenuation properties. They selected hard materials that had minimum water content and different tissue densities such as fruits of South American Palm (*Syagrus flexuosa* Mart), English oak wood (*Quercus robur* L.), and soft objects with more water content and lesser tissue densities such as pineapple (*Ananas comosus* L.), tulip flower (*Tulipa*), and an inflorescence of *Leucospermum tottum* (R.Br.). Their results showed that in regions with no tissue density differences such as pineapple, tulip flower, and *L. tottum*, the technique detected minimum contrast between void space and tissue, yet visualization of external morphology, volume, and surface area could be easily quantified. In hard objects such as oak wood, various plant tissues such as periderm, xylem, and phloem are easily differentiated by the differences in X-ray attenuation even at lower resolution.

8.3.1.7 Grain

The rate of cooling or drying of grain is determined by the rate of airflow through the grain bed. The airflow resistance is influenced by variables such as moisture content of grain, velocity of air, viscosity, shape and size of grain kernels, and various other features. Neethirajan et al. (2006a) conducted studies to explain the airflow resistance variation between vertical and horizontal directions of grain bulk using X-ray CT. Five varieties of grain—barley, wheat, flax (oblong), peas, and mustard (spherical)—were selected for the study and images were obtained using a high-resolution X-ray CT at 420 kV and 1.8 mA (Austin, Texas). The images were analyzed using image processing techniques such as image cropping, thresholding, blob coloring, skeletonization, and feature extraction. In the horizontal direction, smaller area airpaths are uniformly distributed compared to vertical airspace, which makes it possible for air to travel along the grain with lower resistance in the horizontal direction compared to the vertical direction of the grain bulk. When compared with the vertical direction, the airpaths were 145%, 92%, and 187% more in the horizontal direction for barley, wheat, and flax, respectively. For mustard and pea, the increase in air path in the horizontal direction was 17% and 28%, respectively. The difference in resistance of airflow between both directions was explained by the number of airpaths. Also, a nonuniform distribution of airpaths was seen in the vertical direction than in the horizontal direction for barley, wheat, and flax, which may be the cause for the variation in airflow resistance. X-ray CT proved to be a useful technique to explain the airflow resistance in grain bulk. Macedo et al. (1999) examined the corn seeds for mechanical injury during heaping in silo using X-ray micro-CT with a spatial resolution of 100 μm. The determination and study of mechanical injury is important in genetic selection because the injury can affect the seed germination and also it increases the possibility of contamination by microorganism through the fracture.

8.3.2   Food

8.3.2.1   Fruits

8.3.2.1.1   Quality assessment.   Herremans et al. (2012) studied watercore in apples using X-ray CT. X-ray CT images were acquired from the Skyscan 1173 system operating at 80 keV and 100 μA, and apples of cultivar Verde Doncella were used for the study. The CT images of apples showed watercore disorder by density differences. Healthy tissues showed proper organization of cells and intercellular voids with a porosity of 30%, whereas in the affected tissue, values of porosity were as low as 10%. The study showed that X-ray CT images provided valuable information on the microstructural changes that occur in the affected apples.

Mendoza et al. (2007) studied the 3D quantification of pore space in apple tissue using X-ray micro-CT. Since pore space structural geometry has a crucial role in carrying gas and fluid through any cellular tissue, the objective of the study was to perform an experiment to acquire high-quality tomographic images at micrometer resolution of apple tissue using advanced image processing technologies. Apple cultivars Jonagold and Braeburn were selected and samples were collected from the fleshy part of the fruit. Images were obtained from the Skyscan 1072 high-resolution micro-CT system (Belgium). From the scanned image, a small region of interest for each sample was extracted and analyzed using image segmentation and medial axis analysis. From the image analysis, it was evident that porosity distribution for the two apple varieties was heterogeneous and variation in the size, orientation, and organization of air channels contributed to the heterogeneity of fruit tissue. The results of the study provided valuable information that could be used for extracting a quantitative description of the pore space. Mendoza et al. concluded that resolutions greater than 13.7 μm/pixel were appropriate for quantitative evaluation of apple tissue.

Woolly breakdown is a chilling injury caused by low temperature, which may result in abnormal degradation of cell wall pectin. Woolly breakdown disease is common in peaches and nectarines and is not visible until it reaches an advanced stage. Conventional monitoring is performed by cutting a large number of fruits which is time consuming and destructive. Sonego et al. (1995) studied the woolly breakdown in nectarines using X-ray CT. The X-ray CT images of nectarines with 10 mm slice thickness were obtained at 80 kV and 40 mA with an acquisition time of 2 s on a CT Hilight Advantage. The regions affected by woolly breakdown appeared dark under X-ray CT indicating the presence of gas inclusions. In fruits with mild or no woolliness, gas inclusions are less or absent.

8.3.2.2 Ripening assessment

Harvesting of fruits at proper maturity is a critical factor that determines the quality of the fruit. External factors related to fruit maturity are very subjective and may result in immature fruit being harvested. Immature fruits that are harvested do not ripen well or take a very long time to ripen as they may not have the potential to develop a desirable flavor. Fruits that are left too long after maturity do not withstand shipping and handling and become very soft and have reduced shelf life. The potential of X-ray CT in assessing fruits maturity has been studied by many researchers.

Ripening assessment of mango was studied by Barcelon et al. (2000) using the TOSCANER-20000 (Toshiba Co., Japan) X-ray CT at 150 kV and 3 mA. Mangoes were analyzed 2 days after harvest, and groups of 10 fruits were scanned and ripened at 25°C and 75% relative humidity. Images of the same set of fruits were obtained every week for 2 weeks. Physical structural changes of the mango resulted in decreasing CT number values to −46 from an initial value of 24. Density and moisture content also decreased from 0.99 to 0.96 g/mL and from 90% to 85%, respectively. The seed portion had higher X-ray absorption resulting in brighter portions on the image because seed was denser than the flesh tissue. The images showed the changes in the internal sections of fruit showing defects and ripening were clearly visible. Barcelon et al. concluded that X-ray CT has the potential to monitor internal changes and ripening of fruits.

Barcelon et al. (1999) explored the ability of X-ray CT for quality evaluation of peaches at various physiological maturity stages. They determined the X-ray absorption and internal changes in images at different levels of maturity in peaches and also determined the changes in CT number, physical, and chemical contents at different maturities and post-harvest ripening time. The CT number is the unit to measure X-ray absorption and is also called the Hounsfield unit. The CT number of air is −1000 and the CT number of water is zero. The equipment used for the study was the TOSCANER-20000 (Toshiba Co., Japan), and the CT number range was from −1000 to 4000. Peaches were harvested at 92, 97, 104, 111, and 1222 days after flowering and were marked as maturity stages 1 to 5 where maturity increased with numbers. The images were obtained through the central region and at two different locations, 15 mm from the center of the fruit. The CT images with increased brightness showed an increase in density, and dense portions mean higher CT numbers. In newly harvested peaches, the flesh that constitutes larger portions absorbed X-rays evenly. After 2 weeks of ripening, regions surrounding the stone become dry containing void spaces, resulting in lower absorbance and lower CT numbers. The authors concluded that CT numbers significantly decreased with increasing maturity. X-ray CT images showed the changes occurred at the inner regions of the peach at various maturity levels, and hence the X-ray CT technique can be used to monitor changes of peaches during ripening and different maturity levels.

Predicting the tomato maturity by locular gel formation and seed development as criteria for harvesting requires destruction of the fruit. Brecht (1991) studied the possibility to determine the maturity of green tomatoes using X-ray CT. The equipment used was an EMI 5005 scanner (Hayes, Middlesex, United Kingdom) with 120 kV and 1881 mA X-ray intensity. The fruits were placed individually in a wooden holder specially constructed to hold the fruits, and, after scanning, the fruits were cut in half for visual observation. The fruits were classified into four maturity classes and 12 fruits per maturity class were selected for scanning. About 92%, 58%, 75%, and 83% of the fruits were correctly classified in maturity class 1, 2, 3, and 4, respectively. The results suggest that X-ray CT has good potential to monitor maturity in tomatoes, but classification accuracy needs to be improved in order for X-ray CT to be useful for maturity sorting for commercial purposes.

8.3.2.3   Cereal products

X-ray CT was explored by many researchers to study the internal structure of various food products, including bread (Falcone et al., 2005; Lape et al., 2008; Miri and Fryer, 2008), aerated chocolates and muffins (Lim and Barigou, 2004; Frisullo et al., 2010b), bakery products (Chevallier and Bail, 2012), and biscuits and bread sticks (Frisullo et al., 2010a).

Chanvrier et al. (2009) used X-ray CT to characterize the structure of extruded rice. Rice flour was processed to obtain pellets of 10 mm diameter and placed on the sample holder. The moisture content (m.c.) tested was 17%, 20%, and 23%, and temperatures were 120°C, 135°C, and 150°C. X-ray CT scans were obtained with the Skyscan 1172 micro-CT at 40 kV and 100 μA. Scans of samples were performed over 180° for every 0.4° and scanning time was around 45 min. 3D image analyses were performed, and distribution of cells and cell walls and the structure thickness were obtained. The cross-sectional images of the samples revealed that samples at 120°C and 23% m.c. appeared less expanded than at 17% m.c. The range of cell size at 17% and 20% m.c. was higher (500 to 2000 μm) than at 23% m.c. (500 to 1400 μm). The images also revealed that porosity of the 23% m.c. sample was lower (84%), while it was between 87% to 91% for the 17% and 20% m.c. sample. By using X-ray tomography, good contrast could be obtained between the cells and the cereal matrix, and hence X-ray CT is a potential technique to determine the expanded structure of cereal food products.

Multicomponent food products comprised of dry and moist products, such as biscuits with fruit filling, is of great interest, and a technology to prevent moisture migration from moist to dry product is important. Hence knowledge of the microstructure of food components and its relation to water mobility is very crucial in the development of such products. Dalen et al. (2007) studied the uses of micro-CT to visualize the internal cellular structure of crackers with various porosity biscuit shell and soup inclusions. Images were obtained using Skyscan 1072 desktop micro CT at 50 kV and 100 μA. Micro-CT images of biscuit shell coated with lipid clearly showed the lipid barrier layer as a homogeneous gray area. The images of crackers produced with five different proofing times of 10, 25, 60, 115, and 130 min showed that proofing time in the range of 10 to 60 min produced lower porosity and small pore size, whereas 115 and 130 min proofing times resulted in larger pore size and higher porosity. Also, the image analysis showed that most of the void space was connected in 3D and the number of connections increased with increasing pore size. They concluded that micro-CT is a potential technique for visualizing the internal structure of cellular products.

Lim and Barigou (2004) studied the microstructure of various cellular food products, such as honeycomb chocolate bar, aerated chocolate bar, mousse, marshmallow, and chocolate muffins, using high-resolution X-ray micro-CT (Skyscan 1072) at 100 kV and 96 μA. Images were obtained through rotation of the sample at 180°. X-ray CT image of the chocolate bar revealed fewer and larger air cells at the center than at the bottom and top surfaces. For the semiliquid foam strawberry mousse, the variation between the air density in the cells and the enclosing semiliquid material resulted in a high contrast in the reconstructed image. Quantitative information such as number of air cells, average cell size, and relative and total cell area was extracted from 2D horizontal slices. The cell wall thickness distribution was obtained from the 3D models and the average thickness of cell wall for aerated and honeycomb chocolate was 0.660 and 0.240 mm, respectively. The thickness value indicates the mechanical strength of the cellular microstructure and its potential to resist loading forces. The measured values indicate that compared to aerated chocolate, honeycomb has a crumblier microstructure. Lim and Barigou concluded that this noninvasive technique needs no preparation of sample and provides complete 3D microstructure of the sample. This could be very valuable and useful for the analysis of aerated food materials and could open new perspective for the mathematical model development that connects microstructure of the product to its mechanical properties and rheology.

8.3.2.4   Bread

The textural characteristics of food products are very important, which are dependent on the microstructure of the food. Especially in bakery products, the texture plays an important role. Although many techniques are employed to determine the microstructure of bakery products, there is a need for a method capable of explaining the microstructure in three dimensions and it needs to be a noninvasive technique. X-ray CT could prove a new method to determine and investigate the microstructure of bakery products (Miri and Fryer, 2008). Miri and Fryer (2008) prepared bread dough samples and investigated the microstructure during the bread-making process. They obtained detailed data on various parameters describing the microstructure, such as pore size distribution, thickness of cell wall, interconnectivity of pores, and development of crust during baking.

The quality attributes of bakery products depend on the crispy texture of crust, softness of the crumb, and color. Chevallier and Bail (2012) explored the capability of X-ray micro-CT to evaluate the microstructure of bakery products, especially the crust and crumb interface of bread. The images were acquired using Skyscan 1174 (Skyscan, Kontich, Belgium). The 20 mm thick bread sample was kept on a plate and evaluated starting from the crust surface. The crust was characterized by many small pores with low connectivity, whereas crumb was made of fewer and larger, highly connected pores. The results showed that X-ray microtomography is a powerful tool to characterize the microstructure of bakery products.

The sensory attributes and consumer appreciation of biscuits and breadsticks strongly depend on the texture and crunchiness of the product. Although information on 3D structure of the food can be obtained by various techniques, such as light microscopy, electron microscopy, atomic force microscopy, and magnetic resonance imaging, these techniques are invasive and need extensive sample preparation. X-ray microtomography allows high-resolution 3D visualization and characterization of internal food structure without requirement for any sample preparation and is noninvasive. Frisullo et al. (2010a) studied six types of Italian biscuits and three different varieties of breadsticks using the Skyscan 1172 X-ray microtomography system (Skyscan, Belgium). The results of the study showed that a correlation exists between microstructural data such as degree of anisotropy, object structure volume ratio, percentage object volume, and crunchiness of the sample. Hence, analysis of bakery products at the microstructural level could be used to improve the sensory characteristics of various food products.

Lape et al. (2008) used X-ray CT to analyze the inner crumb structure of three varieties of bread having distinct characteristics such as nutritional component (flax and fiber wheat bread), mouth feel (artisan bread), visual appeal, and consistency (white Wonder Bread). Conventional analysis of bread crumb structure was performed with a scanner or

CCD camera, but the 2D images obtained may not characterize the overall bread morphology. But X-ray micro-CT provides more accurate details to analyze the density characteristics of bread. The frozen bread was cut into 1 cm^3 cubes and used for the study. Images were obtained with the Skyscan^{TM} 1072 X-ray microtomograph at 60 kV and 100 mA. The important parameters that were analyzed were cell wall thickness, percent density, percent object volume, and air cell size. Their results showed differences in characteristics based on type of bread. For instance, the fiber wheat bread had the highest solid structure volume of 27% among the three bread varieties studied, which reflects the higher density inclusions in fiber bread. The visual uniformity of Wonder Bread was correlated to the consistent cell wall thickness. In case of artisan bread, the broad cell wall thickness and the differences in size of air cell corresponds to the desirable rustic handmade characteristics.

8.3.2.5   Frying of potato

Microstructure of food provides the desired textural characteristics and for deep-frying of potato strips, frying time and temperature are very important. Miri et al. (2006) explored the potential of X-ray micro-CT to study the internal 3D microstructure of potato strips during frying. In this technique, tomographic scan was obtained by rotating the sample perpendicular to the X-ray beam and radiographs of the object were acquired at narrow angular increments. Reconstruction of radiographs provide a series of 2D slices, which are then transformed into a 3D image either as a complete image or as slices of samples at various depths and in different directions. Potatoes were cut in cylindrical shapes (11.5 mm diameter and 40 mm length) and frying was conducted at 160°C, 170°C, and 180°C temperatures for a period of 2, 3, 5, and 7 min. High-resolution X-ray CT scans were obtained using Skyscan 1072 (Skyscan, Belgium) at 100 kV and 96 µA. From the micro-CT images, significant changes in the sample occur in the structure of the sample between 5 and 7 min of frying, and void areas could be seen due to steam entrapped during frying. The images also revealed that there was a broad distribution of pore sizes ranging from a few micrometers to millimeters and fewer larger pores contributed to the void area and limited interconnectivity between the pores were observed. The study showed that X-ray micro-CT could be a potential technique to obtain complete microstructural characterization, and it was also possible to determine crust size and the crust increased with increase in temperature and frying time.

8.3.2.6   Chocolate

Frisullo et al. (2010b) studied the microstructural characterization of 12 varieties of Italian aerated chocolates using X-ray microtomography. The high-resolution Skyscan 1172 desktop X-ray microtomography system (Skyscan, Belgium) was used for the study at power settings of 37 kV and 228 µA. The various quantitative 3D parameters such as structure thickness (ST), object structure volume ratio (OSVR), percentage object volume (POV), fragmentation index (FI), structure model index (SMI), structure separation (SS), and degree of anisotropy (DA) were measured. Micro CT uses the difference in X-ray attenuation, which arises due to difference in density of the sample. The microstructural information acquired by CT is the same as those obtained by chemical analysis. The results demonstrate that micro-CT is an efficient tool for quantitative and qualitative evaluation of product composition and has showed that the technique has the ability to estimate the sugar content of chocolate.

8.3.2.7   Bouillon

Unilever, a global manufacturer of consumer goods, produces bouillon cubes that need to be strong enough to survive transport and handling but also should be easy to crumble by hand. Bouillon cubes are made of sodium chloride, fat, seasonings including monosodium glutamate (MSG), and flavoring. These ingredients are compressed and made into cubes and the microstructure was studied using X-ray micro-CT because mechanical behavior such as cracking depends upon the composition and microstructural parameters such as size and shape of the particles and porosity of the matrix (Dalen et al., 2008). The Skyscan 1172 X-ray micro-CT was used and the parameters were set at 50 kV and 200 μA, or 100 kV and 100 μA. The length, breadth, and thickness of the particles measured by image analysis were compared to those obtained by manual measurements of micro-CT image using the interactive 3D measurement tool. In the X-ray micro-CT images, salt (sodium chloride) particles are clearly visible as dark objects in a light gray fatty matrix. But salt cannot be distinguished from MSG by difference in gray level; they can only be identified by a difference in morphology because salt particles are generally cubic shaped whereas MSG has a plate or needle structure. They concluded that X-ray CT is a useful, noninvasive technique to study the 3D visualization and microstructure characterization of bouillon cubes.

8.3.2.8 Meat

In any processed meat product, total fat content is a critical factor and the most commonly used method to analyze fat content is chemical analysis (AOAC, 1995). But this method is expensive, tedious, destructive, and sometimes uses harmful, flammable solvent that is considered a health and environment hazard. X-ray microtomography, a noninvasive technique, could be used to analyze fat content and Frisullo et al. (2009) determined the fat content of five varieties of Italian salami (Milano, Ungherese, Modena, Norcinetto, Napoli). The 3D parameters that describe the fat structure such as structure thickness (ST), percentage object volume (POV), and the object structure volume ratio (OSVR) were calculated. Salami samples were prepared with 28 mm in diameter and 18 mm thickness and wrapped in parafilm (plastic paraffin film) to avoid moisture dispersion and imaged using Skyscan 1172 X-ray micro tomography (Skyscan, Belgium) with a power setting of 82 kV and 125 μA. The contrast in micro-CT images are due to variation in X-ray absorption by sample constituents such as fat, protein, and air, and the contrast is due to differences in density and a variation in sample composition. The highest fat content was seen in Ungherese and Norcinetto, whereas Napoli salami had the lowest fat content. The images obtained from reconstruction software clearly showed the fat, protein, and air matrix. Also the average POV values obtained by both CT and chemical analysis are similar without any significant statistical difference. Hence, they concluded that X-ray microtomography could be an efficient technique to examine the quantitative distribution of fat in meat products.

To produce high-quality fried food, a good understanding of microstructure of the food is essential. X-ray micro-CT is a unique noninvasive imaging technique with little or no sample preparation and results in 3D rendition of high-resolution images. Adedeji and Ngadi (2009) studied the potential of X-ray micro-CT for 3D imaging of fried chicken nuggets. The samples supplied by a local producer (OLYMEL Co., QC) were stored at −50°C and kept at refrigeration temperature for 24 h prior to frying. The nuggets were fried at 180°C for 0, 1, 3, and 4 min, brought to room temperature and cut into 5 mm × 5 mm × 7 mm by a knife, kept in parafilm to prevent drying, and placed in a sample holder for imaging. The X-ray micro-CT (Skyscan 1072, Belgium) was set at 100 keV, 98 μA and 6 s exposure time. The images were reconstructed into a series of 2D images and quantitative assessment such as binarization, cutting the region of interest, and image processing of the reconstructed raw image were achieved using the CT analyzer and CT vol software (Skyscan, Belgium). The 3D model clearly showed the air space within the fried sample as a solid network of interconnected spaces within a transparent body fat, protein, and carbohydrates.

In unfried samples, almost 90% of the pores were less than 65 micron in diameter and a high percentage of small micropores could result in decreased oil absorption during frying. Even distribution of pore volume within the pore size range was observed in fried samples. The 3D images showed the degree of interconnectivity of pores, pore shape, and pore count under different conditions of frying and porosity changes were confirmed with varying frying time. They concluded that X-ray micro-CT has a great potential in analyzing the microstructural characteristics of fried foods by providing quantitative information on pore size distribution, porosity, and connectivity of pores.

In meat processing, curing is an important process but due to the absence of nondestructive methods to analyze the diffusion and distribution of curing ingredients, development of new and desirable curing methods is very limited. Vestergaard et al. (2004) investigated the use of the X-ray CT method for quantification of concentration of salt in cured pork. Eight pork loins of different pH and different days of aging were obtained for the experiment and after initiating the curing process, CT measurements were made from day 1 to day 5. CT measurements were made using the Siemens Somatom AR whole body scanner (Norway). The results showed that a strong correlation exists between sodium chloride measured by chemical methods and that determined using X-ray CT. Vestergaard et al. concluded that X-ray CT could be used as an efficient and nondestructive technique for quantification of salt content in meat products and the technique could be of great value for research and product development.

8.3.3   Aquaculture

In Norwegian smoked salmon, the average sodium content ranges between 2 and 4 g/100 g of product. The daily recommended intake for sodium is 5 g, whereas the actual daily intake of a Norwegian adult is 10 g (Norwegian Directorate of Health, 2009). But reducing the sodium chloride content in smoked salmon may reduce the shelf life and alter the texture and taste. The only change that could be made is to reduce the duration of dry salt contact because raw fillets of Norwegian salmon are dry salted. The salt diffusion depends on water content, but negative correlation exists between water and fat content, so with increasing fat content the salt content generally decreases. Hence, to meet the minimum requirement of salt content, some parts of the fillet are over salted. To monitor the salting process and control the salt content, it is important to understand the salt diffusion dynamics, and nondestructive imaging techniques such as X-ray CT could be useful (Segtnan et al., 2009). Segtnan et al. (2009) studied the potential of X-ray CT for noncontact analysis of fat and salt distribution in salted and smoked salmon fillets. The Siemen Somatom Emotion CT scanner (Siemens AG, Germany) was used for the study at 106 mA and 1 s rotation time and at three voltages (80, 110, and 130 kV). The analysis showed that higher fat content was observed on the belly and the fat content variation within a fillet was much higher than the variation between the fillets. In most parts of fillet except the belly portion, the correlation between salt and fat is high (–0.78). For the belly portion, the correlation between salt and fat is almost zero because of physiological differences within the fillet. Since the belly region is thinner than the back, the salt diffusion in belly part was not affected by lower water content (or high fat) compared to the rest of the fillet. The correlation between predicted CT and reference values were between 0.78 and 0.8 for one or two voltages, and with all three voltages the correlation coefficient went up to 0.92. Segtnan et al. concluded that X-ray CT could be used to determine the analysis of sodium chloride in salmon fillet during salting and smoking.

Folkestad et al. (2008) determined the fat and pigment concentration in slaughtered and live salmon using visible/near-infrared (VIS/NIR) spectroscopy and digital photography and chemical analyses and X-ray CT were used as reference methods. The salmon were anaesthetized and analyzed live using VIS/NIR spectroscopy and then slaughtered and gutted, and CT images were acquired. Within 2 h of CT examination, salmon were again imaged using VIS/NIR, filleted by hand, and digital photograph images were obtained. The results showed that prediction of fat content was less accurate with digital photography compared to VIS/NIR, and the NIR spectroscopy provided accurate results of fat percentage as compared to the CT method. A new method of VIS/NIR spectroscopy has been used successfully to estimate the pigment and fat percent of live and slaughtered salmon. NIR spectroscopy and digital photography methods are both suitable to estimate the pigment contents in salmon, and digital photography is more economical compared to NIR spectroscopy.

In fish production, fat composition is an important characteristic from the feeding cost of fish as well as meat quality. Body composition is most commonly performed by chemical analysis, which is a destructive method. A nondestructive method to determine fat composition is gaining popularity and Romvári et al. (2002) studied the possibility of X-ray CT to determine the fat content of fillet and protein content of anaesthetized live fresh water fish. The study included 48 fish samples: 18 common carp (*Cyprinus carpio* L.), 10 grass carp (*Ctenopharyngodon idella* Val.), 10 silver carp (*Hypophthalmichtis molitrix* Val.), and 10 pike-perch (*Stizostedion lucioperca* L.). A strong correlation between the outcome of chemical analysis and pixel density data could be used to develop prediction equations. 3D volumetric estimation of fat tissue was calculated based on fat index displaying good correlation with the measured fat content. X-ray CT is a potential method to determine fat composition of fish fillet and also enables one to determine the body composition during a period of growth or under various feeding conditions.

Starvation of Atlantic salmon before slaughtering is practiced to make sure that the fish has an empty gut, which improves the freshness and quality of fish. Unfortunately, documentation relating to quality characteristics and production loss due to starvation before slaughter is very limited. Hence slaughter yield and fillet yield are of economic importance for processors, and it is important to study and evaluate these criteria. Since consumers of Atlantic salmon look for body shape and fat content as important features, Einen et al. (1998) investigated the effect of starvation time on shape of body, weight loss, product yield, and fat composition. Experiments were performed with seven groups of 0, 3, 7, 14, 30, 58, and 86 days of starvation before slaughter and the images were acquired using X-ray CT body scanner (Somatom 2CT, Siemens, Germany). The results showed that weight loss percentage significantly increased with starvation time except between 30 and 58 days of starvation, when no significant difference in weight loss was observed. A negative correlation was observed between viscera percent and slaughter yield. There was a reduction in body weight with an unchanged or increase in body length indicating vertebrae growth and muscle development are two different processes. The result also suggests that the body reserve could be used by the fish to support vertebrae growth during starvation. The study also showed a higher slaughter yield for 30 days of starvation and fillet yield was reduced after long-term starvation. Based on the results of the study, it could be explained that for slaughterhouses long-term (30 days) starvation would be advantageous, whereas for smokehouses and other filleting applications fillet yield will be reduced after starvation for long term.

8.3.4   Livestock management

In commercial breeding programs, for evaluating the carcass composition, ultrasonic scanning is mostly used in vivo but X-ray CT has demonstrated an improved prediction of carcass traits over ultrasonic scanning. Karamichou et al. (2007) studied the selection of carcass quality in hill sheep using X-ray CT and the results of the study showed that X-ray CT could provide efficient means of selection for improved carcass composition. Kolstad (2001) examined the various fat deposit development in three groups of pigs by repetitive body composition measurement by using X-ray CT to increase the knowledge and understanding of the genetic variation in fat distribution in pigs of various live weights.

The evaluation of live cattle characteristics is significant in the carcass composition analysis and in improving the breeding methods. Although an ultrasonic technique is used, ultrasonic photographs are not very precise to observe visually; hence, Nade et al. (2005) explored the use of X-ray CT to study live standing cattle, and its meat yield, carcass composition, and so forth. The animals were confined at their front, back, and side using air bags and were injected with sedative to limit movement. After scanning, animals were slaughtered and the scanned carcass cross-section was photographed. The correlation coefficient between X-ray CT and photograph image for *Musculus longissimus* and *Musculus trapezius* area were 0.843 and 0.585, respectively, and the correlation coefficient of the back fat thickness was 0.926. The lower correlation coefficient of *M. Trapezius* area may be due to the slight movement of the animals when exposed to X-ray CT. Hence, a more efficient method to confine the animals needs to be developed in the future. The results showed X-ray CT could be of practical commercial use in the study of cattle composition.

8.3.5 Engineering applications

Although X-ray CT was originally developed for medical applications, the potential of X-ray CT was later realized by researchers in other fields and has been widely used for engineering purposes. Researchers started using the term "industrial X-ray CT scanner" from 1996 based on its application in soil mechanics and geotechnical engineering (Otani et al., 2010). The applications of X-ray CT were explored in various engineering industries such as geological, automobile, aircraft, electrical and civil, and construction.

X-ray CT has potential application in civil and geotechnical engineering, and many studies have been conducted to measure the failure pattern and soil behavior during loading. Asphalt mixture with high percentage of air voids breaks down quickly due to stress. Also two mixtures with the same mean air void radius may have significantly different rates of crack propagation and moisture damage due to the difference in the size of the variance of the air void (Luo and Lytton, 2011). Luo and Lytton (2011) established the potential of X-ray CT to accurately estimate the air void and subsequent crack radius distribution. To develop realistic predictive models to determine aging and moisture damage, accurate measurement of initial distribution of air void sizes and distribution of cracks is very essential.

The alloy steel used in various engineering industries experience damage due to various operations, and the last stages of failure are due to creation of voids and cracks. Gupta et al. (2009) explored the potential of employing microfocus X-ray CT to acquire images of voids that occur due to deformation in alloy steel. Scanning was performed using the Skyscan 1172 high-resolution X-ray microtomography at 100 kV and 100 μA. The results showed that X-ray CT has the potential to explain and characterize the process of development of damages that occur in dense structural material such as steel. Mizoguchi et al. (2010) examined the effectiveness of using X-ray CT imaging to detect the propagation of cracks that occur at solder joints during temperature cycling test. Their study showed that X-ray CT images are efficient for detecting and monitoring of defects at the assembly levels such as the connector, printed circuit boards, and solder joints.

In the construction industry, corrosion of steel reinforcement in concrete is a major issue and from the current available methods, such as the electrochemical method, it is not possible to obtain information on the extent and distribution of corrosion without destroying the specimen. Beck et al. (2010) proposed analyzing the surface of steel within the mortar specimen by X-ray CT and the results showed that it is possible to visualize the propagating corrosion on reinforced steel in a mortar with a 35 mm cover thickness. The results showed that X-ray CT could determine the mass loss at different stages of corrosion. Birgul (2008) studied the potential of X-ray CT to determine the macrovoids and to analyze the strength development in mortar specimen. X-ray CT images were acquired on the same sample on various days and image analysis was performed. The results showed that the mortar sample porosity decreased from 3.94 at the initial period to 3.06% at the end of the evaluation period showing that X-ray CT is a powerful technique to determine voids in mortar specimen.

The feasibility of X-ray CT for soil and rock engineering applications was studied by Otani et al. (2000). They determined the fracture toughness of rock by the crack propagation method. The measurement of crack aperture was examined using X-ray CT, and the results showed that crack aperture was propagated in the rock as the load was increased. The use of X-ray CT in soil testing was demonstrated by examining the mechanism of bearing capacity of the ground for vertical pile loading and visualized by the X-ray CT scanner. The authors concluded that X-ray CT is a potential tool for conducting geotechnical analysis of soil and rocks. Otani et al. (2010) studied the use of X-ray CT for quantitative measurement, such as deformation and strain on soil, and compared the results with numerical analysis. Their study showed that X-ray CT could be very useful for geomechanics and geotechnical engineering. Alramahi and Alshibli (2006) determined the internal structure of geomaterials using nondestructive X-ray CT obtaining valuable information on the structure of the geomaterials. But they also suggested that geometry of the scanned sample and surrounding material plays a critical role in the image quality; and artifacts, such as beam hardening, and partial volume effect need to be carefully assessed and minimized.

Measurement of soil properties on the microscale has lots of difficulties, hence geotechnical engineers use macro properties such as porosity, void ratio, and density to determine the behavior of soil when subjected to various stresses. Mokwa and Nielsen (2006) conducted analysis on five different soils and provided a viable method for nondestructively measuring the pore size and grain size distribution and pore characteristics of soil using X-ray CT. Otani et al. (2006) investigated the failure pattern in sand during lateral loading using X-ray CT. Images of the ground acquired by the X-ray CT scanner at several levels of loading that was applied at the pile head and the cross-sectional images were then reconstructed to obtain 3D images, and the failure pattern of the ground during lateral loading was visualized using X-ray CT. Morita et al. (2007) visualized the failure pattern of both laterally and vertically loaded piles using X-ray CT. Their study showed that bearing capacity mechanism of both laterally and vertically loaded piles were visualized and evaluated in three dimensions without any actual destruction, and concluded that X-ray CT is a powerful technique for applications in geotechnical engineering.

Due to increasing economic pressure on the production process in the automotive industry, applications of X-ray CT for nondestructive testing has great potential because of the fast and precise characteristics (Bauer et al., 2004). At the corporate research center of Robert Bosch in Germany, a CT system was tested for the process of reverse engineering to construct computer-assisted design (CAD) models from measured data. The measured volumetric data and the material defect analysis and classification using CT images demonstrated that X-ray CT could be a fast, accurate, and inexpensive technique to enable complete testing of the various automotive components at the end of the production line in the automotive industry.

The major disadvantages of the current inspection technique during castings manufacturing are that the process is subjective and ambiguous and does not correlate well to the actual service requirement of the components. Bossi and Georgeson (1992) evaluated the ability of X-ray CT for inspection of castings. The study showed that the 3D feature definition obtained from CT can be transformed to CAD/CAM (computer-aided manufacturing) files and provide input to finite element models to examine the performance of castings. They demonstrated a dimensional measurement with great accuracy and precision better than 50 microns and a significant cost savings in the manufacture of castings using X-ray CT. Sasaki et al. (2006) studied the microdefects in aluminum castings using X-ray CT and successfully determined the volume and number of microdefects present in the aluminum castings.

8.3.6 Applications of X-ray CT in medicine

The introduction of X-ray CT in the early 1970s significantly changed the practice of medicine, and the advance in the technology from early generation CT scanners to single slice and then to multislice scanners further enhanced their use in medical diagnostics. X-ray CT scanning produces cross-sectional images or slices of the body that are used for a variety of diagnostic and treatment procedures. The ability of CT to demonstrate lesions in the brain, tumors, abscesses, and hemorrhage directly caught the attention of radiologists around the world. In 1975, Sir Godfrey got the attention of the entire world with the announcement of whole body CT at an international conference in Bermuda (Husband and Dombrowe, 2005). Within 5 years, most of the medical centers installed CT systems for investigation of malignant diseases. Today, X-ray CT is used for diagnosis of various diseases, trauma, or abnormalities in the body, and helps in planning or monitoring the whole process of treatment.

Currently tremendous technical improvements have been made to X-ray CT imaging such as development of helical acquisition, multidetector, and large area detector acquisition. Besides these improvements, a recent development is the dual source CT in which a dual source detector has two X-ray tubes and two detector units. This system allows dual energy scanning, that is, two synchronous CT acquisitions at different tube potentials. The dual scanner system offers many advantages such as reduced CT acquisition time, improvement in differentiating various tissues, increased resolution of images, and reduced overall radiation dosage (Grignon et al., 2012).

The whole body X-ray CT scan is performed for various diagnoses and treatment and the most common uses of CT are

- To examine the chest, abdomen, and pelvis, and in patients with severe injuries due to vehicle accidents or work-related accidents
- To diagnose different types of cancer such as lung, liver, kidney, and pancreas; to measure the size and growth of tumor, location of the tumor, and its effect on the nearby tissues

CT scanning has great potential in the diagnosis and treatment process of vascular diseases that may eventually result in stroke or malfunctioning of the kidney. Head CT scan is performed to detect injury to brain, bleeding, skull fractures, blood clot, brain tumors, stroke, aneurysm, and so on. CT scan images provide valuable information to assess and evaluate the extent of damage caused to the bone and soft tissue in patients affected by facial trauma, and in the planning of surgical treatment and planning process for treatment of cancer (Radiological Society of North America, 2012).

Improvements in the increase of gantry rotational speed along with multislice acquisition have improved the performance of CT in medicine in many diagnostic applications, such as CT peripheral angiography, CT abdominal perfusion (kidney, liver) and CT virtual colonoscopy. Ko et al. (2012) studied the dual energy CT for thoracic applications and stated that imaging with dual-energy CT allows tissue characterization along with morphological evaluation of the region of interest. X-ray CT is widely used for diagnosis of tumor and cancer growth in various organs and also used in bone investigations. More than 30% of CT scans are recommended for the chest where high-resolution spiral CT could show chronic interstitial processes in the lung (Morris and Perkins, 2012).

8.3.6.1 Cardiology

Among the applications of multislice CT imaging, cardiac applications are very significant. Applications of the CT scanner in cardiology have tremendously improved after the latest improvements in multislice acquisition and high rotational speed. Within seconds or minutes, the latest CT scanners have the potential to diagnose whether the chest pain is because of coronary blockage or pulmonary embolism or due to aortic aneurism. All of these are critical conditions that require immediate attention but totally different therapeutic interventions. The most advanced and new 64-slice scanners could provide adequate images of the heart in 8 heartbeats and very accurate images of hearts in 20 heartbeats (Deych and Dolazza, 2006). Coronary heart disease (CHD) is an important and critical health care challenge in the United States. The total direct and indirect cost per annum for treatment of CHD is estimated to be around $110 billion and is anticipated to rise by 53% during the next two decades (Heidenreich et al., 2011). Patients affected by CHD are exposed to several imaging tests before a final evaluation is made on their condition. But in ideal conditions, one imaging modality should facilitate rapid and accurate diagnosis. Advances in computed tomography have led to improvement in spatial and temporal resolution, and computed tomography angiography (CTA) has become a single technique for extensive assessment of myocardial function, coronary arterial anatomy, perfusion, and myocardial viability (Sharma and Arbab-Zadeh, 2012). Many studies have been conducted to compare coronary CTA with traditional coronary angiography to detect the accuracy of coronary stenosis in patients with ≥50% stenosis (Budoff et al., 2007; Gaemperli et al., 2008; Ravipati et al., 2008), and the studies revealed that accuracy of CTA was high with sensitivity and specificity of 99% and 88%, respectively.

Advancements in CT technology, including multidetector array, faster gantry rotation, and dual source devices, have made CT angiography (CTA) an alternate to conventional coronary angiography for diagnosis of coronary artery disease (CAD). Gaemperli et al. (2008) studied the accuracy of 64 section CTA with myocardial perfusion single-photon emission computed tomography (SPECT). They examined about 78 patients and analyzed 1093 coronary segments in 310 coronary arteries. The results of the study showed that 64-section CTA could help to rule out CAD in people with intermediate to high possibility although an abnormal CT angiography is not a good predictor of ischemia.

Sharma and Arbab-Zadeh (2012) have stated that CTA provides promising results for characterizing coronary atherosclerotic plaque. CTA could provide more cost-effective treatment and the CTA-assisted examination of patients with severe chest pain has resulted in 54% reduced time for diagnosis and 38% lowering of cost compared to the standard testing procedures. Another interesting development is the modeling of coronary blood flow with the help of CTA based on computational fluid dynamic calculations. With further improvements, CTA may become a potential technique for hemodynamic evaluation of coronary artery stenosis using CTA images without any additional procedures. Compared to traditional angiography, CTA has significant advantages such as noninvasiveness, because a single injection could obtain multiple views, visualization of both extraluminal and intraluminal structures, and high speed of the procedure (Grignon et al., 2012).

8.3.6.2 *Lung and related diseases*

Lu et al. (2012) reviewed dual-energy computed tomography (DECT) acquisition and clinical applications in lung blood volume measurements, detection of pulmonary embolism (PE), and the role of DECT in lung ventilation and characterization of lung malignancies. Based on the various studies, they stated that DECT could provide both functional and anatomical information of the lungs in various pulmonary diseases and could perform better in the diagnosis of both chronic and acute pulmonary embolism, various vascular disorders, lung malignancies, and parenchymal diseases.

Airway-related diseases such as asthma and chronic bronchitis are common worldwide and the prevalence of asthma affects 25 million individuals in the United States and 300 million worldwide (National Heart, Lung and Blood Institute, 2007). Human airways appear to be a treelike branching network of tubes that enable airflow into the lungs through the trachea, and in order to understand the underlying mechanism noninvasive investigation of airways is a subject of great research interest. Pu et al. (2012) reviewed the CT based computerized identification and analysis of human airways. Computerized analysis of airways depicted on CT images covers a number of areas such as airway segmentation, airway identification, matching and labeling, and airway morphometry, which may further provide information related to pulmonary physiology and pathophysiology.

Jong et al. (2006) examined the use of CT to calculate the airway wall, lumen, arterial, and parenchyma dimensions in children during their growth phase to provide data that could be used to study any alterations caused by pulmonary diseases. During birth, about one third to half of adult number of alveoli exists and it increases rapidly until 1.5 to 2 years of age. In this study, CT scans of 50 children between the ages of 0 to 17.2 years undergoing CT investigation for nonpulmonary diseases were acquired and used for parenchyma, airway, and artery investigation. The data exhibited only a small increase in expansion of lung during childhood. The airway wall, lumen, and arterial region were associated exponentially with the height of the subject. Jong et al. concluded that the data from this study provided normative estimates of lumen, airway wall, and arterial and parenchyma dimensions, which could be useful to study in conditions in other individuals.

8.3.6.3 *CT colonography*

Brenner and Georgsson (2005) reviewed mass screening with CT colonography. Computed tomography colonography (CTC) based on a noncathartic technique has potential to improve compliance for screening colorectal cancer, because the geometry of CTC is favorable and could be performed with much smaller radiation doses compared to other types of CT examination. Screening using CTC, also referred to as virtual colonoscopy, has become a vital option for mass screening. But from the technological perspective, sensitivity and specificity of the CTC technique to identify and detect lesions from 5 to 100 mm was lower and standardization of CT parameters should be regulated before used for mass screening. In regard to exposure to radiation, the benefit-risk ratio is potentially large for CTC.

Ascenti et al. (2010) examined the potential of dual energy CT for urinary tract stones detection and characterization. A total of 39 patients (19 women, 20 men) with suspected renal colic were subjected to a preliminary low dose CT acquisition of complete urinary system followed by a dual-energy acquisition of the specific area with the urethral stone. Two radiologists reviewed the images and the results were compared with the results of biochemical analysis. The results of the study proved that use of dual energy CT could characterize all ureteral calculi and could also differentiate between uric acid stone and calcium salt stones. This differentiation of uric acid with calcium stone could allow the former to avoid surgical or interventional treatment for removal of stone, because urine alkalinization can dissolve uric acid stones and also CT exposure is significantly minimized using a limited stone-targeted dual-energy protocol. But the limitation of the study was that only stones with diameters greater than 3 mm were included in the study and the study was conducted on a small number of patients. Boll et al. (2009) evaluated the capability of dual-energy multidetector CT with advanced and improved postprocessing techniques for renal stone assessment. Fifty patients with renal calculi were examined, of which 30 stones are of pure crystalline composition and 20 of polycrystalline composition. The results of the study showed that dual-energy multidetector CT along with advanced image processing techniques performs better in the characterization of renal stone composition compared to single energy multidetector CT, thereby enabling optimization and individual treatment options for patients suffering from renal calculus disease. Graser et al. (2010) examined DECT for characterization and detection of renal masses as benign or malignant by examining a total of 202 patients. The results showed that DECT accurately assessed 96% of patients with malignancy and 93.2% of patients without malignancy with an overall assessment accuracy of 94.6%. The authors concluded that renal masses could be characterized in a speedy and accurate manner by DECT and image interpretation time was significantly lowered by interpretation of color-coded images.

The technical limitations for CT applications, such as prolonged data acquisition resulting in motion artifacts, has been overcome by the recent advances in DECT, which has become an important tool for medical diagnosis. DECT enables image acquisition at two different peak kilovoltages (kVp) and the currently available DECT configurations use a lower value of either 80 or 100 kVp and a higher peak kilovoltage of 140 (Ko et al., 2012). When DECT material differentiation becomes feasible and two scans can be replaced by one, which reduces the radiation dose, it eliminates misregistration artifacts, and saves postprocessing time (Postma et al., 2012). The advantages of DECT over single-energy CT is its ability to differentiate between substances of various X-ray energy attenuation, that is, it enables tissue characterization along with morphological evaluation. Heye et al. (2012) reviewed the applications of DECT for abdominal organs such as liver, pancreas, and kidney including renal stones and adrenal glands. Ma et al. (2010) assessed the possibility of dual-energy bone subtraction in cranial computed tomography angiography (CTA) and concluded that postprocessing time and reading time with dual energy bone removal are shorter. Using DECT, better vessel delineation at the skull base and similar vessel visualization of the intracranial vessels were noticed. Mühlenbruch et al. (2010) examined the carotid and intracranial vessels in 16 patients with symptomatic carotid artery stenosis and concluded that dual-energy CTA was equally good as magnetic resonance angiography and yielded additional morphological information on calcifications. Postma et al. (2012) reviewed the applications of dual-energy CT of brain and intracranial vessels and stated that DECT has not been widely implemented in neuroradiology. Removal of bone at the skull is always a concern, but bone removal in DECT angiography allows easier and faster acquisition compared to CTA. They also stated that detection and follow-up of treated aneurysms are reliable, and the detection of hemorrhage and analysis of underlying pathologic mechanism of hematomas is promising.

8.4 Advantages, limitations, and future of X-ray CT

8.4.1 Advantages

X-ray CT is a nondestructive imaging technique with little or no sample preparation required. In medical examinations, major developments in the CT technology over the last 20 years have reduced the scan time and reconstruction time and improved the image quality. Conventional radiographs cannot distinguish between soft tissues, whereas modern CT scanners could provide accurate details on various tissues and bones. With the advent of the latest improvement in CT scanners, it requires relatively less time to acquire images of patients compared to other techniques. Motion artifacts do not cause big differences as it occurs in MRI, and CT scans can be used for patients having implanted medical devices.

An industrial CT system is enclosed within a radiation shielding cabinet and hence, could be used in any environment without fear of radiation and additional safety concerns. A user-friendly interface, decreased scan time, and increased image quality of internal features have made X-ray CT the most viable tool in many industries. The new GE "speed-scan atline CT" works up to 200 times faster than conventional fan beam CT. The precise control of the geometry and dimension of products ensures that the geometrical and dimensional errors are detected and could be corrected at the early stages in the production line, which could save lot of money and time. The high-contrast resolution of CT enables one to distinguish differences between industrial materials that vary in physical density by 1%. This significant sensitivity in density allows CT to be able to highlight the structural irregularities, thereby increasing the accuracy of the production process.

X-ray CT provides more accurate information in measuring body composition of pigs and cattle compared to ultrasonic methods (Szabo et al., 1999). X-ray CT provides accurate information on the microstructure of various food products, which helps in understanding and development of food products with desired texture, sensory, and organoleptic properties.

8.4.2 Limitations

The resolution of CT image is limited to 1000 to 2000× the cross-sectional diameter of the object, and higher resolution could be obtained with smaller objects. Image artifacts such as beam hardening can create complications in data acquisition and interpretation. The most commonly occurring artifact is beam hardening, which results in sample edges appearing brighter than the center, even when the material is uniform throughout. The limitation for X-ray micro-CT is the penetrating power of X-rays relative to the material density, because dense samples need either very small specimens or very high energy X-rays. Also when the material phases have a huge difference in absorption of X-rays, the resulting image will have very poor image contrast (Landis and Keane, 2010).

In medical applications, the major limitation of X-ray CT is the overexposure of persons to radiation and an effort to reduce the exposure to X-ray would directly affect the image quality. In the mid-1990s CT scan accounted for only 4% of the total X-ray procedures in medicine but accounted for 40% of the total dosage, which provides a clear understanding of the high exposure related to X-ray CT (Wang and Yu, 2008). In micro-CT, the patient's exposure to radiation increases with the fourth power of the voxel side dimension when the image noise remains constant. Hence, higher spatial resolution results in larger exposure to radiation (Ritman, 2011). Another limitation of the CT scanner is that in order to overcome the beam hardening artifact, the X-ray photon energy needs to be monochromatic and tunable, which can be attained with synchrotron radiation, but it is not a practical source for routine medical applications (Natterer and Ritman, 2002). The contrast agents administered to patients to obtain CT images may sometimes cause allergic reactions in patients. For application of X-ray CT in the cattle industry, lack of portability of the equipment is a major drawback, which may limit the application only to research and breeding purposes (Szabo et al., 1999).

8.4.3   Future

The applications of X-ray CT are growing significantly not only in medicine but in other industries, including geosciences, civil, mechanical and electronic engineering, aquaculture, agriculture, and food. In medicine, use of X-ray CT has improved the diagnosis, planning, and treatment of the most severe diseases and in cases of emergency medical care for patients involved in accidents and other unforeseen events. X-ray CT has great potential to offer more benefits in the future in cutting edge technologies such as molecular imaging, nanoimaging, and combined imaging modalities such as CT/PET (positron emission tomography). Wang and Yu (2008) suggest that research and development of X-ray CT will be critical in the following fields: analytic and iterative reconstruction, dual source and multisource CT, flat-panel-based CT, new scanning modes, nano-CT artifact reduction modality fusion, energy sensitive CT, and phase contrast CT. It is expected that advanced X-ray sources such as portable synchrotron radiation devices will be more easily available and used in one or two decades from now.

chapter nine

Magnetic resonance imaging

9.1 Introduction

Edward Mills Purcell, an American physicist, and Felix Bloch, a Swiss physicist working at Stanford University, independently demonstrated the technique of nuclear magnetic resonance (NMR) in 1946 and shared the Nobel Prize for Physics in 1952. The concept of magnetic resonance imaging (MRI) was conceived by Dr. Raymond Damadian in 1969. Later, Damadian and coworkers, Minkoff and Goldsmith, acquired the first scan image of the human body in 1977 and the first commercial MRI scanner was introduced in 1980. The experiments on NMR were one dimensional and deficient in spatial information until 1974 when Peter C. Lauterbur, from the United States, and Peter Mansfield, from England, explained the magnetic field gradients potential for spatial localization of NMR signals and both were awarded the Nobel Prize for Physiology or Medicine in 2003. Until the late 1970s, the technique was referred to as nuclear magnetic resonance, but later, due to the stigma associated with the word "nuclear," it was widely referred to as magnetic resonance imaging.

Initial clinical NMR imaging was very difficult and tedious, and in early 1980, significant interest was developed in the clinical application of NMR imaging technique. In 1980, the future of clinical MRI was predicted by Goldman and his associates from Massachusetts General Hospital and Harvard Medical School in Boston. The technique was accepted as a potential clinical and research tool to examine and analyze congenital heart disease. Once the potential of MRI in the medical field had been understood and explored, researchers from other industries started exploring the potential of MRI. Slowly the applications of MRI started to develop and expand in various industries, including agriculture, soil science, food industry, animal science, aquaculture, and engineering.

9.2 Magnetic resonance imaging

9.2.1 Principle

The basis of magnetic resonance imaging depends on the magnetization properties of atomic nuclei. The MRI is based on the observation of water molecules in the human body. When an external strong magnetic field is applied, the protons present in the water molecules align with the magnetic field as magnetic dipoles and rotate around the axis of the magnetic field. This movement is called precession. The higher the magnetic field, the higher the precession. When electromagnetic radiation such as radio waves of the same frequency of the precessing nuclei is applied, they absorb the radiation that is at resonance and turn back becoming aligned at the opposite direction of the field. When the radio waves are turned off, the nuclei emits back the radiation, and each tissue of the body because of its different chemical composition re-emits radiation at a different rate known as tissue relaxation time. The radiation is absorbed by an antenna and transformed to an electrical current that is then used to construct the image (Secca, 2006). The important advantage of MRI images is that they produce sharp contrast images of soft tissues as compared to X-ray or computed tomography (CT) images.

The MRI system consists of very powerful super conducting magnets that create a static magnetic field. The magnetic field strengths are measured in gauss (G) and tesla (T) (1 tesla = 10,000 gauss). Most magnets used in MRI scanners have a magnetic field strength in the range of 0.3 to 1.5 T, whereas the magnetic field strength of Earth is 0.00005 T. So the magnets used in MRI scanners have thousands of times higher field strength than the Earth's magnetic field strength.

9.2.2   Components of MRI scanner

The major components in a MRI scanner are the magnet, radio frequency coils, gradient coils, and processor (computer).

9.2.2.1   Magnet

The magnet is the important and expensive component of the MRI scanner. The various types of magnets available are permanent, resistive, and superconducting magnets. A permanent magnet is made up of material that has been magnetized and it will never lose its magnetic field. The magnetic field strength lies in the range of 0.064 to 0.3 T. The permanent magnets have low power consumption and low operating cost, but are heavy and have limited magnetic field strength. The resistive magnets are very large magnets and magnetic field strength is generated by a current which runs through a loop of wire and can be switched off when not in use. The advantages of the resistive magnets are that these are light in weight and can be switched off to conserve power when not in use but have limited magnetic field strength (~0.3 T), higher power consumption, and require water for cooling. The most commonly used magnet is the superconducting magnet and the magnetic field is produced by a current that passes through a loop of wire. The wire is surrounded with coolant (usually liquid helium) to lower the electric resistance of the wire. The major advantages are that these have very high field strength of up to 12 T (for medical uses 1.5 T) and high field homogeneity. The disadvantages are high capital cost, acoustic noise, and associated motion artifacts (Blink, 2004). An ideal magnet produces a perfectly homogeneous magnetic field, which can be theoretically accomplished, but a closed structure is not patient friendly. Cylinders (1.5 T scanners) and parallel plate (open scanners) magnets are close to ideal (Steckner, 2006).

9.2.2.2   Radio frequency coil

Radio frequency (RF) coils are essential to receive and transfer radio frequency waves used in MRI scanners. RF coils affect the image quality. The two types of RF coils available are surface and volume coils (Blink, 2004). The surface coil lies on the object surface being imaged. The surface coil produces a small homogeneous field and the penetration depth depends on the coil size. This is the major advantage of using surface coil for imaging areas that are closer to the surface because a good signal-to-noise ratio is obtained by excluding the noise away from the region of interest (Clare, 1997). Volume coils could fit either one specific region or be big enough to fit the whole body and the most commonly used design is the birdcage coil.

9.2.2.3   Gradient coil

The gradient coil is essential to create a linear variation in the field along one direction and to result in higher efficiency and lower resistance to minimize the deposition of heat and current requirements (Clare, 1997). Gradient coils are located inside the magnet, the bore through which current is passed. The flow of current through the gradient coil produces

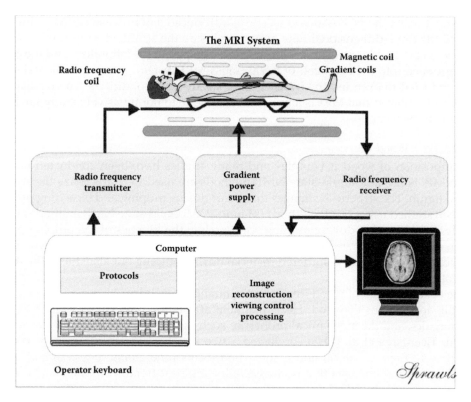

Figure 9.1 Typical architecture of a medical MRI system. (From Sprawls, P., Magnetic resonance imaging system components, in *Magnetic resonance imaging: Principles, methods, and techniques,* Madison, WI: Medical Physics Publishing, 2000b. With permission.)

a gradient magnetic field that has many purposes, including spatial encoding, slice selection, flow compensation, and rewinding. A typical architecture of a medical MRI system is shown in Figure 9.1.

9.2.2.4   Processor

The control operations of the scanner are performed through a computer, which specifies the shape of the gradient and radiofrequency waveforms and transfers the information to the waveform generator that outputs the signal, amplifies it, and sends it to the coil. An analog-to-digital converter transforms the signal to digital form, which is passed on to an image processor to perform Fourier transformation and the image is seen on the monitor (Clare, 1997).

9.3   Applications of MRI

9.3.1   Agriculture

9.3.1.1   Soil

The study of the movement of liquid in porous media is an interesting field, especially important in petroleum extraction and transport of contaminants and water through unsaturated soils. The commonly proposed method is the invasion of porous rock using high-pressure water, but the movement of liquid happens along discrete pathways and this phenomenon is called fingering. It is essential to understand this phenomenon to develop new extraction methods. Posadas et al. (1996) introduced a noninvasive MRI technique to examine the three-dimensional flow occurring inside the stratified soil samples. A cubic $15 \times 15 \times 15\ cm^3$ double layer sand column was developed in the laboratory and the column was positioned into the head coil of a 500 Gauss MRI system. Two experimental studies were conducted to examine the transient and steady-state conditions. The results of the experiments showed that MRI is a potential technique to noninvasively study the 3D soil fingering in the laboratory.

9.3.1.2 Wood

The composition of wood is complex and many studies have been conducted on wood using NMR. Solid- and liquid-state NMR methods are used to characterize the structure of wood lignin. The structural changes that occur during pulping and bleaching processes have been studied using NMR methods (Maunu, 2002). Solid-state NMR methods are used to study delignification during pulping and to study the kinetics of the pulping process. Larsson et al. (1999) showed that higher crystallinity in pulps compared to wood is not only because of the loss of disordered material during pulping but also due to the restructuring of carbohydrates.

The heat treatment of wood improves the quality of wood and has significantly diversified the applications of wood. Heat treatment affects the physical as well as chemical characteristics, and the mechanical properties such as bending strength and elasticity are reduced. Tjeerdsma et al. (1998) conducted a two-step heat treatment process to a hard wood (beech, *Fagus sylvatica*) and a soft wood (Scots pine, *Pinus sylvestris*) and investigated the chemical changes that occurred following heat treatment. The results showed that heat treatment modified the structure of wood components and significant variations were obtained in the amount of amorphous carbohydrates during the process.

9.3.1.3 Cereal grains

9.3.1.3.1 *Rice.*   MRI is a potential tool to analyze the moisture distribution in food samples. Horigane et al. (1999) studied the distribution of water and structural changes in cooked rice grain using MRI. The experiments were conducted on a Bruker DRX300WB (Bruker, Karlsruhe, Germany) spectrometer with a microimaging accessory. Two-dimensional images of both transverse and longitudinal sections of 3D MR images showed dark spots that occurred only within the grain, and lacerations did not occur on the grain surface. The hollows may be due to changes in structure that occurred in grain during the process of cooking because there were no hollows in uncooked rice except for presence of fissures or cracks. The gelatinization of starch results in swelling which prevents penetration of water by cementing crack lacerations resulting in internal hollows within the grain. They concluded that MRI clearly demonstrated the hollow formation in cooked rice.

Takeuchi et al. (1997) studied the potential of MRI for moisture profile measurement in real time during boiling of rice grain. A Bruker AM200WB (4.7 T) spectrometer with radio frequency coils spaced at 20 mm was used for the experiment. The sample used for the study was short japonica rice that was hulled, polished, and cleaned. The multispin echo pulse sequence was used to acquire many magnetic resonance echo signals with various echo times. During boiling, the moisture profile rise was asymmetrical, that is, the increase in moisture content was very rapid in the ventral side (0.1 g water/g grain), and there was a delay on the dorsal side (0.04 g water/g grain). There was no difference in the moisture profile after boiling for 22 min indicating that there was no intake of moisture after 22 min of boiling and the moisture absorption of rice was completed.

Mohorič et al. (2004) studied the MRI of single rice kernels during cooking with the optimized 3D imaging strategy to obtain both high spatial and temporal resolution to develop a relationship between moisture content profiles, microstructure of rice, and level of gelatinization. The experiments were performed using a 0.7 T Bruker Advance MRI system having a 10 mm micro imaging detection coil. The images are useful in assessing the water ingress during cooking of rice kernels and the results confirmed the normal pattern of moisture ingress from the previous studies.

9.3.1.3.2 Moisture distribution in corn and wheat. Song and Litchfield (1990) analyzed the potential of MRI to study the moisture distribution that occurs in an ear of corn during drying. The three-dimensional Fourier transform method and multislice 2D Fourier transform method were used to obtain proton density images of corn. The results of the study showed that mass transfer occurred in individual kernels but the moisture transfer between kernels during drying was negligible compared to the moisture transfer inside the corn kernels. Ruan and Litchfield (1992) determined the water distribution during steeping in the maize kernels using MRI. The MRI equipment used was a spectroscopy imaging system with a 200 MHz, 4.7 T, 330 mm bore diameter (Doty Scientific Inc., Columbia, South Carolina) and a microscopic imaging probe. The corn kernels were steeped in a NMR test tube, and the MRI data acquired were analyzed and reconstructed with imaging software. Using MRI, variation in water content and mobility in various components of corn kernels during steeping was measured, and the technique clearly described principal tissues in corn kernels and valuable information concerning differences in water mobility and distribution.

Knowledge of the moisture distribution profile of wheat kernels is very vital to increase the milling performance and thereby increase the yield. Traditional moisture migration studies involve dissection, which is disruptive and does not allow one to study and examine the diffusion within the same grain. Magnetic resonance imaging could be used to study the distribution of moisture in wheat in situ by nondestructive means. Song et al. (1998) used MRI to measure the moisture distribution in single kernels of wheat at storage moisture content of 12% wet basis. A Bruker MSL-400 (Bruker Instruments, Inc., Massachusetts) spectrometer at 9.4 T was used to obtain images of wheat kernels. To obtain proton density images with high resolution, a 3D projection reconstruction technique was employed. The results showed that at 12% moisture content of grain, the distribution of moisture was nonuniform in the starchy endosperm and the moisture content variation ranged from 7.3% to 16.4% wet basis.

9.3.1.3.3 Stress cracking in maize. Stress cracking induced during drying reduces the mechanical strength of the kernel and results in breakage during handling and yields lower starch recovery when wet-milled. Not many studies have been conducted on the initiation and measurement of stress cracking during drying. Song and Litchfield (1990) used MRI to measure the stress cracking in maize kernels. A 200 MHz, 4.7 T MRI instrument (Spectroscopy Imaging Systems Co., United States) with a radio frequency coil region of 17 mm was used. Based on the MR imaging study, it was found that stress cracks initiated in the vitreous endosperm during drying and cracks propagated from near the maize surface to the center of maize kernels. Also, crack initiation occurred in areas with high moisture gradient and low moisture content. Temperature has an effect on stress cracking and during high temperature drying (71°C and 93°C) cracks appeared earlier than during low temperature drying (27°C), and the maize variety affected the location of initiation of stress cracks.

9.3.2   Aquaculture

9.3.2.1   Effect of freezing

Freezing is an important unit operation to reduce deterioration in quality of fish, but it may also result in irreversible quality changes compared to fresh fish. Protein denaturation and lipid oxidation are the two major processes that occur during freezing that affect quality. Nott et al. (1999b) evaluated the effect of freeze thawing on trout using MRI. The images of fresh and thawed fish were obtained using Bruker BMT imaging console (Karlsruhe, Germany) attached to a 2.35 T, 31 cm horizontal bore superconducting magnet. To study the freezing effect, four trout were subjected to either quick freezing using liquid nitrogen at –196°C and stored in domestic freezer for 4 weeks at –18°C, or slow freezing and subsequent storage at –18°C for a period of 4 weeks. Also, MR images of another 18 trout samples were acquired on the first day when the fish were killed and then kept frozen at –18°C in a domestic freezer and then exposed to any one of the following treatments: 6 were maintained at frozen conditions for 2 days and after thawing images were acquired, 6 were maintained at frozen temperature for 2 weeks and then imaged after thawing, and another 6 were maintained at frozen conditions for 4 weeks and then images obtained on thawed samples. The results of slow and fast freezing showed that few MR parameters displayed a bigger effect on slow freezing than for fast freezing, which could be due to the various physical damages caused by slow freezing. In slow freezing, protein denaturation occurred due to larger ice crystals, which resulted in more cellular disruption. Fast freezing resulted in smaller ice crystals and hence no major water redistribution was observed. On the storage of frozen fish for 2 and 4 weeks, no significant difference was observed and hence it was concluded that significant damage occurred during the initial freezing of fish. The results of the study demonstrated that MRI can achieve great resolution of anatomy of individual organs of trout and explain the difference in quality between frozen and fresh trout.

Nott et al. (1999a) studied the effect of freeze-thawing on the magnetic resonance parameters of cod and mackerel using the same system. Cod and mackerel (16 each) samples were acquired fresh from a market and refrigerated at 4°C until the next day. Sixteen more cod fillets were obtained in an individually quick frozen (IQF) state and were thawed on the examination day, and they were considered as fresh. Each sample was split into five portions, one was analyzed on the same day as fresh and the other four portions were frozen at –18°C for 2, 4, 8, or 12 weeks. The results of the experiments showed that greater variability in water content was observed for mackerel compared to the fresh or IQF cod. Based on MR parameters, fresh and IQF cod could be differentiated because moisture content of IQF cod was lower than the fresh, which might be because of drip loss during thawing. The most significant changes that occurred during frozen storage of fresh and IQF cod and mackerel were provided by the magnetization transfer rate. Among the fresh and IQF cod, an intrinsic difference existed, which became indistinguishable after storage at –18°C for 2 weeks.

9.3.2.2   Evaluation of quality

Low field NMR spectroscopy performs in the frequency between 2 and 25 MHz and is a cheaper and simpler version of conventional NMR spectrometer. Aursand et al. (2006) explored the potential of the low field NMR technique to evaluate the changes in quality that occur in fish processing and storage. Two types of instruments—a stationary (Bruker Optik GmbH, Germany) instrument with a magnetic field strength of 0.47 T and resonant frequency of 20 MHz, and portable NMR analyzer with a field strength of 0.35 T—were used. Atlantic wild salmon were tested for fat and water content using the NMR method and chemical analysis. The results showed that fat and water content measured using stationary low frequency NMR had a good correlation ($R^2 = 0.94$) with the chemical analysis, and the portable NMR analyzer also had a good correlation ($R^2 = 0.95$). Aursand et al. concluded that NMR is a useful tool to nondestructively determine the composition of Atlantic salmon and since portable NMR analyzer results showed good correlation with chemical analysis, real-time quality monitoring may be possible in the near future.

In muscle-based food products like fish fillet, water is the most abundant substance, and the interaction between water and macromolecules are important for the quality attributes such as juiciness and texture. Jørgensen and Jensen (2006) have stated that low field NMR studies can provide information on how the distribution of water can be associated to raw material characteristics such as fat content, fish stock, quality characteristics such as water holding capacity and texture, and changes that occur during processing and storage such as protein denaturation.

The ability of MRI to provide high contrast for soft tissues and nonintrusive procedure gives it a great potential to examine the anatomy of a variety of fish species for nutrition or anatomical investigation. Chanet et al. (2009) performed MRI examination on many species of common carp (*Cyprinus carpio* L.) and images were acquired using a 1 T superconducting magnet (Harmony, Siemens). MRI studies were performed on common carp preserved since 1970 by soaking in alcohol and a fresh dead fish from the same species. The results showed that the images of fresh and alcohol-preserved specimens were identical. No difference in the tissues and sizes of organs were observed in alcohol-preserved fish, and the size, shape, morphology of muscle, digestive tract, bladder, ovary, and nervous systems could be clearly visualized. The study showed that the anatomy of specimens could be easily examined even though they are preserved in alcohol for a long duration of time and hence keeping the sample for a long duration does not affect the quality of the image.

Veliyulin et al. (2008) stated that MRI could be useful to examine the effect of feed composition and determination of water, salt, and fat content including their spatial distribution in fish tissues. In the aquaculture and fish processing industries, MRI could be used for optimization of different unit operations, namely, freezing, salting, and thawing. Research studies have shown that MRI has great potential in monitoring and evaluating the quality of products in the aquaculture industry.

9.3.2.3   Sex determination and gonad development

The investigation of marine animals involves destructive methods since the hermetic shell protects the animal and the techniques are normally time consuming. Davenel et al. (2006) studied the noninvasive sex determination and gonad maturation in Pacific oysters using MRI. The images of live oysters were obtained on several occasions (February to August 2002 and 2003) using the 0.2 T Open Siemens MRI system operating at 8.25 MHz to determine development of gonad and the sex of the oyster. After MRI analyses, dissection of specimen and sex determination was conducted on all individuals and the presence of oocytes or spermatozoa confirmed if the oysters were female or male, respectively. Based on the results of the study they concluded that MRI technique could determine the sex of the oysters without actually opening the shells and this was the first noninvasive method to provide such results in oysters.

Pouvreau et al. (2006) investigated the marine bivalve morphology using in vivo MRI for the Pacific oyster, (*Crassostrea gigas* Thunberg) with the closed shell. Adult oysters (shell length 11–12 cm, 3 years old) kept under controlled conditions were used for NMR imaging without any anesthetics. Images were obtained using the General Electric Signa 1.5 T whole body scanner with actively shielded gradient coils, and oysters were placed in the center of the 12 cm diameter radio frequency coil to enhance signal detection. The images had good contrast to noise level and all the major organs of the oyster were shown with sufficiently good resolution. On the basis of these results it could be stated that MRI has potential applications in aquaculture, such as to detect the condition of broodstock individually, follow gonadal evolution, determine the sex of the broodstock oysters, and provide indication of quality of oocytes and spermatozoa.

Hatt et al. (2009) explored the possibilities and limitations of the MRI technique to evaluate the development of gonad and body growth in the oyster. This was a follow-up work from the studies of Pouvreau et al. (2006) and Davenel et al. (2006). The oysters were scanned five times during February to October 2007 (these oysters were all offspring of the same group of females). The major issue of investigation for this study was whether conclusions based on sexual maturation and the growth of oyster (C. *gigas*) would be different using an MRI technique rather than a common group monitoring method. MR images were acquired with the 0.2 T Open Siemens system and with 4.7 T horizontal magnets. The results showed that when determining the growth of oysters based on gross weight or dry flesh, assessment by MRI provides the same results as group monitoring methods. The 0.2 T MR images quantified the gonad maturation and volume of gamets, whereas 4.7 T MR images provided accurate analysis on the volume of organs such as gonad, digestive gland, cardiac cavity, and labial palps.

Smith and Reddy (2012) explored the potential of MRI to examine the anatomical and reproductive status of live Sydney rock oyster (*Saccostrea glomerata* Gould). Oysters were randomly selected and MRI scans were obtained within 24 h after collection. A total of eight groups with 12 to 30 oysters per group were used for the study. After acquiring MRI images, traditional techniques were followed to compare with the MRI results. MRI images were acquired using Varian unity plus 300 MHz spectrometer equipped with a magnet of 7.05 T and microimaging accessory. The images showed that Sydney rock oysters possess large gills that occupy around half of the cavity volume on the ventral side. The large surface area of gills performed various functions, including establishing water current, gathering food, and transferring them to labial palps. MRI images showed that in oysters gas bubbles were developed that increased in size with time and moved to other places within the oyster during emersion. The bubbles contained higher levels of carbon dioxide indicating that respiration contributes to the process. Based on MRI observation and gas analysis it was stated that gas bubbles are produced by oyster tissue to remove CO_2 from soft tissue. Based on the results it was concluded that MRI technique could provide hatchery operators with a better technique to image the reproductive state of potential broodstock oysters.

9.3.3 *Meat*

9.3.3.1 *Body composition*

In livestock production, the major goal is to improve the body composition of the animals when subjected to a variety of genetic and environmental conditions. In the livestock and meat industry, it is very important to determine the body composition of live animals and carcass, respectively. Since MRI could provide high contrast cross-sectional images, it should be feasible to estimate the quantity of fat and lean tissue in livestock. Baulain (1997) used an MRI (Bruker Medspec BMT 15/100) whole body scanner with a magnetic field strength of 1.5 T and an opening of 50 cm diameter and 2 m long to scan animal bodies. Animals were immobilized prior to scanning because movements could produce artifacts that affect the quality of the image. After imaging, animals were killed and carcasses were cut into lean, fat, and bone. The MRI scan results showed a good correlation coefficient for lean ($R^2 = 0.87$ to 0.95) and for fat content ($R^2 = 0.84$ to 0.91). The results showed that MRI could be a very useful tool to determine the body composition of livestock and also a potential tool for three-dimensional reconstruction of single muscles and organs of animals.

9.3.3.2   Fat content and quality evaluation

Fat content is an important meat quality parameter and although several methods are available to determine the fat content, MRI has the advantage of being a nondestructive method that provides clear contrast between muscle, fat, and connective tissues. Ballerini et al. (2002) determined the fat content of beef using MRI technique. The equipment used was a Bruker Biospec horizontal magnet at 2.35 T to acquire images of eight heifer *longissimus dorsi* muscle from beef meat. The fat percentage calculated by MRI was compared with the chemical method, and the results showed that a good correlation ($R = 0.77$) exists between the average fat content determined by MRI and chemical method. The preliminary results showed great potential for the MRI technique to estimate the fat content of meat, although many improvements are possible in the current method. Tingle et al. (1995) investigated the distribution of muscle and fat in retail quality meat using MRI and stated that MRI is a potential technique to noninvasively determine fat and water distribution in meat.

Beauvallet and Renou (1992) reviewed the applications of NMR in meat research and stated that NMR is a good technique for assessment of meat quality, which could be very useful in breeding and animal research. NMR technique could be used for determination of diffusion rates of injected products and water in muscle, which would be helpful in understanding the changes in meat structure. Laurent et al. (2000) explained the potential of NMR in understanding meat characteristics. In the evaluation of meat quality characteristics, the amount of fat and connective tissue and its distribution are important factors, and MRI is a noninvasive technique that provides great insight in the various structural components such as muscle fiber, fat, and connective tissues.

Collewet et al. (2005) determined the percentage of lean meat in pig carcasses using MRI. The objective was to develop MRI as a potential method with high correlation to the reference dissection method to estimate the percentage of lean meat in pig carcass. Images were obtained using the 1.5 T Siemens Vision plus apparatus. For each carcass, the left side was dissected and the right side was evaluated based on indirect methods. From the dissection results, the two variables, weight of lean meat on the left half carcass, and the total weight of carcass on the left half were computed. The results obtained from MRI study showed that image analysis on the right part of carcass could predict the dissection results from the left portion with an accuracy of 586 g for lean meat weight and 1.1% for lean meat percentage. The result of the study has shown that MRI has the potential to be used as a reference method.

Kato et al. (2007) examined the potential of MRI to monitor the quality of various kinds of meat. Meat with significantly varying fat content and tenderness, including chicken thigh, chicken breast, porcine fillet, porcine stomach, and porcine thigh, were selected for the study. Chicken breast is soft and contains low fat compared to chicken thigh. Porcine fillet is soft and consist of lesser fat compared to other porcine parts and porcine stomach contains the highest fat content among all the samples. MR images were acquired using the spin echo method with 1.5 T MRI System ExcelArt (Toshiba Medical Systems Corp., Tochigi, Japan). The mean intensity of porcine fillet was significantly different from that of porcine thigh and the mean intensity of chicken breast was significantly different from that of chicken thigh. The results indicated that mean intensity is associated with the structural organization, which in turn is associated with the eating quality. They concluded that MRI is a potential technique to evaluate the quality characteristics of various meat samples. Renou et al. (2003) studied the water interaction in meat using MRI because different dynamic phenomena that occur during processing and storage of meat could be explained by MRI. By measuring the diffusion coefficient in meat both axially and radially, MRI could explain the influence of intracellular diffusional barriers or postmortem structural changes.

9.3.4 Food

Important food product characteristics are quality, safety, and stability. Food quality is dependent on many characteristics that are governed by functional and rheological properties of individual components. NMR has become a potential tool to explore and understand the structure and dynamics of various food constituents. Yan et al. (1996) studied the NMR applications in complex food systems. Liquid-state NMR is a potential tool to evaluate the liquid components and they studied the lipid spectra extracted from pretzels of various ages: fresh-made pretzels, prepared 6 months before experiments and pretzels prepared 2 years before experiments. The spectra clearly showed the loss of vinyl protons due to oxidation of lipid resulting in decreasing intensity of the peak of lipid spectra, which demonstrates that NMR could be used to quantitatively measure the rancidity of food at the molecular level. The liquid NMR is also used to compare the distribution of sucrose in fresh and aged cookie. The concentration of key compounds were determined by high-resolution liquid NMR, which showed that fructose and glucose levels were similar; however, the sucrose level was doubled in old cookie. Yan et al. also studied the MRI application in food by examining the oil distribution in two varieties of crackers. The MRI images were studied to explore the laminating effect of the dough during the cracker manufacturing process. Laminating is the process of applying shortening or filling to form separated layers of dough and the knowledge of oil distribution is important for determining the eating quality as well as for the shelf stability of the cracker. The MRI images showed a similar trend in the oil distribution between laminated and nonlaminated crackers with maximum oil content in the top layer, second most in the bottom layer, and least oil content in the inner layers. But the inner structure of laminated layers was easier to differentiate than the internal structure of the nonlaminated layers.

Koizumi et al. (2008) constructed a small, lightweight MRI apparatus that could be used for quality determination of food and agricultural products. The system consisted of a small MRI spectrometer (MRTechnology Inc., Tsukuba, Japan) with a 1 T permanent magnet. The materials tested were margarine, frozen pork and beef, fermented soybean (*Glycine max*), natto (a fermented food), blueberries, and sweet cherries. The images of frozen margarine were obtained during the thawing process. The intensity increased with thawing partially due to mobile oil molecules and partially due to higher molecular mobility with increase in temperature. The frozen pork and beef were naturally thawed at 28°C, and time-lapse images were acquired at 5 min intervals. At the beginning of acquisition, weak signals were obtained in the fat tissue region and the fat tissue signals intensified in the final stages of thawing for pork. Images of similar trend were obtained for beef. Natto (fermented soybean) was measured by emphasizing signals of the internal structures and oil concentrations. The MRI images of sweet cherry showed that vascular tissues joining the seed with the peduncle exhibited strong signals because of low mobility of water.

Koizumi et al. concluded that the small MRI is easy to operate, costs less than one-fifth of usual micro MRI units, and is useful for quality evaluation and research purposes for agricultural and food materials.

Amin et al. (2007) studied the use of MRI to quantify the heating of commercially available jarred baby food using microwave heating or immersion in a warm-water bath. Three-dimensional MRI temperature mapping showed the nonuniform heating and presence of hot spots in the samples heated using a microwave. Therefore, caution should be taken when feeding the babies with microwave-heated foods. The study demonstrated that MRI measurement of temperature quantifies the spatial and temporal progression of heating of food either in a microwave or in warm water.

9.3.4.1 Confectionery

In the food industry, MRI is used to measure moisture and fat content, determine adulteration, measure the solid-to-liquid ratio of fats and oils, and measure microbial spoilage. MRI has been used in two major ways: to directly evaluate the internal structure and to determine parameters that characterize the physical properties of the material. McCarthy et al. (2000) studied the analysis of confectionery products and processes using MRI. Since MRI could be used to evaluate the spatial distribution of oil in crackers, MRI was used to understand the mechanism of oil transport in crackers by determining whether the oil should be sprayed on the cracker when it is hot or cold. Experiments were performed by spraying oil on the crackers and allowing them to cool to various temperatures and the MR images were obtained at 1, 5, and 15 min and several days after oil application. The images showed identical oil coverage and oil depth with time and temperature of the cracker having no effect on the oil content or distribution in the crackers. Based on the study, they concluded that the major mechanism responsible for oil transport is the capillary forces arising from the small pores developed during baking, and the oil is pulled into the pores and held in place by these physical forces.

Wagner et al. (2008) studied the process of bread baking using MRI. The objective was to design and develop an oven suitable for continuous measurement and to investigate whether similar behavior was observed in products baked using an MRI oven and domestic or industrial oven. MR images were obtained using a Siemens open 0.2 T imager, and temperature and MR images were acquired continuously for 45 min. The bread temperature kinetics was similar to the previous reports, and during the first few minutes, bottom temperature increased quicker than the top surface because of solid contact and due to lesser cooling effect of water evaporation that was significant on the upper surface. An oven especially meant for MRI measurement was developed and tested, and the results showed that baking conditions produced by an MRI oven were similar to traditional ovens. The study also highlighted the sensitivity of MRI signals to different factors that vary during baking. They concluded that with the actual baking environment provided by an MRI oven, it would be possible to produce interesting information that aids in better understanding of various mechanisms involved in the process of baking.

9.3.4.2 Dairy food

The sensory and textural characteristic of feta cheese largely depends on the brining process. The duration of brining has an impact on the salt and moisture content of feta cheese, which is very critical for the end quality of the product. Altan et al. (2011) monitored the uptake of salt and loss of moisture in feta cheese during the process of brining using nondestructive MRI and NMR relaxometry. Cheese was produced from pasteurized cow milk and brining was carried out by suspending a cheese sample in a 50 ml container with 4.8%, 13.0%, or 23.0% (w/w) Nacl solution at 20°C for about 169 h. MR images were acquired with the 1.03 T Aspect Al magnet equipped with solenoid coil at 43.85 MHz frequency. The MR images showed higher signal intensity corresponding to the higher water content at the beginning of the brining period. With an increase in brining time, a decrease in signal intensity was observed along with a decrease in water diffusion outside the cheese and salt diffusion into the cheese. The signal intensity change was the highest for cheese brined at 23.0% salt and lowest at 4.8% salt concentration. A good linear correlation existed between the magnetic resonance signal intensity and cheese water content. They concluded that MRI could be a useful tool to assess the structural changes and salt and water content in cheese, and could be used for implementing the optimization process for quality control of cheese.

Whey protein is a valuable by-product from the cheese industry and can be used in various types of foods. Gels made from whey protein absorb water and swell when kept in aqueous environment. The conventional method to determine swelling is to calculate mass uptake or to determine the change in dimensions, which provides very little information. Oztop et al. (2010) used MRI technique to monitor the swelling of whey protein gels in solution at three different pHs. The images were acquired using a 1.03 T (43.8 MHz) NMR spectrometer (Aspect-AI, Netanya, Israel). Whey protein isolates with 95.6% protein were used for gels and were kept in metal baskets with fine mesh to allow swelling. The baskets were placed in distilled water adjusted to pH 2.5, 7, or 10. The final swelling ratios was 30.11%, 91.19%, 123.73% for pH of 2.5, 7, and 10, respectively, indicating that pH influences swelling ratio with more swelling observed at higher pH. The results of the experiment proved that MRI could be used to assess the swelling rate of whey protein gel at various aqueous environments. The MRI images showed extensive details about the spatial resolution of water in gels and the images at low pH showed that water uptake results in microstructural changes in the gel, which could be used in product formulation of gastric juices.

9.3.4.3 *Moisture migration*

One of the challenges in food industries is to understand the water movement and its distribution in low moisture content foods. Cornillon and Salim (2000) studied the mobility and distribution of water in foods with low and intermediate moisture content, such as cereals, cookies, and candy. Their study showed that MRI has the potential to examine how moisture interacts in various food products and provides an understanding of the moisture uptake mechanism, moisture migration kinetics, and moisture interaction with various food components in low moisture food. Microstructure of cereal is an important quality attribute in cereal because moisture rehydration and milk diffusion depends on the microstructure, which in turn is responsible for texture and crispiness of the cereal. Melado et al. (2011) studied the rehydration and milk diffusion using noninvasive MRI techniques in cereals of different varieties (var03, var09, var14) coated (with sucrose, dextrose, water) and noncoated, and used different kinds of milk (3.6% and 1.55% fat). The high water composition and fat content in milk provides good signal detection using MRI to study the mobility of milk and rehydration in cereals. To acquire real-time images, an injection system with 5 ml and 10 ml syringes and a capillary tube connecting the syringes was designed. Cereal pellets were placed inside a 5 ml syringe and 10 ml syringe filled with air, and a capillary tube filled with 5 ml milk. The milk was forced to enter the syringes filled with cereal and MR images were acquired a using Bruker BIOSPEC 47/40 (Ettlingen, Germany) spectrometer operating at 200 MHz. Image processing algorithms were applied and the average gray level showed how much each sample was rehydrated. The results showed that fiber addition seems to refrain the liquid penetration in the pellets. Based on the rehydration level, no clustering behavior was seen, and when coating had an impact, gray level variance for coated cereal was greater than for noncoated cereals.

Moisture migration within the components of a food with varying water activity is critical in understanding the microstructure of food and in preservation of food to maintain its quality. Weglarz et al. (2008) studied the moisture migration mapping in real time for cereal-based food with contrast water activity using MRI. The study was comprised of two extreme cases: high water activity contrast with fast hydration and low water activity contrast with slow hydration. To monitor water distribution, the fast spin echo and single point imaging (SPI) methods were used. In the fast spin echo imaging method, based on signals received from echoes measured at various echo times, a single image is produced. SPI is based on frequent measurements of a specific point on the free induction decay (FID) signal in the presence of gradients. The samples selected were crunchy inclusions and biscuit shell with apple filling. Wheat-flour-based crunchy inclusions with different internal microstructures (A, B, C) were prepared and all samples were made in coated (vegetable fat) and uncoated forms. Figure 9.2 shows two different situations: rapid non-uniform hydration and slow homogeneous hydration. Experiments on two non-coated samples showed two different cases: in the first sample, rapid water ingress occurs and at a certain point led to the sudden failure of sample structure and quick rehydration. In the next sample, the integrity of the sample's outer part significantly delayed the hydration and the variation in rate of hydration may be due to internal structural differences. The measurements on coated samples showed some fast catastrophic hydration, but in general it was not frequent as compared to noncoated samples. The moisture migration effect on biscuit shells with apple pie were monitored for 3 months. The highest intensity signal was observed at the middle of the sample corresponding to apple pie and the outer part had significantly lower intensity. During the course of time, changes in signal intensity between barrier and shell appeared, and the water activity of shell at the final stages increased to 0.64 from 0.35, while water activity of apple filling reduced from 0.98 to 0.92. The results of the study showed that MRI has a great potential to study and monitor the moisture migration in multicomponent food systems.

Ready-to-eat and multicomponent food products are gaining popularity with consumers. In the multicomponent food system, variation in water activity within the food may result in moisture redistribution phenomena thereby affecting the textural quality of the product during the shelf-life period. A major issue in the design of multicomponent food system is to develop strategies to regulate moisture migration. When the moisture migration could be studied noninvasively, it could result in development of novel multicomponent foods and MRI is a feasible noninvasive technique to study moisture status in food materials. Ramos-Cabrer et al. (2006) studied the moisture distribution in multicomponent food using MRI. MR images were acquired using a 4.7 T horizontal bore magnet (Oxford Instruments, Abingdon, United Kingdom). Two types of multicomponent food were studied: the first one was composed of a layer of soft bread containing two sausages and creamy cheese; and the second was composed of two sandwiches, each with two slices of bread, a piece of cheese, a cured ham slice, a tomato slice, and a lettuce leaf. The scanning was done within two hours after their preparation and the first sample was monitored at two temperatures (7°C and 25°C) for 2 weeks. In the second sample, a moisture barrier was applied to one sandwich and regarded as the treated sandwich, while the other was considered untreated. In the untreated sandwich, significant moisture loss was observed in tomato and minimum moisture loss was observed in ham and cheese compared to the treated one. In the untreated sample, higher moisture absorption was detected especially for the lower slice, which shows that in an untreated sandwich, moisture transport

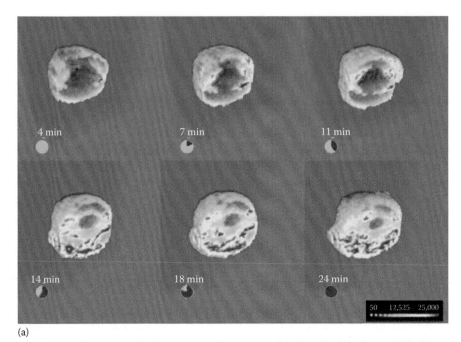

(a)

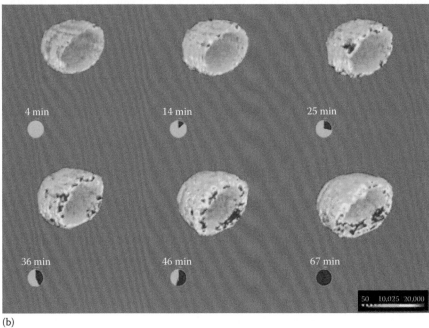

(b)

Figure 9.2 3D visualization of MR images of crunchy inclusions hydration: (a) fast, catastrophic water ingress, (b) slow homogeneous diffusion of water into inclusion structure. Color scale from green to red corresponds to A_w range between ~0.85 and 1.0. (From Weglarz, W.P. et al., *Food Chemistry*, 106, 1366, 2008. With permission.)

is gravity driven. Less moisture migration was observed in the treated sandwich demonstrating that the pesto layer acted as a barrier for moisture. Ramos-Cabrer et al. concluded that MRI techniques could be used to noninvasively quantify dynamic moisture changes in multicomponent foods.

The most important factor affecting the texture of spaghetti is the internal moisture distribution, and frozen and dried pasta have a distinctive moisture distribution with a lower moisture region in the center referred to as the al dente state. The pasta texture deteriorates quickly after cooking and during distribution because of the homogenization of moisture distribution. Horigane et al. (2006) explored the internal moisture distribution using a DRX300WB MRI (Bruker, Karlsruhe, Germany) with a high spatial resolution. Fresh spaghetti was prepared from semolina flour and the spaghetti was dried at 74°C for 12 h. Fresh or dried spaghetti was cut into 7 cm lengths and boiled in 400 ml water for a period of 2 to 14 min at an interval of 2 min. Cooked spaghetti was cut 1 cm long, covered in polyethylene film to avoid moisture loss, and placed in a NMR tube for MRI measurements using spin echo sequence. The images depicted that water penetration occurred concentrically towards the center of the spaghetti. After boiling for 10 min, a small area at the center was at <35% moisture content, which indicates the cooking time for al dente texture and at 12 min, moisture content at the center was >40%. The moisture content at the center after 2 h of holding went up to 55% to 60% and the MRI map clearly explained the variation in moisture content distribution toward homogenization maintaining concentric distributions. The dried spaghetti had a lower diffusion coefficient compared to fresh spaghetti showing the tighter structure formed during drying. The drying also prevents moisture homogenization during the holding period of cooked spaghetti. The results also showed that after 2 hours of holding time, the moisture profile hardly changed.

Troutman et al. (2001) explored the potential of MRI to study the moisture migration during engrossing and aging in soft-panned confections. Conventional MRI techniques could produce moisture maps for high moisture content food but as the moisture content decreases, conventional methods are not efficient in providing moisture information. Single point ramped imaging with T_1 enhancement (SPRITE) is a MRI technique based on SPI, which could be useful for imaging short-signal lifetime systems. The sample tested was jellybean and around 20 samples were chosen for determination of water activity. Samples were collected instantly after panning and after every 2 h for a 48 h aging period. SPRITE and spin echo techniques were carried out using the Nalorac (Nalorac Cryogenics, Martinez, California) system with a 2.4 T superconducting magnet. The results of the experiments showed that a reduction in moisture content and water activity was observed during aging time in the presence of the coating material of jellybean. MR images displayed a hydration front entering the center of jellybeans at the time of the aging process.

9.3.4.4   Detection of spoilage

In commercial production, quality monitoring of yogurt is usually performed by destructive sampling. Ye et al. (2004) has shown that MRI offers a rapid and noninvasive alternative method to monitor the yogurt fermentation process. Plain yogurt was prepared using standard procedures and MR relaxometry and imaging were performed during the process of yogurt fermentation to obtain data of free induction decay (FID) curves, relaxation time and distribution, and diffusion coefficient. For spoilage detection using MRI, yeast, mold, and *E. coli* were inoculated in to the standard sample and the same monitoring procedures were followed. The results of the study clearly indicated that microbial growth was highly correlated with MR signals and images, and microbial growth and contamination could be revealed from FID data, relaxation time distribution, and diffusion coefficient.

The study thus investigated and provided fundamental information about the interaction between microorganisms and their environment, and MRI could be used for online detection of spoilage of yogurt and other food products.

Most commonly used methods for spoilage detection are statistical sampling, manual inspection, or ultrasonic inspection. The limitations of these methods are that statistical sampling requires destruction of a few batches; manual inspection requires more time; and ultrasonic inspection needs a transducer, which contacts each container introducing considerable packaging/repackaging (Schenz et al., 1999). Schenz et al. developed a successful spoilage detection technique using MRI, which has several advantages including noncontact, sensitivity to many types of food contamination, rapid processing, and bulk inspection ability. As food products spoil, proteolysis of proteins and hydrolysis of carbohydrates results in a decrease in the pH of food, which is the major indicator of food spoilage. The MR system is a low field (0.15 T) clinical imaging system that utilizes a permanent magnet that is well suited for commercial production, as it uses neither cryogens nor cooling water and has low power consumption (150 W). A special MR inspection sequence based on a multislice, multiecho sequence was developed to collect spatial information from a case of product. The detection of spoilage depends on a statistical method called control charting in which the running average of items analyzed is kept and compared to the newest data point. The results of the study showed that a viable MRI technique to detect spoilage in packed food containers was successfully tested.

9.3.5   Fruits and vegetables

MRI has become a potential technique in the study of microstructure of fruits and vegetables due to various reasons. MRI is a nondestructive technique that allows the study of intact samples such as fruits and vegetables. Due to presence of high water content in fruits, MRI could differentiate various tissues because of the sensitivity of MRI in predicting water distribution and migration. MRI could provide three-dimensional high spatial resolution data on the internal structure of fruits. Also various parameters related to microstructure, moisture distribution, and mobility can be measured, which often provides complimentary information. Different substances such as oil, water, and sugar could be distinguished by MRI (Defraeye et al., 2013).

9.3.5.1   Apple

MRI has been used to study and analyze apple by many researchers, including texture analysis during storage and ripening of apple (Létal et al., 2003), detection of quality characteristics such as voids and bruising (Chen et al., 1989; McCarthy et al., 1995; Zion et al., 1995), deterioration of apple quality due to watercore (Wang et al., 1988; Cho et al., 2008), monitoring of internal browning (Clark and Burmeister, 1999; Gonzalez et al., 2001), evaluation of mealiness (Barreiro et al., 2000; Marigheto et al., 2008), and evaluation of quality during drying (McCarthy et al., 1991; Hills and Remigereau, 1997; Nguyen et al., 2006). All these studies were conducted with entire apples in which a complete range of fruit structure (i.e., vascular bundle, voids, pits, inner and outer cortex tissue) is included in the image. The objective of Defraeye et al. (2013) was to perform MRI (AVIII 500WB, Bruker Biospin, Germany) at higher resolution with smaller field of view in small samples to acquire more detailed information. Hence, the main objective of the study was the characterization of tissue based on outer and inner cortex tissue, different fertilization treatments, and various storage times. For tissue characterization, proton density, T_2 value, and self-diffusion coefficient were measured. The results of the study showed that no clear differentiation was observed between samples with various fertilization treatments. Increased proton density was observed for samples with more storage time. Inner tissues showed an increase in proton density and diffusion coefficient compared to the outer tissues. The results of the study showed that MRI has a great potential to detect the microstructure of fruits with respect to various treatments.

Gonzalez et al. (2001) evaluated the ability of MRI to estimate internal browning in apples during controlled atmosphere storage. They also monitored the progress of damage in fruits subjected to two different controlled atmosphere storage conditions: 18% CO_2 at 20°C and 3% CO_2 at 0°C. The images were acquired using a 0.6 T Oxford magnet connected to a General Electric CSI NMR imaging spectrometer (Fremont, California). The results of the study showed that MRI could detect early development of internal browning in apples. In monitoring the progression of damage, MRI could detect injury as early as 3 days when exposed to 18% CO_2 at 20°C, and by the ninth day all the apples developed internal browning at this storage condition. At storage condition of 3% CO_2 at 0°C, no internal browning was observed until 21 days, whereas after 21 days, signal intensity at the core area decreased indicating the development of internal browning. The study concluded that MRI could be used to monitor and detect internal browning in apples.

Mealiness in apples is considered a negative attribute of texture, which gives a sensation of a lack of juiciness. Barreiro et al. (1999) determined the mealiness in apples using nondestructive MRI techniques to assess the internal quality of samples. Eight fruits of Top Red variety were tested using mechanical and MRI techniques. Four fruits were stored under controlled atmospheric conditions for 6 months, and another four fruits were stored at 2°C for the same period. MRI experiments were conducted using a Bruker Biospec 47/40 (Ettlingen, Germany) spectrometer. The fruits stored under controlled atmospheric conditions had higher soluble solids than those stored at 2°C and three out of four stored under controlled conditions had a firmness value higher than 16 N, while all fruits stored at 2°C had firmness values less than 16 N. The important MRI characteristic for mealy apple is the presence of skew histograms with a tail located at the extreme of the histogram when compared to nonmealy apples.

Zion et al. (1995) examined bruise detection in apples based on analysis of 2D magnetic resonance images. Apple varieties Jonathan, Hermon, and Golden Delicious bought from a store were used for the experiments. Images of Jonathan apples were acquired once before damage and then a single bruise was inflicted manually. Image were acquired 1.25 h after a inflicting bruise. For the other two varieties, images were acquired before and after 2.25 to 41 h inflicting bruise. Images were obtained using a 4.7 T Bruker Biospsec imaging magnet (Bruker, Fremont, California). The MR images of bruised tissues appeared brighter than firm tissues, and detection of bruised and nonbruised apples was achieved using MRI. The method required only two scans: one for determination of geometry and centers of samples by thresholding the background pixels, and the other scan to calculate the number of pixels with higher intensities than the threshold and whose distance from the center is larger than preset value. They concluded that MRI is a fast and efficient method, but the algorithm needs to be extended to analyze 3D low-resolution magnetic resonance images to be of value for practical on-line applications.

9.3.5.2 Pomegranate

Black heart is a major disease affecting pomegranate. It develops in the inner regions of the fruit without affecting the rind. For detection of black heart, visual inspection is inefficient due to the absence of any external symptoms in the affected fruit. Zhang and McCarthy (2012b) evaluated the use of MRI to determine black heart in the pomegranate variety Wonderful. The samples harvested at maturity were obtained from an orchard and prescreened to ensure the fruits were affected only by black heart and had no other defects. The images were acquired using a 1 T spectrometer (Aspect AI, Industrial Area Hevel Modi'in, Shoham, Israel). Image histogram features, including median, mean, mode, standard deviation, kurtosis, and skewness, were analyzed using partial least square discriminant analysis. The model was successful in detection of the black heart disease in pomegranate with 92% accuracy.

9.3.5.3   Tomato

Maturity of tomato is a critical factor in determination of the quality of processed tomato products. Zhang and McCarthy (2012a) evaluated the maturity of tomato using MRI. Tomatoes were obtained from ConAgra Foods (Oakdale, California). The tomatoes were harvested at six different maturity stages (green, breaker, turning, pink, light red, and red) and equilibrated at room temperature (22°C) prior to analysis. The images were obtained using a 1 T permanent magnet MRI system (Aspect AI, Industrial Area Hevel Modi'in, Shoham, Israel). As tomatoes mature and ripen from green to red color, changes were observed in the structural characteristics and volume element (voxel) intensity of the images. The classification accuracies were around 90% and the authors concluded that at various maturity stages, physiological changes in tomato were observed from the MR image signal intensity.

The canning of peeled tomatoes consists of various steps that may result in mechanical damage to the product. Steam peeling of tomatoes may result in severe bruising causing disintegration resulting in loss of the product. Milczarek et al. (2009) developed an MRI-based imaging method to identify damaged pericarp tissue during commercial processing of tomatoes. Samples of eight heavily bruised and eight nonbruised California tomatoes were selected for the study. Images of individual tomatoes were acquired by a 1 T industrial grade MR imaging system (Aspect AI, Netanya, Israel). Thirteen images were obtained for each sample, and multivariate image analysis was performed to make classification more efficient. The results of the study proved that MRI provided a contrast between the sound and bruised image pixels, making it possible to detect damaged pericarp tissue in tomatoes.

Ciampa et al. (2010) examined the variation of internal structure and physical and chemical characteristics of cherry tomatoes (*Lycopersicon esculentum* cv. Shiren) using MRI. Samples were collected in two seasons: January–May 2005 and June–July 2005. MRI measurements were obtained using a Bruker Avance 300 MHz spectrometer (Bruker Biospin GmbH, Ettlingen, Germany). The results of the study showed that cherry tomatoes harvested in different seasons exhibited different morphological and chemical–physical characteristics.

Ishida et al. (1989) investigated the changes in movement and distribution of water in tomatoes using MRI. Common tomato (*Lycopersicon esculentum*) was cultivated in a growth chamber at two stages: immature green and mature red were selected for the study. An NMR spectrometer with a superconducting magnet operating at 270 MHz (GSX-270, JEOL USA, Inc., Peabody, Massachusetts) was used for acquiring images. The images showed that water distribution was different among tissues in immature and mature fruit. In immature fruit, a large amount of water was present in the seeds and seed envelopes, and a minimum amount of water was found in dissepiments and columella. In mature red fruits, a higher amount of water was present in the pericarp, dissepiments, and columella, while not much water was detected in the seeds and seed envelopes. Thus NMR images, precisely detected the variation in water distribution among various tissues in immature and mature tomatoes.

9.3.5.4 Pears

Internal browning is a postharvest disorder in pears that results in cavity development and softening and browning of tissues. Since the appearance of the fruit is not externally affected, it is difficult to identify the affected pears. Hernández-Sánchez et al. (2007) explored use of MRI as a nondestructive method for on-line identification of internal browning of pears. Pears (*Pyrus communis* L. cv. Blanquilla) bought from local market were separated into healthy and affected samples. For macroscopic NMR, magnetic resonance images and T_2 maps were acquired from whole fruit with various stages of damage including healthy samples. For microscopic studies, samples were cut in half and pieces of extracted tissues were placed in tubes and sealed to avoid dehydration. A Bruker Biospec spectrometer that operates at 200 MHz was used for dynamic experiments. The microscopic changes due to abnormal development are visible in the NMR responses and such changes responsible for magnetic resonance image contrast of whole fruit. MRI provided a higher sensitivity in detection of browning and a good contrast between affected and healthy tissues compared to X-ray imaging. Based on the results of this study, an on-line MRI monitoring has the potential to evaluate internal browning in pears at the rate of 30 fruits/min with 96% accuracy.

Core breakdown is a storage disorder in pears resulting in tissue browning and cavity development. It was not possible to identify the affected fruits because it does not show any external symptoms. Lammertyn et al. (2003) studied core breakdown for a course of time in pears (cv. Conference) using MRI and X-ray CT methods. The pears were collected from a commercial orchard, and core breakdown was induced by cooling the pears at 1°C for 7 days, and stored in controlled atmosphere (CA) conditions (1°C, 10% CO_2 and 1% O_2) for 6 months during which MRI (Bruker Biospec, Karlsruhe, Germany) and X-ray CT system (AEA Tomohawk Philips, Netherlands) measurements were performed. The results of the study showed that browning could be detected after a period of 2 months with the two techniques, but the contrast between the healthy and affected tissues was higher on the magnetic resonance images compared to CT scans. The browning of tissues does not increase spatially over a period of time but only increased in the contrast between healthy and affected tissues during storage.

9.3.5.5 Wine grapes

The maturity of grapes is measured based on sugar content (measured in Brix), acidity, color and fruitiness. Harvesting of grapes at maturity depends on various factors: sugar content, weight, acidity, tannins, anthocyanins, and total phenolic contents. Andaur et al. (2004) used MRI to examine the growth and maturity of three varieties (Cabernet Sauvignon, Carmenere, and Chardonnay) of wine grapes. The equipment used was a clinical MRI Philips T5-Intera (Philips Healthcare, DA Best, The Netherlands) of 0.5 T magnet. Clusters of grapes were scanned on the same day, but when they could not be analyzed within the same day, they were frozen, stored, and later thawed before using for the experiments. No change in sugar content was found in the sample before and after freezing. For estimation of volume, since freezing significantly changes the shape and volume of berry, only fresh berries were used. One of the interesting results obtained was the homogeneity in sugar content inside the berries, which is shown by low deviation in Brix values among the pixels. They also determined the size distribution with a fair accuracy, which is important in predicting extractability in grapes that is a function of skin to flesh ratio. The MRI could also visualize the seeds and seed size, which are important in the prediction of impact of tannin on wine astringency. The results of this study showed the potential of MRI for analysis of wine grapes, which could provide information about the ripening of berries, berry size, and sugar content, which are valuable inputs for selection of grapes in wine making. Standard laboratory analysis of grapes takes hours to estimate sugar content and size of berries, whereas MRI technique could obtain such information within 20 minutes.

9.3.5.6   *Avocado and cherry*

To evaluate the quality characteristics of agricultural products, various techniques, such as acoustical, electrical, optical, and X-ray are being explored by researchers. But most of these techniques are suitable for evaluating only certain quality characteristics; X-ray and gamma rays have radiation hazards, and optical and sonic techniques have limitations in the penetration depth of tissues. NMR has a better ability for use in agricultural materials because NMR is sensitive to oil, mobile water, and sugar, which are the important composition in agricultural materials. S. Kim et al. (1999) examined the potential of NMR to determine the oil-to-water ratio in avocados to assess maturity and to detect the presence of pits in cherries. A 2 T NMR spectrometer (General Electric CSI-2) working at 85.5 MHz frequency attached to a conveyor system was used for the experiment. For avocado, 10 sets of spectral data were obtained at 3 conveyor speeds and 5 different positions with respect to the coil center. The correlation between percentage dry weight and ratio of oil-to-water magnetic resonance peaks were examined. The results showed a good correlation of $r = 0.970$ at 50 mm/s conveyor speed and minimum correlation coefficient of $r = 0.894$ at 250 mm/s, between oil-to-water resonance peak ratio and dry weight. For testing cherries, magnetic resonance projections were obtained for whole cherries with increasing speed and then for pitted cherries. It was possible to discriminate whole cherries from pitted ones regardless of the speed of the conveyor, and as the speed of the conveyor increased, the signal intensity of samples became weaker. The results demonstrated that NMR has the potential to study the internal quality characteristics of fruits.

Harvesting of avocado fruits should be done on maturity because immature avocados do not ripen properly and become rubbery, flavorless, and shriveled. But no external changes appear in the fruit to indicate maturity. Oil content is the most common criteria for maturity determination, because it is high enough and closely related to the development of fruit. The common methods to determine oil content are Soxhlet extraction and dry weight analysis, but these methods are destructive, expensive, and time consuming. Chen et al. (1993) explored the potential of NMR methods to evaluate maturity in avocados. Various changes occur during the maturation of avocado such as decrease in water content and increase in oil content, which in turn affects the NMR measurements. Avocado fruits of different maturity were obtained from a commercial orchard and the fruits were evaluated based on three NMR parameters: image intensity, ratio of oil and water resonance intensities, and T1, T2 relaxation times. NMR images were acquired using a General Electric CSI-2 NMR spectrometer operating at 85.5 MHz resonant frequency. The NMR spectrum of an avocado sample shows that the water and oil resonances ratio correlates well with percentage dry weight of the fruit. The technique of measuring resonance peak ratio is desirable because measurements can be rapidly done, and the quality index, which is the ratio of two resonance peaks, will minimize the effect of instrument variability. The use of surface coil not only facilitates testing intact fruit but also reduces the effect of factors such as size of fruits and presence of seeds. The results of this study showed that NMR could be useful for internal quality monitoring of various fruits.

9.3.5.7   *Courgettes (zucchini)*

Duce et al. (1992) examined the potential of NMR to detect changes in the food that occur with the state of water in the food. The sample used was frozen and thawed courgettes, and the images were acquired using an Oxford spectrometer operating at 84.7 MHz connected to 2 T superconducting magnet. The images of fresh courgette displayed fine anatomical features such as vascular tissue, skin, cortex, seeds, and seedbed. The signal from vascular tissue, skin, and seeds displayed a greater intensity than that from the seedbed and cortex. The images of fresh and frozen courgette differed in two aspects: First, the overall intensity of thawed courgettes was greater than that of fresh courgettes, and the image contrast between various tissues was less distinguished in thawed courgettes than the fresh samples. The results of this study provided significant information about the courgettes' internal anatomical structure and also provided information about how freezing affects the cells and alters the morphology of the plant tissue.

9.3.5.8   Strawberry

Osmotic dehydration is used as an alternate method for air-drying of fresh fruits and vegetables by immersing the samples in sugar or salt solution. Osmotic dehydration can enhance the texture of the product and increase the vitamin retention in the product. MRI has been used to noninvasively measure the moisture content and provide moisture profiles of drying models in apples (McCarthy et al., 1991) and potatoes (Ruan et al., 1991). Evans et al. (2002) examined strawberry slices during air-drying and osmotic dehydration with the help of MRI. The objective was to measure the one-dimensional map of MR parameters T_2 (water proton spin-spin relaxation time) and M_0 during drying of fresh slices of strawberry, where T_2 indicates the molecular mobility of water and M_0 is the proton density determined from the magnitude of magnetic resonance signal. Two drying regimes were followed: first was osmotic dehydration with 60% aqueous sucrose for 2 h followed by air drying at 20°C, 30°C, 45°C, or 60°C for 30 min; the second was the air drying of untreated slices at 20°C, 30°C, 45°C, or 60°C for 1 h. MR images were acquired using 2.35 T super magnet (Oxford Instruments, Oxford, United Kingdom), connected to a Bruker BMT imaging console. The results showed that during shorter osmotic rehydration, water diffusivity was rapid enough to supply water lost at the surface, hence maintaining molecular mobility in the strawberry slice. The MRI revealed important parameters corresponding to water molecules in sample tissue during osmotic dehydration. Air-drying above 20°C resulted in variation in water movement related with a heterogeneous collapse in sample tissue.

Hall et al. (1998) studied the potential of MRI to determine the textural changes in fruits such as cucumbers, pineapples, melons, and peaches. Cucumbers infected with *Mycosphaerella* sp. were bought from a local producer and pineapples (unripe and ripe), yellow melons (overripe and ripe), and peaches (bruised and healthy) were obtained from a local supermarket. Images were acquired with a 2 T Bruker BMT (Bruker Medzintechnik Biospec II, Karlsruhe, Germany) with a 100 cm bore magnet. Images of healthy cucumbers showed good contrast compared to the images of cucumber infected with *Mycosphaerella* sp. (Figure 9.3). The gradient echo images of overripe melons showed a decrease in signal intensity, which clearly demonstrates the internal necrosis (Figure 9.4). Also, bruised and unbruised gradient echo images of peaches showed increased contrast between healthy and damaged tissues, because the region of bruised tissue holds greater quantity of air than the undamaged area (Figure 9.5). The results of the study suggested that MRI could be a potential tool to examine the texture of various fruits and vegetables that are fresh and those affected by pathogen infection, damaged or over ripened.

9.3.6   Medical applications

MRI has revolutionized the medical imaging and diagnosis process because MRI could provide images of internal organs without any incision and without the use of any ionizing

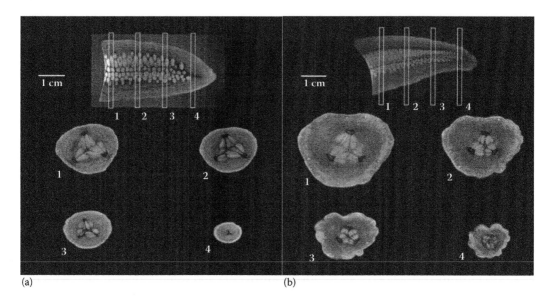

(a)   (b)

Figure 9.3 (a) Multislice images from a healthy cucumber. (b) Multislice images from a cucumber infected with *Mycospharella* sp. (From Hall, L.D. et al., *Magnetic Resonance Imaging* 16, 485, 1998. With permission.)

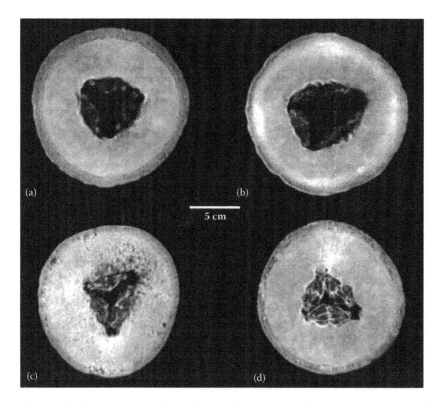

Figure 9.4 Spin echo image from (a, b) healthy melons and (c, d) melons with internal necrosis. (From Hall, L.D. et al., *Magnetic Resonance Imaging* 16, 485, 1998. With permission.)

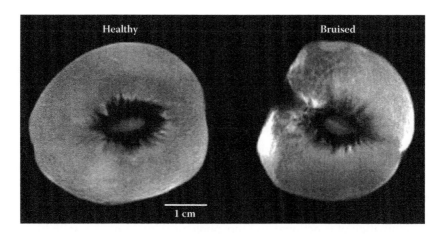

Figure 9.5 Spin echo image from healthy and bruised peaches. (From Hall, L.D. et al., *Magnetic Resonance Imaging* 16, 485, 1998. With permission.)

radiation. MRI could be used to monitor and diagnose a variety of medical conditions, such as abnormalities in the brain or spinal cord, tumors or cysts in various parts of the body, injuries to the joint, diseases of the liver and other abdominal organs, and problems associated with the pelvic region (U.S. Food and Drug Administration, 2012b). MRI can be used to detect and estimate the excess amount of iron in various parts of the human body such as the heart, liver, pancreas, spleen, and pituitary gland. Excess iron is toxic and may cause endocrine, cardiac, and hepatic dysfunction (Chavhan et al., 2009). Functional MRI (f-MRI) is performed to determine which part of the brain is handling critical functions such as speech, thought, and sensory functions by asking the patient to perform active motor, language, or cognitive tasks or passive tasks and the brain is then imaged. The scanner could determine the increase in blood flow to certain parts of the brain by detecting the difference between hydrogen nuclei in oxygenated and deoxygenated blood.

Intraoperative MRI is widely accepted as a valuable tool for image guidance during neurosurgery. Intraoperative guidance of MRI was easily accepted because it uses the same imaging modality for localization during surgery as is done for preoperative diagnosis, and also has improved the navigation during real time and interactive with frequent volumetric updates (Jolesz, 2005).

The introduction of high-field MRI imaging at 3 T resulted in a great expectation in medical imaging and Dahmoush et al. (2012) studied high-field MRI use in the pediatric population. The use of high-field MRI provides a great potential for improving the image quality and provides exquisite details, which facilitate diagnosis of numerous issues in clinical applications. Especially in the pediatric population, increased spatial resolution is sometimes essential to delineate small structures and subtle diseases. Use of high-field 3 T imaging could achieve faster scan times and hence help to reduce the need for sedation or anesthesia in younger population. But having a high-field magnetic field strength results in challenges such as altered T_1 contrast, and increased susceptibility and safety issues related to specific absorption rates. Many medical devices that have been declared safe for a 1.5 T system may not be safe for a 3 T system.

9.3.6.1 Lung diseases

Wielpütz et al. (2013) examined the magnetic resonance imaging of cystic fibrosis (CF) lung disease. Cystic fibrosis is a common lethal hereditary disease among the white population, and pulmonary complications constitute the major cause of death due to cystic fibrosis. MRI is considered an ionizing-radiation-free technique to assess CF, and MRI could display several components of lung function such as ventilation, respiratory movements, and perfusion. MRI could provide relevant clinical information that is better than any other diagnostic method. CF is the first lung disease for which clinical applications based on MRI have been developed. Functional MRI of the CF of lung is being considered as a routine application to support early diagnosis and improve the survival rate of patients affected by CF.

Wielpütz and Kauczor (2012) reviewed the technical aspects of MRI and its role in the evaluation of disorders related to lungs, such as airway diseases, ventilation, respiratory mechanics, perfusion, pulmonary vasculature, and hemodynamics. According to the authors, lung MRI is very challenging because of the low proton density and rapid signal decay of lung parenchyma and other challenges such as loss of tissue and hyperinflation. However, combination of functional and morphological lung imaging with high temporal and spatial resolution at the scale of the whole organ is a major advantage of MRI that distinguishes it from other imaging techniques. In pulmonary diseases, such as CF, bronchopulmonary dysplasia, congenital cardiopulmonary vascular anomalies, and Pancoast tumors, MRI has been developed as the most important imaging method. Also MRI is of great value in patients suffering from locally or systemically advanced lung cancer when the decision for surgery is critical.

Ohno et al. (2011) reviewed the pulmonary MR imaging for airway diseases and stated that pulmonary MRI provides not only information associated with morphology but also information related to pulmonary function. Liu et al. (2010) examined the ability of diffusion-weighted magnetic resonance imaging (DWI) for evaluation of pulmonary lesions. DWI is a noninvasive technique with an ability to probe biological tissues at the molecular level and expressed by apparent diffusion coefficient (ADC), which represents the specific diffusion capability of biological tissues. Sixty-two patients with pulmonary lesions were subjected to conventional MRI and DWI, and the apparent diffusion coefficient values of lesions were measured. The signal intensities of benign and malignant tumors were not significantly different but the benign lesions had a significantly higher ADC value compared to malignant tumors. Based on the study the authors concluded that quantitative analysis of ADC values could be used to diagnose pulmonary lesions and hence DWI could be used to evaluate pulmonary lesions.

9.3.6.2 Cancer

Lung cancer is difficult to efficiently diagnose and treat, and is one of the common causes of cancer-related death worldwide (Parkin et al., 2005). Koyama et al. (2013) reviewed the developments in MRI related to lung cancer focusing on detection and characterization of solid pulmonary nodules (SPNs), prediction of lung function after surgery, and response to tumor treatment. Based on the review of various studies they stated that the potential of MRI to identify SPN is lower compared to CT, but the capability to detect malignant SPN without ionizing radiation seems to be advantageous than CT. There are emerging applications of dynamic MRI to differentiate between nodules that require further treatment and those that need no treatment. The ability of MRI was on par with CT and positron emission tomography (PET)/CT in terms of T staging, which represents the size of the tumor, and MRI is more accurate than CT at N staging (N stands for lymph nodes) and shows whether the tumor has spread to lymph nodes or how far they are from the tumor. They concluded that further research on medical applications of MRI is important to improve the diagnosis and treatment of lung cancer. Ohno et al. (2007) examined the postoperative lung function in patients affected with lung cancer and compared the ability of CT, MRI, and single photon emission computed tomography (SPECT). The study was performed on 150 lung cancer patients and everyone was subjected to preoperative contrast enhanced multidetector computed tomography (MDCT), dynamic perfusion MRI, and perfusion SEPCT. Based on the results of the study, they concluded that compared to qualitative CT and perfusion SPECT dynamic perfusion MRI displayed higher accuracy in predicting the postoperative lung function.

Yoshida et al. (2011) examined the potential of diffusion weighted MRI (DWI) for detection of cancer in the upper urinary tract. DWI is a functional imaging technique that achieves image contrast between tissues based on differences in water molecule movement. The cancer-affected tissues display high signal intensity on DWI due to disorganization of tissue and increased extracellular space tortuosity that restricts water diffusion. DWI does not require any contrast agent and could be applied to patients suffering from contrast agent allergies or those with conditions of renal insufficiency. Seventy-six patients suspected of suffering from upper urinary tract cancer were examined using DWI by two independent radiologists. The sensitivity, specificity, and accuracy of DWI of the first radiologist were 92%, 96%, and 93%, respectively, and that of second radiologist was 94%, 81%, and 89%, respectively. The interobserver agreement of DWI between two reviewers were excellent, and Yoshida et al. concluded that DWI provides useful and precise information for noninvasive diagnosis of upper urinary tract cancer.

9.3.6.3 Cardiac diseases

Coronary heart disease is the major cause of mortality in developed countries and can be present during acute myocardial infarction or end up in ischemic cardiomyopathy with heart failure and ischemic valvular disease. Knobelsdorff-Brenkenhoff and Schulz-Menger (2012) reviewed the cardiovascular magnetic resonance (CMR) imaging in heart disease, which is an important imaging modality due to its versatility. CMR is a potential technique to assess myocardial function both during stress and at rest and allows stress perfusion analysis with high temporal and spatial resolution. CMR provides information on cardiac dimensions, function, and myocardial perfusion with high degree of accuracy, and provides insight into myocardial tissue alterations during acute and chronic ischemic disease. With the use of CMR, detection of ischemic disease is possible at an early stage, could also differentiate nonischemic disorders, and improve the patient monitoring and provide guidance during therapy. Beek and Rossum (2013) reviewed the medical applications of CMR in patients with acute myocardial infarction (AMI). For patients with AMI, CMR is very safe and could be carried out without any risk after implantation of coronary stent because artifacts due to stents are lower and do not affect the image quality. Nandalur et al. (2007) evaluated the diagnostic performance of stress CMR imaging for the detection of coronary artery disease (CAD) and stated that stress cardiac MRI demonstrated good specificity and sensitivity for diagnosis of CAD in patients with high prevalence of disease, however minimum information is available for use of the technique in low disease prevalent population.

The use of cardiac magnetic resonance and magnetic resonance angiography (MRA) is increasing in infants with complex congenital heart disease (CHD). Rangamani et al. (2012) investigated the safety of CMR and MRA in neonates and infants less than 120 days of age and reported the adverse events from the three types of sedation: general anesthesia (GA), deep sedation (DS), and comforting methods during a period of 10 years (June 2001 to 2011). The study was based on 147 children of which 143 children with complete information were analyzed including cardiac diagnosis, anesthesia type and agents, prostaglandin E1 (PGE1) dependence, and gadolinium (Gd) use. CMR utilized GA in 86 children, DS in 50, and comforting methods in 7, and MRA was performed in 136 children. In CMR, 12 children had adverse events, 1 major respiratory arrest, and 11 minor events; no adverse events occurred during MRA. They concluded that CMR and MRA can be performed safely in infants and neonates for a broad range of presurgical cardiac conditions.

9.3.6.4   Kidney

Zhang et al. (2013) evaluated the applications of various techniques of MRI to assess the renal function and evaluation of renal diseases using MRI. The serum creatinine is the commonly used measure for renal function, however, it becomes insensitive especially in chronic disease. In the past decade, MRI has been examined as a versatile technique to assess the kidney function, and various techniques such as diffusion weighted MRI (DWI), dynamic contrast enhanced (DCE) MRI, blood oxygenated level-dependent (BOLD) MRI, and arterial spin labeling (ASL) enable assessment of various aspects of renal function. MRI shows promising potential in assessing physiological aspects of renal functions including perfusion, glomerular filtration, interstitial diffusion and tissue oxygenation. Chandarana and Lee (2009) reviewed the fundamentals of renal imaging and elaborated some medical applications. Acute rejection and acute tubular necrosis (ATN) are the common causes difficult to discriminate and often require renal biopsy for diagnosis. Due to the risks involved in biopsy, MRI was explored and MR renography could be used for the diagnosis in early transplant dysfunction. Major advantages of DWI are the potential to examine the performance of each kidney separately and thereby one could obtain split function data. However the concentration of serum creatinine does not provide split renal function separately and hence the ability of affected kidney is overestimated and that of the healthy one is underestimated. Nikken and Krestin (2007) evaluated the role of MRI in renal imaging and stated that due to excellent soft tissue contrast, MRI becomes a superior technique in renal lesion detection and characterization. According to the authors, the role of MRI is differentiating between malignant versus benign lesions in patients on whom CT scanning based on iodinated contrast media cannot be performed and in patients with nondiagnostic CT results. The accuracy of MRI in identification and characterization of lesions is equivalent to CT, and MRI has more diagnostic value in the examination of lesions with minimum amount of fat or intracellular fat. MRI shows superior sensitivity in examination of complex cysts and greater accuracy compared to CT in the diagnosis of lymph node spread.

Crohn's disease affects the complete gastrointestinal tract including all layers of bowels and is a chronic disease. Fiorino et al. (2011) reviewed current and future clinical applications of MRI in Crohn's disease. MRI and CT imaging techniques have been recommended for evaluation of small intestines, detection of complications, and assessment of Crohn's disease. MRI provides an accurate visualization of the whole gastrointestinal tract and is less operator dependent. In detecting small bowel disease, MRI is more accurate than ultrasonography, and extremely sensitive and specific in detection of complications related to Crohn's disease. Since MRI does not involve any radiation exposure, it is a very safe and better option for repeated assessments. In patients affected with Crohn's disease, a critical challenge is the distinction between intestinal inflammation and fibrosis because pharmacological treatment is provided for inflammation and surgical treatment is required for fibrosis. MRI helps to differentiate between patients with inflammation and fibrosis. They concluded that MRI should be the first choice along with endoscopy for assessment of complications in Crohn's disease and MRI provides complete evaluation and monitoring and it could be useful for tailoring therapeutic strategies.

9.3.6.5 Arthritis

Rheumatoid arthritis (RA) is an inflammatory joint disease that is chronic and impacts all aspects of life due to pain and impaired physical function. Conventional radiographs are considered common methods for detection and quantification of joint damage, but they do not indicate the bone marrow and synovial tissue changes that occur much earlier. Hence, a need exists for an imaging modality capable of detection of inflammatory joint diseases at an early stage. Troum et al. (2012) evaluated the MRI applications in early rheumatoid arthritis diagnosis and management, and stated that MRI has the advantage of detecting both joint inflammation and damage. Hence, MRI could provide more unique data that could be used for early and accurate diagnosis and to monitor response to therapy. MRI enables detailed visualization of bone marrow, synovium, cartilage, and tendons, and provides high resolution, soft tissue contrast, and reproducibility. Boesen et al. (2009) evaluated the current knowledge and future perspectives of MRI for diagnosis and treatment of rheumatoid arthritis. The first study comparing MRI and CT for RA was published in 1988 and now MRI is accepted as the noninvasive imaging technique for visualization of inflamed synovium in people affected by RA. MRI has the capability to detect changes in volume and contrast enhancement after anti-inflammatory drug treatment. MRI could be used for detection of bone erosions, which are visible on radiographs only after around 2 years and about 20% to 30% of bone is affected. Also, MRI is the only imaging technique that detects bone marrow edema, which is a predictor of bone erosions in the future.

Osteoarthritis is an important cause of disability for people over 65 years in the industrialized world. Kornaat et al. (2005) developed a scoring system for knee osteoarthritis as identified by MRI. The authors determined its inter- and intraobserver reproducibility to monitor the therapy because MRI has been successfully used to visualize osteoarthritic changes that are not displayed by conventional radiographs. The study involved 25 patients with knee osteoarthritis and images were acquired using MRI. Two observers, one a skilled musculoskeletal radiologist and the other a research fellow, evaluated the MR images. The authors' extensive magnetic resonance knee osteoarthritis scoring system had a very good inter- and intraobserver reproducibility and hence can be utilized for standardized evaluation of osteoarthritic changes to monitor medical therapy.

Since MRI is sensitive in detection of early inflammation related to RA, all MRI examinations have been conducted using a high-field expensive whole body scanner. Economic low-field MRI systems specially designed for assessment of peripheral joints are available. Lindegaard et al. (2006) investigated the potential of a low-field extremity MRI (E-MRI) system to detect joint inflammation and destruction of finger and wrist joints by performing the follow-up study for one year. Twenty-five patients with RA for less than 12 months were selected for the study and an MRI of the wrist and metacarpophalangeal joints was performed at the beginning, after 6 months, and after 1 year using a 0.2 T Artoscan system (Esaote Biomedica, Genoa, Italy). Their results showed that low-field extremity MRI was highly suitable for assessment and prediction of early RA. The advantages are low cost and because positioning of patient was easy and comfortable, claustrophobia was avoided. But the limitations of E-MRI are a smaller field of view and a longer imaging time and a lower spatial resolution. Savnik et al. (2001) performed a similar kind of study comparing the extremity MRI of 0.2 T with high-field MRI of 1.5 T for arthritic joints. They confirmed that E-MRI was as good as high-field MRI for assessment of small joints in hands. Assessment based on quantitative and qualitative measures of joint enhancement exhibited a significant relation with good to moderate agreement and was readily accepted by the patients.

9.3.6.6 MRI in tissue engineering

In the human body, organ failure is treated by either transplanting tissue or by mechanical or electrical replacement devices such as artificial joints, pacemakers, or stents. Tissue engineering provides an alternate option of regenerative medicine where new sources of replacement tissues are used. Xu et al. (2008) studied the potential of MRI for monitoring tissue engineering. MRI could be a sensitive method to visualize the biological tissues. As biological tissues grow, die, or regenerate, the tissue water content changes, which is the source of the MRI signal. Such changes in tissue water are captured and reflected in MR images. X-ray micro-CT of bone provides high resolution and contrast, but X-ray contrast is not clear enough in the marrow and newly formed bones prior to mineralization. However, MRI with superior soft tissue contrast provides greater detail of images at the beginning stages of bone growth. MRI provides a flexible, safe, and noninvasive way to monitor the parameters related to the structural, biochemical, and functional changes that occur in the developing tissues. MRI has the capability to visualize the development of tissue during initial in vitro stages and subsequently during tissue implantation development in vivo, where the final integration of the implant with the surrounding tissues must be monitored. In the future, MRI could play a major role in tissue engineering and ultimately develop the speed of the regenerative medicine.

9.3.7 Engineering applications

Desalination is a standard method for treating water, and reverse osmosis is a membrane separation process mostly used in desalination applications. Fouling is a major challenge in reverse osmosis because fouling of membrane decreases the production capacity and quality of water, and increases the cost of production. Various cleaning techniques are performed to remove foulants and increase the effectiveness of the process but assessment of such cleaning efficiency is mostly difficult. Creber et al. (2010) evaluated the chemical cleaning of biofouled reverse osmosis membrane using MRI. A membrane fouling simulator (MFS) was fouled by providing a continuous stream of dechlorinated tap water, and several cleaning tests were performed under various conditions. Two types of images were made: 2D structural and 2D velocity. The structural images of the unfouled MFS cell show brighter regions indicating stronger water signal intensity, whereas the fouled cell image show several dark regions attributed to biofilm growth. Velocity images of the unfouled cell exhibited a relatively homogeneous flow distribution, whereas the fouled cell showed a significant flow disruption with narrow flow channels due to biofilm growth. The results of the study proved that chemical cleaning broadens the flow channels by attacking the biofilm, however, none of the cleaning methods were able to completely remove the biofilm present. The study has shown that MRI could be successfully employed to visualize and quantify the efficiency of various membrane cleaning procedures in reverse osmosis.

Water plays an important role in hydration of cement to produce concrete, but it may also have a detrimental effect. When temperatures fall below the freezing point, water present in the concrete freezes, creating an internal tension that results in the development of internal cracks in the concrete. In colder regions, deicing salts are applied during winter and water acts as a medium to transport chloride ions into the reinforcement initiating oxidation in the steel. To minimize the effect of chloride ions, concrete structures must have proper drainage facilities and the concrete must be designed to prevent excessive permeability. Hence, to assess the long-term performance of concrete, it is essential to quickly and accurately determine the permeability of concrete. Although there are various methods available to determine the permeability, Estrada et al. (2004) determined the potential of MRI for quantifying permeability of concrete. Many experiments were conducted using an MRI scanner and standard chloride ion testing machine, but the results were inconclusive because of the ferromagnetic materials. Hence, MRI testing was conducted on each of the ingredients used to make the concrete and the source of ferromagnetic material was found to be aggregates. The authors concluded that further testing using nonferromagnetic aggregates is necessary to obtain a conclusive correlation between the MRI results and those from chloride ion testing.

In industries such as automobile, chemical, pharmaceutical, and manufacturing, particulate matter removal from fluid suspension is of great significance, and a variety of filter applications has resulted in a broad range of filter design. Although MRI is primarily used in acquiring high-resolution images of internal structures of the human body, it could also be used to visualize the presence of water in a broad variety of porous media such as rock or food. Dirckx et al. (2000) have shown that MRI has the ability to measure in three dimensions, and the velocity of flow of fluids such as oil or water as they pass through opaque media. MRI data acquisition was carried out using Oxford Instruments with a 100 cm bore and 2 T superconducting solenoid magnet. The experiments were split into two groups: to identify the position of the deposited iron-oxide particles, static imaging of the filter with no flow was conducted; the second was the dynamic imaging to estimate the velocity of the fluid flowing through the filter. This study shows that MRI could be used to study filtration problems and it is feasible to observe and estimate the interior structure in 3D of a filter filled with aqueous medium, provided it does not contain any ferrous materials.

La Heji et al. (1996) studied filter cake formation during sludge mechanical dewatering based on one-dimensional NMR imaging of porosity profiles. Sludge samples were obtained from a wastewater treatment plant in Eindhoven, The Netherlands. The filtration expression experimentation was conducted with a NMR scanner having a magnetic field of 0.7 T corresponding to 30 MHz frequency. At the initial stages of study, a uniform porosity was present, and then a porosity gradient rapidly developed and slowly disappeared at the expression stage resulting in a uniform porosity at the end. The results of the experiment showed that using NMR imaging, porosity profiles were measured at the time of filtration and expression of solid–liquid mixtures. From the porosity profiles measured, it was concluded that the resistance of filter medium was higher than theoretically expected.

Many engineering equipment, such as heat exchangers and mixing vessels, have abrupt pipe expansion and the flow of fluid through such asymmetric expansion is of practical interest. Arola et al. (1998) examined the wood pulp suspension flow through an abrupt pipe expansion using NMR imaging, and the main focus of the study was the effect of expansion at different volumetric flow rates. NMR images were acquired for different rates of flow and axial positions with respect to the expansion plane. The results showed that the abrupt expansion plane for pulp suspension showed the same kind of behavior as a confined jet. The authors characterized the instability of flow and fluidization of fiber network by examining the intensity distribution and velocity profiles shape as a function of downstream position and NMR observation time.

MRI has provided great insight into various aspects of process engineering. Hall et al. (2001) examined the potential of MRI in three areas of application in industrial process engineering. The evaluated areas were the mapping of temperature distribution in conventional or microwave heating, second was to measure fluid flow through complex geometries, and the third application was the measurement of solid–liquid separation using filters. For temperature measurement, a glass jar was cut into four divisions, filled with gel, reassembled to make the jar complete, and bathed in microwave radiation. Temperatures were measured with an infrared thermal camera. In another jar filled with the same gel and bathed in microwave radiation, three MRI slice images were acquired at the same locations corresponding to the sectioned jar. The comparisons of the results showed that two sets of temperatures were similar thus validating the MRI method. The second study involved an MRI compatible screw thread extruder constructed with polyetheretherketone (PEEK), which can be operated at 100 rpm and at temperatures between –10°C and 60°C for studying flow of fluids. MRI was used to estimate in three dimensions the x, y, and z velocity vector of fluids, and the mixing of fluids as they move through the screw. For filtration studies, a filter was filled with water and a three-dimensional MRI was used to scan its geometry to determine the spatial resolution. The same measurements were made for a filter already used in the field, and a range of MRI protocols was assessed to find out which produced the sharpest delineation of material trapped by filter. The results of the study showed that MRI studies are not just confined to research and academic studies but can be useful in industrial settings and industrially robust MRI hardware exists.

In civil and chemical engineering, a moisture concentration profile is mostly obtained by the gravimetric method. But the gravimetric method is a destructive method, and hence moisture content of every profile has to be determined using different samples. But it is not always possible to exactly duplicate the sample preparation, and it is a laborious and time-consuming method. Kopinga and Pel (1994) explored the potential of the NMR method to determine moisture transport in porous media, such as building materials, in which moisture could result in various kinds of damages. The samples used were cylindrical rods with a diameter of 2 cm and length varying in the range of 2 to 20 cm. The results of the study showed that it was possible to measure a one-dimensional moisture profile in a variety of porous materials with a spatial resolution of 1 mm and an absolute accuracy of a few percent.

9.4   Advantages, limitations, and future of MRI

9.4.1   Advantages

MRI is a noncontact, noninvasive imaging method, and a slice of an image can be obtained in any plane through an object. The spatial resolution of MRI is superior to other imaging techniques. The MRI technique is free of any ionizing radiation, which is of paramount importance for human scans, and hence MRI does not require any radiation protection and safety equipment for the operators or anyone involved in the process. The contrast material used in MRI is safer for kidneys compared to contrast material used in other techniques such as X-ray or X-ray CT (Kwong and Yucel, 2003).

The most potential advantage of MRI lies in determining the real-time in vivo monitoring of various processing operations, including drying, rehydration, heating, frying, curing, draining, and freezing. The ability of MRI to determine moisture mobility and moisture distribution in food samples provide an understanding of various changes that occur during the processing of food. MRI is particularly advantageous for fruits and vegetables because of their high water content. Also MRI has high sensitivity to quality parameters affecting the produce, such as browning, and MRI has the ability to distinguish different substances, such as water, oil, and sugar (Defraeye et al., 2013). MRI requires minimal or no sample preparation and can be used for both homogeneous and heterogeneous food samples.

The most important advantage of MRI compared to X-ray or CT is the excellent contrast resolution. With MRI, it is possible to detect the smallest differences in soft tissues better than X-ray CT. Hernández-Sánchez et al. (2007) have stated that MRI provides higher sensitivity and better contrast between healthy and affected tissues compared to X-ray.

9.4.2 Limitations

A limitation is that spatial resolution of MRI is poor compared to X-ray imaging (Blink, 2004). In measuring the body composition of live animals and carcass, MRI images cannot be obtained for animals bigger in size than human beings without major equipment modification. Based on magnet size, radio frequency probe, and the gradient coil, the size of the sample to be imaged is limited (Baulain, 1997). The higher cost of the equipment and slow speed as opposed to high volume and low cost of fresh produce and horticultural products is the major limitation in adopting MRI technology for fresh produce (Clark et al., 1997). Also, there is only limited design of the equipment especially meant for food purposes.

In medical applications, MRI cannot be used on patients with metal implants because the magnet may cause pacemakers or other implants to malfunction. The commonly used 1.5 T MRI scanners in the medical field are now replaced by 3 T scanners to achieve higher quality imaging, but the limitation is that many implants, such as stents, that are considered safe with 1.5 T scanners are not as safe for 3 T scanners. Also the safe amount of heat induced in human tissue is reached faster with 3 T magnet scanners (Jerrolds and Keene, 2009). The major safety concern while using MRI is the presence of ferromagnetic objects in the vicinity. Due to the strong magnetic field present, the ferromagnetic material if present will be turned into a projectile and may cause serious injury to persons in the area. Any tool or equipment present inside the MRI room should be made of nonferrous material and the subject must be free of objects like chains, keys, belts, pens, or any other metal (Clare, 1997). Compared with X-ray CT, MRI takes a longer time to perform; about 45 to 90 min is necessary to perform most cardiac MRI (Kwong and Yucel, 2003).

9.4.3 Future

MRI has wide applications in the medical industry and many new technologies are combined with MRI to provide more sophisticated imaging. After about 20 years of research the PET/MR scanner was launched in 2010 enabling simultaneous acquisition of PET and MR images (Balyasnikova et al., 2012), which offers the advantages of both PET and MR imaging. However, the technique is still in its infancy and the clinical experience is scarce. Blamire (2008) predicted that in the next decade, there will be a shift toward higher magnetic field imaging (3 T), further improvement in MRI coil technology, introduction of ultra-short echo time imaging, and combined modality methods such as PET/MRI. The global MRI system market, which was estimated at $4.2 billion in 2011, is expected to exceed $6 billion in 2018. Advances in technology including superconducting magnets, high-field MRI, open architecture, and software applications are expected to increase the growth of the market (GBI Research, 2013).

Research studies have shown that in the future, a greater connection could be made possible between food science, food engineering, medical science, and pharmaceutical applications. For instance, applications involving monitoring and characterization of food in the gastrointestinal tract in humans and animals have been studied, and Marciani et al. (2006) used MRI to examine the behavior of lipid emulsions in the human stomach. Other than the commercially available scanners, the MRI system is custom built for the needs of the food industry and research purposes, which opens new avenues of research for various products and increases the potential of commercial MRI applications in various industries. In the food industry, many research studies have been conducted using MRI in the last decade and MRI companies are proposing dedicated MRI systems that are specially designed with smaller magnets and lower magnetic fields for the needs of food industry. The availability of a portable MRI system would increase the research and commercial applications of MRI in the food industry in the next decade.

chapter ten

Optical coherence tomography imaging

10.1 Introduction

Optical coherence tomography (OCT) involves imaging of the inner cross-sectional micro-structure of biological objects based on measurement of optical backscattered or back-reflected light. OCT is high-resolution imaging for transparent and turbid media, and applications are mostly related to biological materials. OCT is a new kind of optical imaging technique that is noninvasive and best suited for in vivo and real-time imaging. Since the spatial resolution of OCT is in the micrometer scale, it is highly suited for cellular-level imaging. Compared to traditional microscopic techniques, OCT has better penetration and provides high-resolution subsurface images up to several millimeters in tissue (Fan and Yao, 2012). The OCT could provide image resolution of 1 to 15 μm, higher than the magnitude of the conventional ultrasound and can be connected with a broad range of imaging probes and image delivery systems (Fujimoto and Brezinski, 2003). The first applications of OCT were demonstrated in 1991, and optical imaging was conducted in a controlled environment in the human retina as well as in atherosclerotic plaque (Huang et al., 1991).

OCT is very similar to ultrasound imaging, but the difference is that OCT imaging uses light rather than sound. In ultrasound imaging, high-frequency ultrasound is directed toward the sample with an ultrasonic probe transducer, and the sound wave is reflected back from the inner structures having various acoustic properties. The ultrasonic probe detects the reflected sound, and the measurements of internal structures are estimated from the echo delay. In OCT, a beam of light is reflected onto the sample material and the backscattered or back-reflected light from the internal structure is measured to determine the microstructure and properties of the sample materials. The major difference between OCT and ultrasound is that the velocity of light (3×10^8 m/s) is a million times faster than sound (1500 m/s in water), and hence measurement of distance using light needs ultrafast time resolution. Direct electronic detection is impossible in this range of time, hence OCT measurements of echo time delay are dependent on correlation techniques. Ultrasound imaging needs direct contact with the material to be imaged or immersion of the material in liquid or other medium for transmission of sound waves, whereas OCT could be performed without making any contact to the material or without any requirement for a transducing medium (Fujimoto and Brezinski, 2003).

10.2 Principle of optical coherence tomography

Optical coherence tomography is an emerging noninvasive imaging technique that can provide real-time three-dimensional subsurface images of biological tissues. The OCT technique could obtain images at a maximum depth of 1 to 3 mm and at wavelengths between 800 and 1300 nm in the near-infrared region with a resolution of 5 to 20 μm. Spatial resolution is an important quality parameter of OCT imaging and there are two types of spatial resolution: axial and transverse. The axial resolution depends on the light source characteristics such as spectral bandwidth and wavelength, whereas the transverse resolution depends on the focusing optics (Leung and Standish, 2013). The OCT image obtained is a false color map that represents bands of relative reflectivity between layers of various refractive indexes (Hrynchak and Simpson, 2000).

Interferometry is a technique that measures the echo time delay and magnitude of backscattered light with higher sensitivity. The OCT is based on the low coherence or white light interferometry phenomenon, and uses a special light source with high spatial and low temporal coherence, which allows high resolution. Figure 10.1 shows an example of an OCT system with a Michelson-type interferometer with a low coherent light source attached to the interferometer. One arm is a reference arm while other arm emits a beam that is directed toward the object to be imaged. The location and magnitude of the back-scattered light from the tissues microstructure are interpreted by the OCT to create an image. The generated image is based on the optical characteristics of the tissue microstructure. The superluminescent diode generates a light beam that is split and directed at the same time toward the imaged tissue and reference mirror. When the backscattered light from the two sources are combined, a phenomenon referred to as interference occurs. The combined signal is received by a photodetector that measures the interference. Depending on the data acquired from the internal reference mirror, the relative position of the back-scattered light from the imaged tissue is determined (Arevalo et al., 2009).

In OCT, the illumination of the sample is by near-infrared light. The light source should possess high spatial and low temporal coherence, that is, a large spectral bandwidth. The choice of light source is critical in OCT imaging, because it determines the axial resolution and the depth of penetration. The light sources commonly utilized in OCT imaging are of three types: superluminescent diodes, femtosecond lasers, and supercontinuum lasers. Of the three light sources, superluminescent diodes are the most commonly used because they are very economical, provide good spectra, and are available at various wavelengths. Higher bandwidth (approximately 200 nm) and higher optical power are provided by femtosecond lasers, but they are very expensive. Supercontinuum laser light sources provide a broad spectrum of bandwidth in the range of 400 to 2400 nm and hence make it possible to acquire very high resolution images (Nemeth et al., 2013).

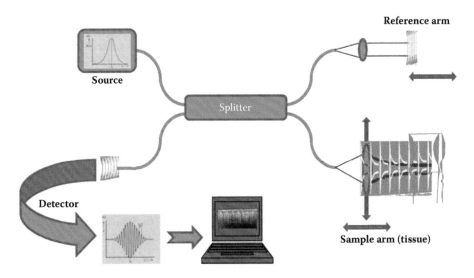

Figure 10.1 Optical coherence tomography system. (From Cauberg, E.C.C. et al., *European Urology*, 56, 287, 2009. With permission.)

OCT images are acquired in a 2D or 3D data set that represents the variation in optical backscattering in a cross-sectional plane or volume of any material. A 2D image is obtained by carrying out consecutive axial measurements of optical backscattering at various transverse locations by scanning the optical beam (Fujimoto and Brezinski, 2003). To increase the speed of the image acquisition process a Fourier domain OCT (FD-OCT) approach could be adopted. In FD-OCT, the reference mirror is kept fixed and the light from the object and reference is detected by resolving spectrally (Nemeth et al., 2013). In time domain OCT (TD-OCT), the depth of the region where measurement is observed is altered by the variation of optical path lengths of both arms of the OCT interferometer. In contrast, FD-OCT utilizes a fixed reference mirror and the photons from different depths simultaneously contribute to the measurement. The major advantage of FD-OCT over TD-OCT is the increased sensitivity of FD-OCT permitting high data acquisition rates. The Fourier domain is further classified into spectral domain OCT (SD-OCT), which uses a spectrometer with a multichannel analyzer, and swept source OCT (SS-OCT), which uses a narrow-band laser source (Stifter, 2007). FD-OCT is the best choice for low light conditions, such as imaging in high speed, because it has the ability to monitor fast dynamic physiological processes and has sensitivities well above 80 dB (Leitgeb et al., 2003). In TD-OCT about 400 axial scans/s could be obtained with a resolution of 8 to 10 μm, whereas in FD-OCT about 25,000 to 50,000 scans/s could be obtained with a resolution of 5 to 7 μm. In the next generation of FD-OCT and SS OCT, 70,000 to 100,000 axial scans/s and 200,000 axial scans/s could be acquired, respectively (Schuman, 2012).

10.3   Applications of OCT

10.3.1   Agriculture

Although the first applications of OCT were in the medical field of ophthalmology, the potential applications of OCT were eventually explored in many other areas. Since OCT involves imaging of cross-sectional microstructures of biological systems, OCT has been explored for assessing the detection of viral infection, studying the structure of seeds and plant tissues, monitoring the defects in various agricultural produces, and evaluating the quality characteristics of different produces. The various applications of OCT in the field of food and agriculture are listed in Table 10.1.

10.3.1.1   Detection of viral infection

Viral infection is a major issue in the orchid industry, because the quality of flowers and plants are significantly affected decreasing the exportability of orchid plants. Chow et al. (2009) studied the possibility of detecting virus infection in orchid plants using high-resolution OCT. The experimental setup of FD-OCT to achieve high-resolution OCT images is shown in Figure 10.2. Leaf samples from *Oncidium* orchid plants were collected from both plants that were healthy and infected by cymbidium mosaic virus (CymMV). After completing OCT images, part of the leaf samples were subjected to standard histological preparation and the ELISA test. The OCT images showed that infected leaves had a characteristic of a highly scattering epidermal layer, and the significant increase in scattering of epidermis may be associated with cell death processes such as autophagy, which involves degradation or breakdown of intracellular components. The highly scattering characteristic in the epidermal layer was not observed in the leaves of stressed plants, which were healthy even though they showed symptoms of virus infection. The results showed that the highly scattering feature of the epidermal layer of infected leaves shown

Table 10.1 Applications of Optical Coherence Tomography in Agricultural and Food Materials

Material of interest	Application	Type of OCT	Reference
Apple (*M. domestica*)	Assessment of peel structural properties	TD-OCT	Verboven et al., 2013
Apple leaves	Diagnosis of fungal disease	TD-OCT	Lee et al., 2012
Onion (*A. cepa*)	Detection of fungal or bacterial infection	SS-OCT	Landahl et al., 2012
Apple (*M. domestica*)	Quality control by assessing thickness of wax layer	TD-OCT; SD-OCT	Leitner et al., 2011
Breakfast cereal	Microstructure analysis of extruded breakfast cereals	TD-OCT; SD-OCT	Leitner et al., 2011
Onion (*A. cepa*)	Monitor defects and rots in onion bulbs	SS-OCT	Meglinski et al., 2010
Rice (*O. sativa*)	Investigate the structure of rice and distinguish rice varieties	TD-OCT	Jiang et al., 2010
Flowering tobacco (*N. sylvestris*) and tobacco (*N. tabaccum*)	Analyze the hypersensitive response of plants due to pathogen attack	TD-OCT	Boccara et al., 2007
Fresh orach (*Atriplex* sp.), tomato (*L. esculentum*), spiderwort (*T. pallida*), starwort (*S. media*)	Morphological and functional state of plant tissue	TD-OCT	Kutis et al., 2005
Purple heart (*T. pallida*)	Monitoring physiological and morphological states under different water supply conditions	TD-COT	Sapozhnikova et al., 2004
Flowering inch plant (*T. blossfeldiana*)	Visualization of plant tissues	TD-OCT	Sapozhnikova et al., 2003
Kiwi (*A. chinensis*), orange (*C. sinensis*), red-leaf lettuce (*L. sativa*), cranberries (*V. macrocarpon*)	Imaging morphology of tissues	TD-OCT	Loeb and Barton, 2003
Foils used in packaging industry	Quality control of foil	SD-OCT	Hanneschläger et al., 2011

in OCT was not visible under histological observation. Based on the results of the study, Chow et al. concluded that OCT imaging is suitable for fast, nondestructive diagnosis of orchid viral infection, which can result in better control of the spread of virus in the orchid industry and resulting in significant cost savings.

10.3.1.2 Seed structure
The OCT has been used by few researchers to conduct plant imaging. Fan and Yao (2012) studied the 3D imaging of cherry tomato seeds using FD-OCT. To acquire the entire 3D structure of tomato seed, it took 10 s and the OCT imaging allowed visualization of the

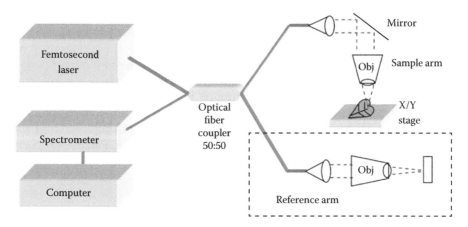

Figure 10.2 Experimental setup of the OCT system. (From Chow, T.H. et al., *Journal of Biomedical Optics* 14, 1, 2009. With permission.)

architecture of subsurface tissue layer. Several important seed structures (e.g., seed coat, endosperm, embryo, and radical) could be identified. The seed radicle at the embryo tip had relatively stronger backscattering than other parts of the embryo. Fan and Yao evaluated the SD-OCT system to visualize the inner seed structures with a depth and lateral resolution of 6.7 μm and 15.4 μm, respectively. They concluded that OCT can be a potential technique to acquire high-resolution structural images of seeds.

Disease caused by cucumber green mottle mosaic virus (CGMMV) is commonly found in cucumber, muskmelon, melon, and pumpkin, and it causes significant economic losses. Biological or serological sensing methods used for diagnosis of viral diseases are destructive and time consuming. Lee et al. (2011) investigated the potential of OCT to determine the morphological changes caused by virus infection in melon seeds. About 140 normal and viral infected seeds were obtained from Seongju, the largest melon-producing region in Korea. From the real-time polymerase chain reaction (RT-PCR) analysis, the seeds were verified for CGMMV infection. Five seeds were collected from each sample and images were acquired using OCT. OCT B-mode scans were obtained at 500 μm depth and A-scan analysis was conducted to obtain more information about normal and infected seeds. By comparison of B-mode OCT images, morphological changes were observed in healthy and infected seeds and 3D OCT images showed that the infected seed has a distinct layer beneath the surface. A fragile second boundary was observed in the OCT image of healthy seeds between the aleurone and pericarp layer, whereas a very distinguished change was seen in the OCT image of infected seeds. According to Bennett (1969), in the infected seed, the presence of a second layer is due to the relationship between plant viruses and their host that provides protection of embryos against viruses attacking the plant. The distinct layer seen in abnormal seed is the barrier that represents the specific host resistance mechanism. The authors concluded that OCT is a promising technique to noninvasively assess infected melon seeds and to monitor the presence of any morphological changes in the seeds.

10.3.1.3 Hull thickness

Hull thickness is a seed quality attribute that determines the dehulling potential, nutritional aspects of food or feed and the cooking times. The major objective during breeding of blue lupin (*Lupinus angustifolius* L.) is to minimize hull thickness. A faster method to screen germplasm for choosing new lines with lowered hull content is desirable, but the regular methods to measure hull content includes manual removal and weighing and use of dehulling devices. Other techniques, such as MRI and confocal microscopy, have been limited due to lower resolution, longer acquisition time, and limited depth of penetration. Clements et al. (2004) studied the potential of OCT for nondestructive measurement of lupin seeds hull thickness, because the technique has displayed significant promise in the micron-resolution subsurface imaging of semitransparent and turbid media. Cross-sectional images were acquired and 12 frames were acquired for each seed and averaged to create an image. The thickness of hull layer determined by OCT had high correlation with original hull thickness observed by scanning electron microscopy and allowed accurate differentiation between mutant and parent genotypes of *L. angustifolius*. Clements et al. concluded that OCT is a rapid nondestructive method that can be used for selection of thin hull lines for lupin seeds and other species.

10.3.1.4 *Plant tissue*

Most of the techniques used for studying internal plant structures are destructive. Numerous attempts undertaken to implement a nondestructive technique have been based on OCT. Sapozhnikova et al. (2003) examined the possibility of visualization of plant tissues by OCT. An experimental OCT system comprised of a single-mode fiber-optic Michelson interferometer, and the light source emission splits into two beams, one directed toward the sample and the other toward the reference mirror. The sample for the study was taken from a flowering inch plant, (*Tradescantia blossfeldiana* Mild), and the tomographic images were compared with conventional microscopy data for the same tissue. The OCT images clearly identified tissue structures located at a depth of 1.5 to 2 mm, and the cells were clearly visualized based on different scattering properties due to difference in their constituents. The cell wall produced stronger scattering of radiation due to dense multilayer structure than the aqueous cell content. The comparison of microscopy and OCT images proved that OCT provided reliable images of tissue structure, and dark structures in OCT images correspond to weakly scattering cells with an abundance of water. Based on the study, it was stated that OCT could be used to visualize tissue structures in plant materials and it is different from other plant imaging methods. The probing radiation is emitted by a low source and hence the radiation power incident on a sample does not exceed 0.5 mW, and this low intensity radiation does not produce injury to plant tissues. The acquisition time for OCT image is between 1 and 3 s, whereas the acquisition time for optical coherence microscopy (OCM) is around 5 to 6 min. Also the penetration depth of OCM is restricted to 500 μm, whereas OCT allows visualization of tissue structure to a depth of 1 to 2 mm from the surface. Hence the authors concluded that OCT is a new prospective imaging method for studying plant structures and tissue. Sapozhnikova et al. (2004) monitored the morphological and physiological states under various water supply conditions for *Tradescantia pallida* (Rose, D.R. Hunt). Comparison of leaf surface grown under standard watering to that of the same plant after deficit water supply showed that there was a significant variation in the palisade parenchymal layer thickness. Under normal conditions two to three palisade parenchyma cell layers were observed in OCT images, but after conditions of drought, only one layer and a few times two layers of cells were observed. Similarly during rehydration, cell size increase in the parenchymal layer was observed and the images of the leaves acquired 24 h after watering did not differ from the leaves observed 2 h after watering, leading to the conclusion that cell size remains unchanged for 2 to 24 h after watering. Based on the study, they concluded that OCT technique can provide a visual monitoring of the dynamics of drought and rehydration of plant tissues and hence OCT is a potential noninvasive technique to monitor variations in leaf physiology and morphology under water stress conditions.

Monitoring the internal structures of biological tissue is difficult by routine optical methods due to high light scattering in biological media. Kutis et al. (2005) compared OCM and OCT techniques to study the functional and morphological state of plant tissues. The samples used were leaves of fresh orach (*Atriplex* sp.), spiderwort (*Tradescantia pallida*), tomato (*Lycopersicon esculentum* Mill), and starwort (*Stellaria media* L.). The characteristics of optical tomography used were 1.3 µm wavelength, 15 µm spatial resolution, 2 mm probing depth, and 1 s acquisition time for tissue images of 200 × 200 pixels. Images acquired with OCT revealed that the method enabled visualization of structure of plant tissue at 1 to 2 mm depth and individual cells could be distinguished clearly because of different scattering properties. However, the resolution of OCM exceeded that of OCT and images from OCM could clearly distinguish and visualize smaller cells of 10 to 20 µm in size, whereas the depth of scanning is restricted to 500 µm. Kutis et al. concluded that the two techniques have advantages and limitations. OCM has a higher scanning rate and superior spatial resolution, whereas OCT provides tissue images at a greater depth, which permits one to visualize the conduction bundles in the mesophyll layer at a lower resolution. Both methods are promising, noninvasive methods to study plant tissues.

Attack of a plant by a pathogen results in hypersensitive response (HR) of plants characterized by necrosis at the infection site. Interferometric techniques, such as OCT, can be used in the analysis of plant tissue during hypersensitive response. Boccara et al. (2007) studied the potential of OCT to analyze the initial events in the establishment of harpin-induced HR in tobacco, and compared the results with confocal fluorescence microscopy (CFM). Harpin produces a HR-like response in many plants including Nicotiana species. *Nicotiana tabaccum* and *Nicotiana sylvestris* grown in a greenhouse were used for the study at the stage of 2 to 5 leaves. The experimental setup of OCT was based on a bulk Michelson interferometer. In both methods (OCT and CFM), a modification in the distribution or structure of chloroplast was observed. In CFM, earlier modification happened 5 h after harpin infiltration and corresponds to redistribution of chloroplast from the inner to the mesophyll cells. In OCT, a reduction in the chloroplast scattering signals was observed within 30 min of harpin infiltration. The authors suggested that OCT observations were correlated with a reduction in photosynthesis, highlighting the chloroplast structural changes as the initial indication of hypersensitive cell death in plants.

10.3.1.5   Rice varieties

There are basically three types of rice (*oryza sativa*)—japonica, indica, and glutinous—and many other varieties are produced by hybridization. Electron and optical microscopy has been used to analyze the rice varieties, but it requires slicing, which may damage and result in inaccurate results. Jiang et al. (2010) examined the waxy rice endosperm structure with OCT and differentiated four rice varieties with an attenuation coefficient derived from the OCT signal. Four rice varieties—indica waxy (IW), indica nonwaxy (INW), japonica waxy (JW), and japonica nonwaxy (JNW)—were selected for the study. A time-resolved OCT imaging setup was used for the study. The optical source was a superluminescent diode (SLD) at a wavelength of 1300 nm, and the axial and transverse resolutions were about 12 µm and 15 µm, respectively. After images were acquired in OCT, rice was sliced and images were acquired with a microscope. The waxy and nonwaxy rice images from OCT were different because in waxy rice, the space between starch granules was larger than nonwaxy rice, which resulted in a higher scattering coefficient for waxy rice compared to nonwaxy rice. The waxy and nonwaxy rice displayed obvious differences in OCT images, whereas it was inappreciable in the microscopy image. Jiang et al. concluded that OCT could provide images of the internal structure and successfully differentiate between four varieties of rice and could be used as a noninvasive, high-speed imaging technique for quality testing of rice grains.

10.3.2   Fruits and vegetables

10.3.2.1   Botanical samples

For studying the botanical samples at the cellular level, microscopic devices (electron and light microscopes) need wide sample preparation, such as dehydration, sectioning, and staining, which are mostly destructive and may modify the structure of the tissue. In high-moisture samples, histological processing is difficult, and noninvasive techniques such as X-ray, X-ray CT, and MRI have relatively lower resolution and difficult to detect character-istics at the cellular level. Loeb and Barton (2003) investigated the possibility of imaging botanical objects using OCT. Based on the instrument configuration and the sample's opti-cal properties, OCT images can be acquired at 1 to 2 mm depth with 5 to 20 μm resolution. Kiwi fruit (*Actinidia chinensis*), red-leaf lettuce (*Lactuca sativa*), orange (*Citrus sinensis*), and cranberries (*Vaccinium macrocarpon*) were selected for the study. Imaging of orange and kiwi was acquired on a cut surface, a section of lettuce leaf including both vein and blade was selected for imaging, and berries were imaged along multiple planes. The preliminary study on botanical samples showed that important morphological characteristics such as cell size, seed characteristics, and vacuole shape can be clearly visualized, and the high resolution of OCT resulted in very accurate morphological measurement compared to any other imaging techniques. But noninvasive imaging of OCT was only possible with thin-skinned fruits such as grapes and cranberry, whereas it was not possible to image through other samples such as orange. Samples that possess high backscattering contrast such as large fluid-filled vacuoles (appears dark) embedded in highly scattering tissues (appears white) are best suited for OCT imaging. Samples lacking this contrast where the tissue structure is homogeneous at the tens of microns level are not suitable for OCT imaging.

10.3.2.2   Defects in onion

Onion (*Allium cepa* L.) is a fresh vegetable consumed globally and storage losses are a major challenge for the onion industry. Many tomography techniques, such as X-ray CT, positron emission tomography (PET), ultrasound, and MRI, have been explored as nonin-vasive techniques for rapid screening of fresh produce but are still not commercially avail-able due to the cost factor and in mobility of the unit. Meglinski et al. (2010) investigated the application of OCT to evaluate defects and decay in onion bulb and to visualize an alive onion internal laminae tissue in situ. The Thorlabs SS-OCT setup (Thorlabs Swept Source OCT System, United Kingdom) was used for acquiring images of internal tissue of an alive onion bulb. The onion cell structure (i.e., outer tissue layer, dried skin, roots) and defects such as bruising were clearly visible in the OCT images at the near-surface zone up to around 0.5 mm. Also, the absorption of radiation was highly variable due to variation in the chemical constituents especially in the defective regions. The authors concluded that OCT technique could be applied to detect histological and temporal microstructural changes that occur due to internal defects in onion and this technique could be extended to other fresh agricultural products.

Rejection of onion lots due to internal defects is a major concern in onion production and current testing is destructive. Landahl et al. (2012) investigated the potential of OCT technique for detection of cell changes due to fungal or bacterial infection in stored onion bulbs. The OCT system used for the study was a Thorlabs 930 nm (Thorlabs Ltd., United Kingdom) based on a broadband, near-infrared superluminescent diode source. Images were acquired from dissected onion samples from outer to inner lamina containing either healthy or infected tissue. The OCT provided high-resolution images at a depth of about 0.5 mm. The OCT images clearly showed the differences between healthy and diseased tissue. The detachment of inner cell wall was seen in regions of neck rot-infected tissue. In the infected regions the average cell size was smaller and cells were less in number compared to the healthy regions. Based on the study, Landahl et al. concluded that diseased onion bulbs could be identified by using OCT. Ford et al. (2011) investigated the potential of OCT for monitoring diseases in several cultivars of stored onions. OCT images revealed the cell level structure of healthy tissues and provided clearly distinguishable images of onions affected by fungal neck rot (*Botrytis allii*) and bacterial soft rot (*Pseudomonas* spp.).

10.3.2.3   Wax coating in apple

Quality control and analysis of fruits are very important during storage. Apple (*Malus domestica* Borkh) is usually stored for a longer duration and the thickness and homogeneity of the wax layer determines the apple's protection and quality maintenance during storage. Leitner et al. (2011) introduced OCT as a novel tool to maintain and control the quality of apples. The experiments were performed with two different setups: an ultrahigh-resolution TD-OCT and a SD-OCT. The advantages of spectral domain are sensitivity and speed, which enable video rate imaging, while the time domain permits application of dynamic focusing and displays a constant sensitivity over the entire range of depth. Braeburn apples obtained from an experimental station (Sint-Truiden, Belgium) were used for the study. The OCT images showed many layers of paring that could be clearly differentiated. Lenticels are important features that act as bypass mediums for gas exchange between fruit and the environment and are also clearly visible in the OCT images.

10.3.2.4   Microstructure of apple peel

The apple peel is important to protect the fruit against several environmental factors and reduces fruit permeability and transpiration. The apple peel also provides protection for the fruit against microorganisms and insect invasion. Any defect on the apple surface or peel reduces the commercial value of the fruit. Verboven et al. (2013) investigated the potential of nondestructive OCT to evaluate the structural characteristics of apple peel. Peel structural properties were compared for different cultivars (Royal Gala, Braeburn, Arlet, and Ida Red). The images were obtained with three OCT setups: a lab-based TD-OCT system working at 800 nm, a prototype SD-OCT working at 800 nm, and a commercial SD-OCT operating at 1300 nm. The results from OCT were compared with confocal microscopy and micro-CT. For all three OCT methods, various layers of the apple peel, namely, the epidermis, cutine, and hypodermis, could be recognized, although differences in contrast and resolution were observed for the three methods. The lowest resolution was obtained for commercial SD-OCT, but it also provided the better penetration depth than the other two methods. The TD-OCT and prototype SD-OCT provided images with higher resolution and a better differentiation between near peel layers, but the increased resolution also resulted in reduced penetration depth (100–200 μm). Compared to confocal microscopy, the lateral resolution of the three OCT systems was lower. OCT images provided a clear picture of deeper tissues, whereas confocal microscopy was restricted to a very small volume. Micro-CT provided images of higher contrast of pores in tissue but failed to analyze the different surface layers, whereas OCT images visualized the surface topology including surface roughness, lenticels, and cracks in wax and revealed the cellular structure up to a few hundred micrometers into the fruit. The authors concluded that OCT is a noninvasive technique that could be used to observe the structural differences between apple peel and to determine the changes in structure that occur during storage.

10.3.2.5   Fungal disease detection

Marssonina blotch is a fungal disease in leaves of apple trees caused by *Marssonina coronaria*, which significantly affects the quality of apples. It is difficult to diagnose the disease with the naked eye and usually takes 3 to 5 weeks to be detected. Fungicide is not effective after the disease has appeared on the leaves. Many techniques, including microscopy, X-ray tomography, PET, and MRI, have been studied and there are limitations with each technique. Lee et al. (2012) studied the potential of OCT for diagnosis of Marssonina blotch in apple leaves. Leaves of both diseased and healthy trees were collected, and experiments were performed within 3 h of sample collection to minimize tissue damage. The OCT system was constructed in the lab with a superluminescent emitting diode with a 3 db band width covering 150 nm. The OCT system produces a microresolution image with axial and lateral resolution of 6.7 µm and 17.3 µm, respectively. The distinction of layers in fungus-infected leaves was not clear, and this is probably because as fungus penetrates the leaf during infection, many components of the leaves are destroyed. Each component has a unique refractive index and if a certain compound is destroyed due to fungal or viral infection, the refractive index is lost. However, when an OCT beam is focused on healthy tissue, a highly sensitive scattering signal is detected, which represents the normal layers. The experiments confirmed that OCT images revealed a broken layer structure in areas of surface lesions and also proved that OCT can reveal not only lesions but also infested areas that are impossible to distinguish with the naked eye. The OCT images can also distinguish between fungus-infected leaves and those that are abnormal for other reasons such as those eaten by worms. Lee et al. concluded that OCT technology can be used as an early diagnosis tool to reveal Marssonina blotch in apple leaves.

10.3.2.6   Extruded cereals

Analysis of microstructure is an important aspect of quality monitoring in the food industry. Leitner et al. (2011) examined the potential of the OCT technique for microstructure analysis of extruded breakfast cereals. Two different experimental setups—an ultrahigh-resolution TD-OCT system and an SD-OCT—were tested for cereals. A comparison of quality for coated and noncoated cereals was performed. They also investigated the rehydration process of cereals in milk showing the ability of OCT for real-time monitoring of the dynamic processes. The rehydration process was tested with the SD-OCT system and a 50 mm probing lens. Sugar-coated breakfast cereal from Nestle was placed on the bottom of the cylindrical jar and milk added up to around 80% of the cereal height. The cross-sectional OCT images were acquired for the whole rehydration process. In the initial images, the surface of the cereal was visible with no milk and gradually milk started appearing along the surface, resulting in surface morphology reformation. And the shrinkage of the cereal height occurred as the structure of the extruded cereal collapsed when kept immersed in milk. Based on the study, capability of OCT for real-time imaging of dynamic processes like rehydration during immersion of the sample in a liquid was demonstrated.

10.3.2.7   Quality control of foil

The nondestructive nature of OCT is best suited for in-line analysis and quality monitoring of multilayered foils that are often used in the packaging industry. Hanneschläger et al. (2011) tested the potential of OCT for quality monitoring of multilayered foils. Films with few micron

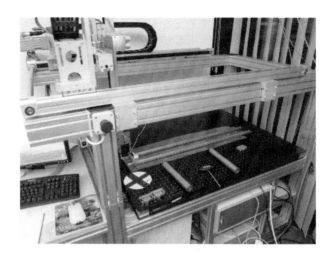

Figure 10.3 Photograph of the off-line testing OCT system. (From Hanneschläger, G. et al., Optical coherence tomography as a tool for non-destructive quality control of multi-layered foils, in *6th NDT in Progress, International Workshop of NDT Experts*, Prague, Czech Republic, October 10–12, 2011. With permission.)

thicknesses can be easily resolved with the OCT system, thus providing inline control of film thickness homogeneity and impurities detection. The experiments were conducted with a portable, high-resolution and high-speed SD-OCT system. To test the capability of OCT systems to image individual layers in a moving multilayered foil, off-line tests were performed (Figure 10.3). Foils were attached to the upper portion of an optical bench and the OCT probe was moved at various speeds in the range of 5 to 800 mm/s, and OCT measurements were carried out at the center of the system. The sample consisted of 10 layers and the overall thickness was 290 µm. Even when the probing head was moving at a high speed, images clearly showed distinction of different layers of foils. The results of the study showed that in-line and off-line measurements of multilayered foils could be performed, and hence OCT could be used for quality monitoring of multilayered foils during the production process.

10.3.3   Applications of OCT in engineering

10.3.3.1   Aerospace materials

P. Liu et al. (2012) performed quality evaluation of aerospace materials with OCT. A custom-built TD-OCT system based on the Michelson interferometer was used for testing two aerospace materials: glass–fiber composite and an epoxy coating. Epoxy coatings are used for protection against corrosion of steel pipes and metal containers, and quality assessment includes testing thickness, adhesion, and coating layer roughness along with identification of defects in the coating and substrate. Glass-fiber reinforced polymer (GFRP) composites are used in the manufacture of aerospace components such as helicopter rotor blades, and defects such as delamination or cracks could seriously affect the safety of the aircraft. In this study, three epoxy-coated samples—a healthy coated, uncoated, and one with substrate defects—were tested. The results of the study showed that compared to the healthy epoxy-coated sample, significant differences could be observed from the images of the other two samples. The authors stated that the results of the study are an early work to validate the hypothesis that OCT could be a promising technique for aerospace material applications. Further development in OCT, such as Fourier domain and ultrahigh-resolution OCT with higher speed and higher resolution, could result in OCT being developed as a standard measurement technique for applications in aerospace engineering.

10.3.3.2   *Printed electronic board*

Czajkowski et al. (2010) evaluated the potential of OCT for quality monitoring of printed electronics products. An ultrahigh-resolution TD-OCT system was used for the study, and the technique was tested on an RF (radio frequency) antenna, an example of printed electronics products. Measurements were conducted at axial resolutions of the submicron level, because such high resolution is essential owing to the thickness of material layers utilized in printed electronics. The measurement results were compared with commercially available measurement devices. The results of the study presented different modalities of OCT such as noncontact and noninvasive cross-section imaging, surface profilometry, and complete 3D volume reconstruction. The study showed that OCT could be an accurate technique that could be used in product testing of printed electronic materials.

Numerous electronic and printed devices are developed with new materials and new fabrication methods for various applications. A thin protective film is used to provide proper operating conditions and to separate the devices based on organic components from the environment. The thin films referred to as encapsulation layers are based on polymers, range from hundreds of nanometers to single micrometers, play a greater role in the process of fabrication, and assure a proper lifetime to the device. Czajkowski et al. (2011) evaluated the potential of the OCT technique for quality inspection of encapsulation, because other techniques such as scanning electron microscopy (SEM), atomic force microscopy (AFM), and X-ray microscopy are either complex or destructive methods. The use of the OCT technique is based on the principle of low coherence interferometry and its sensitivity for changes in refractive index. The authors stated that the advantages of the OCT technique in quality inspection are no sample preparation, nondestructive and noncontact method, high accuracy, and short measurement times.

10.3.3.3   *Glass fiber-reinforced polymer*

Fiber-reinforced polymers have applications in many areas such as aeronautics, aviation, and automotive industries due to their lesser weight compared to metal structures. The structural integrity of the material during impact is a critical issue in the research. Various techniques, such as ultrasonics, thermography, and shearography, employed for testing have advantages and limitations, but these methods do not have the potential to image the structures to the scale of single fibers. Wiesauer et al. (2007) investigated the potential of ultrahigh-resolution OCT to monitor defects and stress in the internal structure of glass-fiber reinforced polymers (GFRP). The specimen used for the study was a preimpregnated composite fiber sheet with fiber diameters of about 9 μm. In the superluminescent diode (SLD) image, the internal structure was only coarsely visible, whereas in the ultrahigh-resolution image, perpendicular and parallel fiber bundles were clearly visible. The authors stated that ultrahigh-resolution OCT is a potential tool for structural investigation of polymer materials, and transverse scanning OCT demonstrated the benefit of providing in-plane information that cannot be acquired by a conventional cross-sectional OCT imaging. Wiesauer et al. (2005) investigated en-face (transversal) scanning OCT with very high resolution for material investigation. They stated that en-face scanning OCT is an effective tool for material analysis and characterization, and might be a potential technique for statistical random sampling in production, for product and process development, and in material research for rapid and nondestructive characterization.

10.3.3.4 Subsurface defect detection

Duncan and Bashkansky (1998) demonstrated the applications of OCT for determination of subsurface defects in nonbiological materials such as lead zirconate titanate (PZT) ceramic material, crystal silicon carbide (SiC), and Teflon-coated copper wire. The PZT ceramic material has multimillimeter-sized discoloration and abnormalities that cannot even be seen with light microscopy because of the material's scattering nature. In the OCT scans, the defects appear at 20 to 30 μm depth, increase slightly in size, and disappear at 140 μm depths. For SiC, 15 individual X-Y scans, at a depth interval of 10 μm from the surface to 140 μm into the sample, were combined to form a 3D representation of the sample for understanding of various defects in the sample. The authors stated that when using OCT, subsurface defects along with their spatial position could be determined in nonbiological materials.

Swanson et al. (1996) demonstrated that OCT is well suited for nondestructive evaluation in the field of polymer processing, especially for the design, processing, and durability of new polymer blends, alloys, and multilayer sheets, which depend on the morphological character of the material. The OCT technique could provide insight into the real-time microstructural characterization of structures beneath the surface and enable monitoring of the functional relationship between morphology and process variables such as temperature and applied stress. Other applications of OCT include assessing adhesion and delamination in electronic packaging and ceramics; assessing state of cure for polymers, composites, and various coatings; and assessing subsurface damage.

10.3.3.5 Paper making

Paper making technology has expanded tremendously and new methods are tested for diagnosing and characterizing paper. Paper can be described by various characteristics, such as porosity, density, roughness, and thickness, and these characteristics can be used to classify the various types of paper suitable for different applications. Alarousu et al. (2005) investigated the potential of OCT for measurement of paper properties. The OCT system consisted of a Michelson interferometer with an illumination of a low-coherent light source such as a superluminescent diode. The experimental result showed that OCT has the ability to become an important method in paper characterization and could be a feasible alternative for traditional methods that are either slow, labor intensive, or invasive. The ultimate goal of incorporating this technology is to create a method suitable for on-line measurements of paper as it passes through a paper machine. Prykäri et al. (2010) evaluated the quality characteristics of the coating layer of the premium photo paper and stated that ultrahigh-resolution OCT is a multifunctional tool for the quality monitoring of various paper products. They also suggested that along with tomography and topography images of objects, additional information similar to gloss could be obtained by recording the magnitude of individual interference signals in OCT.

10.3.4 Medical applications of OCT

The technique of OCT was initially used in ophthalmology and has had great clinical impact. The initial in vivo tomograms of optic disc and macula were studied and demonstrated in 1993 (Fercher et al., 1993). Advancement in OCT has made it possible to image nontransparent tissues, thus enabling a wide range of medical applications. The various applications of OCT in biomedical imaging other than ophthalmology include dentistry (to image the gum and teeth structure), dermatology (to acquire subsurface structural image and blood flow information), gastroenterology (to image the gastrointestinal tracts with endoscopic probes), intravascular (to obtain images of plaques in the blood vessels), cancer diagnosis (to discriminate between malignant and normal tissues), and surgery (to differentiate between normal and malignant tissue for removal of malignant tissue during surgery) (Ali and Parlapalli, 2010). Numerous in vivo and in vitro studies were conducted using OCT in major human systems including applications in cardiology (Brezinski et al., 1997; Jang et al., 2002), gastroenterology (Bouma et al., 2000; Das et al., 2001; X.D. Li et al., 2001), urology (Zagaynova et al., 2001), dermatology (Podoleanu et al., 2000), and tumor diagnostics (Boppart et al., 1998b; Fujimoto et al., 2000).

The OCT has been used for monitoring and diagnosis of a wide range of retinal disorders, including macular edema, glaucoma, macular hole, macular degeneration related to age, optic disc pits, epiretinal membranes, and choroidal tumors. For diagnosis and detection of diabetic macular edema or glaucoma, OCT is very promising because it provides specific information about retinal pathology based on disease progression. OCT can detect the disease at an early stage before loss of vision or any significant physical symptom occur. The use of OCT is significant where traditional excisional biopsy is risky or not possible and where retinal biopsy cannot be performed. OCT has the potential to provide high-resolution images compared to any other technique, and is also used for assisting surgical intervention, which provides the ability to observe below the tissue surface in real time and guide the surgery (Fujimoto, 2001).

Cryosurgery is a technique for destruction of malignant lesions, and real-time visualization of the freezing front boundaries is necessary for optimization of cryosurgical procedures. Choi et al. (2004) evaluated the potential of OCT to monitor biological tissue freezing during cryosurgery. Deionized water and Intralipid were used as biological tissue simulating materials. Water was used to simulate the high water content of skin. Intralipid, a suspension of lipid globule, and hamster skin were used for the experiments. OCT images were acquired during liquid-nitrogen-enhanced cooling of water, Intralipid, and in vivo hamster skin. With OCT, local variations in the refractive index served as the primary source of contrast. The OCT images of water are characterized by a relatively strong surface reflectance signal intensity and negligible subsurface signal intensity, whereas Intralipid, being a heterogeneous lipid suspension, is characterized with a high scattering coefficient. The OCT images had a relatively strong subsurface OCT signal. The results of the study showed that OCT is capable of imaging phase transition dynamics of water, Intralipid, and in vivo skin during freezing. Using an interstitial probe, minimally invasive OCT monitoring of tissue freezing during cryosurgery could be achieved.

10.3.4.1 Cancer

The OCT has shown promising potential for diagnosis and detection of cancer. OCT can provide functional information such as blood flow and tissue birefringence, which could be used for diagnosis to replace biopsy and to guide and monitor therapy. Iftimia et al. (2009) explored the potential of OCT for diagnosis of pancreatic cancer and therapy guidance. A major challenge for a gastroenterologist is to distinguish between benign pancreatic cysts and malignant cyst. An OCT setup with minimally invasive probe appropriate for pancreatic cyst examination was developed. A total of about 60 excised tissue specimens were tested and an overall specificity and sensitivity of 92% and 88% was achieved, respectively. The accuracy of differentiation between benign and malignant cancer tissue was 97%. Iftimia et al. concluded that preliminary studies suggested that OCT could be a potential tool to differentiate between various cystic lesions of the pancreas.

Cauberg et al. (2009) reviewed various technologies, including OCT, for diagnosis of bladder cancer. They stated that the OCT technique could distinguish between the three layers of bladder wall (e.g., urothelium, lamina propria, and muscularis propria) in healthy tissue because of varying scattering properties of each layer resulting in various intensities. However, in cancer-affected tissues, these layers are not visible. Hermes et al. (2008) investigated 142 human bladder samples ex vivo and showed that OCT could distinguish between healthy carcinoma in situ and urothelial cell carcinoma (UCC) with a sensitivity and specificity of 83.8% and 78.1%, respectively, for malignant bladder tissue. Using the OCT technique, Manyak et al. (2005) examined the bladder tissue samples and grouped them as malignant or benign with an overall sensitivity of 100% and specificity of 89%.

OCT has significant potential for assessment of breast cancer, but the major restricting factor is the limited imaging depth, typically about 2 to 3 mm. McLaughlin et al. (2012) studied the feasibility of imaging breast cancer with OCT needle probes, because with limited imaging depth, it is not possible to obtain images at a depth required to evaluate status of tumors in situ. By using OCT needle probes McLaughlin et al. acquired 3D data of breast cancer margins and lymph nodes, and the results were verified against the histological standard. Their study showed that OCT needle probes possess a significant potential for in situ assessment of tumor and lymph node condition in breast cancer, and established a basis for assessment of pathologic features in larger clinical studies involving OCT.

Barton (2012) developed an OCT technique for early detection of cancer with the focus on three organs—skin, colon, and ovary—which represent increasing challenges of access. Handheld probes could be used for skin imaging, and colon imaging can be done by incorporating miniature endoscopes during conventional surface imaging colonoscopies. The system developed for ovarian imaging had a resolution of about 15 μm in both the axial and lateral directions, and was able to visualize normal structures, malignant and benign cysts.

10.3.4.2 Cardiology

OCT is a very high resolution imaging technique that offers the potential to visualize coronary plaques at microscopic levels. Kubo et al. (2011) stated that OCT is useful for the diagnosis of coronary atherosclerotic plaques and for evaluation of plaque rupture, erosions, thin-capped fibroatheroma, intracoronary thrombus, and calcified nodule in patients affected by acute coronary syndromes. With the ability to observe the atherosclerotic lesions in vivo with very high resolution, the OCT technique has provided cardiologists with a technique to have better understanding of the vulnerable plaque and acute coronary syndromes. The biggest advantage of OCT is its very high resolution (10 to 20 μm) that is around 10 times higher than intravascular ultrasound (IVUS), which used to be the gold standard for vessel wall and stent imaging. OCT could differentiate three layers present in the coronary artery wall. Related to tissue characterization, the OCT technique could detect three different types of coronary plaques—lipid, fibrous, and fibrocalcific.

OCT could overcome the limitations of intravascular ultrasound and angiography when imaging coronary stents in vivo due to the use of near-infrared light with a resolution close to histological examination of coronary artery. OCT has provided a great understanding of coronary atherosclerosis with the potential to visualize plaque (Barlis, 2009). In comparison with conventional imaging techniques, OCT performs far better in the assessment of vulnerable plaques that are associated with a higher risk of myocardial infarction, such as thrombus, plaque rupture, and thin-capped fibroatheroma. The OCT technique could also be used to visualize when the stent is not properly positioned against the arterial wall and tissue prolapse after stent deployment, thus providing new insight for the evaluation and treatment of coronary artery disease with stent placement (Shinke and Shite, 2010).

Gutierrez-Chico et al. (2012) analyzed the advantages and limitations of OCT in comparison with other intravascular imaging techniques for a variety of clinical applications, including evaluation of severity of lesion, characterization of severe coronary syndromes, assistance during coronary stenting, and assessment of long-term healing after stenting. The authors stated that intracoronary OCT has provided a greater understanding of plaque morphology, but considerable work is required to establish clinical factors and biomarkers for risk stratification. Even though OCT was initially considered a research tool, it has a potential to become a standard tool for diagnosis and guidance of therapeutic intervention.

Kubo et al. (2011) stated that the limitation of TD-OCT is that it requires vessel occlusion using balloon inflation and vessel flushing with saline infusion during image acquisition because near-infrared light signals are lowered in intensity by red blood cells and hence evaluation of the long coronary artery might be restricted. Insufficient blood displacement can be an issue in vessels greater than 3.5 mm diameter. Another limitation is the low penetration depth of 2 mm and hence OCT signals cannot reach the rear wall of thick atherosclerotic lesions. The depth of penetration is dependent on tissue characteristics, and lipid-rich plaque results in signal attenuation that interrupts the observation of deeper layers of the coronary artery wall. But recently, FD-OCT has been developed to solve the current limitations in TD-OCT by imaging at higher frame rates, which enables imaging of 3D microstructure of coronary arteries. Kanovsky et al. (2012) stated that the maximum acquisition speed of 20 mm/s is achievable in frequency-domain OCT, whereas the maximum speed of time-domain OCT was only 3 mm/s.

Kanovsky et al. (2012) reviewed and summarized the main milestones of OCT in the research field as well as in routine practice. OCT imaging has opened new horizons in coronary interventions. Introduction of micro-OCT systems is expected to be available in the future, which could provide extreme image resolution up to 1 μm, which could bring such a level of detail that the cellular structure of endothelial tissue could be assessed. They also stated that an ideal system in the future should display 3D reconstruction of the vessel along with automatically analyzed structures of the vessel wall, their diameters, and volumetric assessment.

10.3.4.3 Dentistry

Freitas et al. (2006) investigated the potential of detection of caries-affected human dental tissue with OCT and obtained three-dimensional images of a dental microstructure used for qualitative and quantitative assessment. They were able to detect caries in third molars of human teeth and identified the lesion located below the surface of 10 μm with a maximum depth lesion of 50 μm. Melo et al. (2005) evaluated the enamel dental restoration by OCT and stated that OCT images were comparable with X-ray and optical microscopy and the results were promising; hence OCT could be a potential technique for clinical evaluation of dental restorations. Kyotoku and Gomes (2007) employed OCT to image the areas of fracture initiation and propagation of cracks in fiber-reinforced composite. Their results suggest that the OCT technique has demonstrated the potential to produce images of fracture initiation and crack propagation, which could be used for quantitative analysis. The most important advantage is that the technique is nondestructive and noninvasive.

Modern dentistry emphasizes preventive procedures to control caries disease. Braz et al. (2011) evaluated the integrity of dental sealants with OCT. An important feature in the assessment of the clinical success of sealant material is the marginal adaptation because presence of marginal gap leads to staining, which is the first stage of sealant failure. Traditional methods to evaluate sealant, such as visual and probing inspection, do not have ideal performance and cannot detect failures or gaps in the inner structure of sealants. For the study, five human third molars were obtained from a teeth bank. For evaluation of fissure and pit sealant, 20 images before and after sealant treatment were acquired. From the

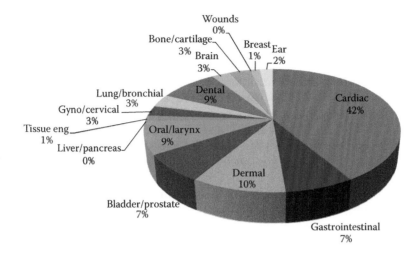

Figure 10.4 Research publications in nonophthalmic biomedical field using OCT technique. (From Holmes, J., *Journal of Biophotonics*, 2, 347, 2009. With permission.)

images, the internal structure of sealant as well as the enamel could be detected. Good differentiation between sealant and enamel was observed and the failure at the surface and the interior was identified through OCT images. Using the OCT technique, it was possible to visualize whether the enamel cavities were present or absent, thereby limiting the use of an invasive technique. Braz et al. concluded that OCT could reveal failures and fissures in the adaptation of sealants and hence could be used for assessment of sealant application and retention for longer term.

Holmes (2009) analyzed various commercial applications of OCT (not taking in to account ophthalmic imaging, which has already reached successful commercial application). Figure 10.4 shows the research studies conducted to explore the potential of OCT applications in various biomedical fields. The data showed that OCT application in cardiac imaging was explored most, followed by research into cancer, specifically cancer of the oral cavity, skin, bladder, and gastrointestinal tract. The rapid growth in the number of research works and papers published about OCT is mostly because of the impact of the FD-OCT, which has the ability to provide video imaging with a higher signal-to-noise ratio compared to TD-OCT.

10.3.4.4 Pharmacy

In the pharmaceutical industry, a film coating is used for different purposes ranging from improved product stability, taste masking, increased shelf life, and regulated release of pharmaceutical ingredients. Tablet coatings are an important aspect in the drug manufacturing process. The coatings allow the design of products with a delayed or regulated release profile, and hence the chemical and physical structure of the coating is critical for product performance. There are still challenges in the coating process due to insufficient knowledge on how material and operating variables affect quality and cause issues such as picking (part of tablet coating pulled off and stuck to another), twinning (two or more tablet cores stuck together), bridging, and cracking. Koller et al. (2011) evaluated the OCT technique for characterization of pharmaceutical tablet coatings. The samples were collected at 15 stages of the coating process consisting of tablets with various thickness of coating ranging from uncoated to a coating thickness of around 70 µm during the industrial spray coating process. OCT images were obtained with an SD-OCT setup consisting of a multifocal length probe head. The coating thickness of cracked tablets obtained using OCT was compared with scanning electron microscopy (SEM). The images acquired during the progress of the coating process clearly showed the increase in thickness, and even thin layers were visible at the beginning of coating. The defects in the coating due to air inclusions or density variations resulting in increased light scattering were also visible in the images. It was also possible to assess coating properties such as homogeneity and thickness using OCT images. Koller et al. concluded that SD-OCT could be used as a noninvasive technique for pharmaceutical tablet coatings characterizations.

Zhong et al. (2011) investigated the potential of OCT and tetrahertz pulsed imaging (TPI) for quantitative characterization of tablet coatings with thickness between 10 and 140 μm. Their study showed that the OCT system has the ability to quantify very thin coatings in the 10 to 60 μm range, while TPI could be used for quantifying thicker coatings between 40 and 140 μm and beyond. Zhong et al. stated that OCT and TPI are two complimentary nondestructive techniques for characterization of pharmaceutical tablet coatings.

Mauritz et al. (2010) assessed the potential of OCT for analysis of pharmaceutical tablet coatings. Various types of tablets with different shapes, coatings, and formulations were tested using OCT. The OCT systems used were the spectral radar OCT (OCP930SR), which operates at 930 nm; and the swept source OCT microscope (OCM1300SS systems, Thorlabs, ELY, United Kingdom), which operates at 1325 nm. Based on the results of the study Mauritz et al. stated that OCT could identify structural characteristics in tablet cores and coatings, although accurate differentiation between various coating layers is based on the strength of refractive index discontinuities between the layers. The images at 930 nm provided better contrast and spatial resolution than at 1325 nm, while differences in penetration depth were insignificant. They concluded that OCT technique could be used as a promising technique in the quality control of pharmaceutical tablets.

10.4   Advantages, limitations, and future of OCT

10.4.1   Advantages

The major advantage of OCT is its ability to provide high sensitivity, high resolution, and noninvasive imaging at the cellular level. The greatest advantage is that OCT can provide high-quality images for physicians and researchers to allow them to visualize, examine, and understand biomedical structures at microscale levels. OCT has revolutionized many fields of medicine, including dermatology, ophthalmology, and cardiology, and has better performance compared to other techniques such as microscopy, ultrasound, CT, and MRI. Microscopy can be used for examining small tissues, but cannot be used for investigating tissues inside the body, and the resolution of ultrasound, CT, and MRI is not high enough to capture the tissues at the cellular level. Electron microscopy can reveal very minute details of cellular structure, but it is not possible to observe living samples inside the body (Subash and Wang, 2013). The limitations from other imaging techniques are overcome by OCT. Another advantage of OCT in medical imaging is that it can be easily incorporated into a variety of clinical imaging devices such as microscopes, surgical imaging probes, fiber optic endoscopes, catheters, laparoscopes, and needles.

The FD-OCT imaging provides 10 to 100 times faster imaging speeds compared to conventional TD-OCT. In addition to advancement in optical imaging, high-speed electronics and real-time algorithms for various operations, such as data acquisition, processing, and recording, have enabled real-time OCT imaging in endoscopy (Zhang et al., 2009). The spectral OCT can provide 40,000 A scans per second, it allows point-to-point registration, and provides an accurate volumetric analysis (Latkany, 2006). Higher imaging resolution of OCT has enabled the visualization and analysis of individual cells and various cellular processes, namely, mitosis and cell migration (Boppart et al., 1998a). The OCT technique allows the imaging of microstructure of tissue at or near the histopathology level without the necessity for tissue removal. Although the penetration into the tissue is confined to a few millimeters, higher resolution of around 4 μm could be achieved while using a longer wavelength source, which is about 25 times higher resolution compared to high frequency ultrasound, MRI, or CT (Hrynchak and Simpson, 2000). Another important advantage of OCT technique in the biomedical field is that imaging can be performed in situ, in real time without the necessity to cut out the specimen.

The OCT imaging devices are low cost, mobile, and compact. The high speed operation of OCT imaging and acquisition of images in real-time makes OCT useful for intraoperative use (Gladkova et al., 2012). The OCT technique could actually eliminate the need for biopsies in the surveillance of precancerous conditions or could at least reduce the number of biopsies required in standard protocols (Zhang et al., 2009).

The noncontact and noninvasive nature and its potential to acquire images in turbid and transparent media make OCT attractive for nondestructive testing and monitoring of nonbiological materials such as manufacturing parts for industrial applications. The technique is very useful for inspection of silicon and plastic microelectromechanical systems (MEMS); quality monitoring of solar panels and devices manufactured from composite materials such as turbine blades and microengineered prototype parts; for product development of miniature components; and inspection and testing of advanced materials. The major benefits of OCT compared with the most common technique computed tomography (micro-CT) are lower price, accuracy, and speed. Compared to conventional IR microscopy methods, OCT offers a much higher speed of imaging (Goode, 2009). To operate an OCT system, an operator needs only minimal training and does not require specialized training.

10.4.2 Limitations

The major limitation of OCT imaging is the small depth of penetration. The penetration depth depends on the optical properties of the tissue being investigated. In tissues of a highly scattering nature such as muscle or skin, penetration depth is about 2 to 3 mm, whereas in more transparent regions such as the eye, an imaging depth of 10 to 20 mm is possible with micron-scale resolution (Boppart, 2003). A major disadvantage of using the OCT technique for intravascular imaging is that the imaging is attenuated by blood. Saline flushes and balloon occlusion are used to overcome this limitation; however, concerns include fluid overloading resulting in pulmonary edema. Another limitation is the depth of penetration, which may be adequate for imaging some of the arteries, whereas with large necrotic cores, the complete core length cannot be imaged (Brezinski, 2006).

OCT technology could not be used for every type of material. The material must be either transparent or translucent to the wavelength at which OCT is available and the technique could not be used for metals (Goode, 2009). Although FD-OCT imaging is faster, the major limitation with FD-OCT is that it is hard to acquire images at the 1310 nm wavelength and hence inexpensive CCD cameras cannot be used at this wavelength. So, expensive InGaAs arrays or swept source systems need to be used, which increases the cost and complexity of the optical sources (BioOptics World Staff, 2011). Irrespective of numerous research going on in the biomedical field, only a few products have reached clinical application outside the ophthalmic sector and not many have achieved significant market penetration.

10.4.3   Future

In 20 years time, OCT has emerged from a new technique to a robustly developed technology. The global market of the technology was less than $10 million in 2001 to more than $275 million in 2009, and it is anticipated to reach around $1669 million by 2019. As of now, there is no technique other than OCT that could be used for vulnerable plaque identification, assessment of calcium amount, and stent monitoring. The potential of OCT in the assessment of atherosclerosis or thickening of walls of arteries are seen as a very important application, and the U.S. Food and Drug Administration's first approval for a clinical OCT system for cardiovascular imaging was obtained in 2010 (BioOptics World Staff, 2011). Hence, OCT has great potential for further development and uses in biomedical and other imaging applications.

Many advances and improvements are expected from the OCT technique, and companies are refining the technology and products for much wider use in the future. The National Institutes for Health's (NIH) funding for OCT increased from around $5 million in 2000 to $60 million in 2010. The funding for research and market applications of OCT is continuously increasing to support research as well as commercialization of OCT systems and devices (Reiss, 2011). Software advances may result in quantitative assessment and display of 3D OCT data, which could enable measurement of subtle changes in pathology and accurate evaluation of progression of disease and response to therapy. In the future, competition between manufacturers may result in rapid innovation of technology, and low cost OCT instruments will enable wider access and usage in the community (Schuman, 2012). The full potential of OCT imaging is still being explored and it will become one of the best potential technologies for use in biomedical applications, and its potential in non-medical applications will increase in the coming decade.

chapter eleven

Imaging-based automation in the food and agriculture industry

11.1 Introduction

The population of the world is increasing tremendously. The current population is 7.13 billion, and it is expected to reach 9 billion by 2042 (Grift et al., 2008). The impact of the population increase can be felt by the increasing pressure on the agriculture and food industry. With 9 billion mouths to feed, there is a great demand in the agriculture and food sector to speed up existing processes to preserve what has been produced, reduce food waste, and increase productivity. However, resources are decreasing with the increasing population. Future predictive models expect that demand for agricultural crops for food and feed purposes will increase significantly in the next decade. This demand needs to be met by improved technology and intensified agricultural practices. Although technological advances occur significantly, the demand for agricultural land in expected to grow by 200 to 500 Mha until 2020, which is very high (Kampman et al., 2008; Jayas, 2012).

The most important challenge of the agri-food industry is to supply safe and healthy food and guarantee food security. The United Nations Food and Agriculture Organization defines *food security* as "when all people, at all times, have physical, social and economic access to sufficient safe and nutritious food that meets their dietary needs and food preferences for an active and healthy life." At present, over 1 billion people are malnourished and 60% of deaths in small children under 5 years old is due to lack of vitamins, minerals, and protein in their food (FAO/OECD, 2012). The situation of food security is expected to further deteriorate due to tremendous population growth, climatic conditions, and reduction of agriculture and natural resources (Langelaan et al., 2013).

Along with the increased demand for food production, the world standards on food safety have also dramatically increased in the last couple of decades. Hence, an increase in agricultural production along with higher quality of processed product is expected out of reduced resources, such as land, water, energy, and human labor. After harvest, raw food materials need to undergo a significant level of processing before being delivered to the consumers. An increase in awareness of food safety among consumers has significantly grown in the recent past. Food contamination and issues related to food safety have led to the need for stringent safety measures to be adopted during the processing of raw materials, and transport and storage of finished products. All these factors have led to an undisputable need for automation in the agriculture and food industries.

The agriculture industry has seen tremendous growth and has transformed into an industry that can continuously adopt changes. In traditional agriculture, most farming practices were performed by human laborers starting with plowing the field, seeding, irrigation, applying fertilizers, weeding, harvesting, and storage. But slowly, agricultural mechanization began and many types of machineries were introduced in the process of farming. In developed countries, agricultural mechanization has completely changed the traditional way of farming and has increased the productivity and reduced the need for labor and resources. But still today, in developing countries, the traditional way of farming is practiced with higher dependence on human labor. The next stage of mechanization is automation in the agriculture sector. Automation can be explained as a technique or method of performing various operations with highly advanced electronic devices resulting in reduced human intervention.

The food industry is a major contributor to the global economy and has developed into one of the major industrial sectors in the developed as well as developing countries. In Canada, the food industry is responsible for more than 9% of the GDP and provides approximately 2.3 million jobs, which is roughly around 13% of total employment in Canada (Grant et al., 2011). In the United States, consumers spend about $1.8 trillion every year on food, which accounts for approximately 10% of the GDP. In the United States alone, around 16.5 million people are employed in food-based industries. The food and agriculture industries are always linked and contribute significantly to the global economy. The processed food chain, which consists of input of raw materials, processing, storage, distribution, and retail of food through restaurants, all combined constitute around 25% of the economy of modern industrial countries (Josling, 1999).

The major contribution of the food and agriculture industry to the global economy is significantly improving due to the incorporation of automation and emerging imaging techniques. The UK food industry spends around £1 billon per year on research and development. Ten years before, there were fewer robots in the food industry and they were considered expensive, complicated, and put people out of work. But today it costs only £5 per hour to operate a robot, whereas it requires £10 per hour to hire a person to perform the same task (Mitsubishi Electric, 2013).

11.2   Need for automation with focus on imaging

Most food processing techniques were discovered many centuries ago, even before development of any civilization. Processing techniques such as salting, drying, roasting, and curing have been practiced since ancient times. The curing of meats with smoke or salt is pre-Christian, baking was evident from excavation of cakes over 5000 years old in the European region, and evidence for baking of wheat breads by Egyptians in 2600 BC has been found. The first processed dairy products were cheese and yogurt, which were developed in West Asia, and more modern processing methods such as canning, freezing, and chemical methods of preservation were introduced in 1800 (Mohamed, 2003). After so many centuries, the basic principle is still the same, but more sophisticated tools and technology have been incorporated in the already existing techniques to meet growing demand.

The need to produce various food products without any compromise on quality and at a higher speed is the most important criterion in the agriculture, food, and beverage industry. As more emphasis is on the quality of the product, the need for automation and machine vision has become mandatory to achieve good and consistent quality. With an increase in population, higher processing capacity is expected in all food processing plants. With an ever increasing demand on speed and accuracy, manual processing cannot meet the demand and the need for machine vision techniques has become crucial.

In the agriculture and food industries, there is a wide range of potential for machine vision applications. From raw material monitoring to various processing and packaging operations, machine vision can be incorporated at most stages. For instance, sorting of materials by shape, size, color, or ripeness could be performed by imaging techniques. Machine vision could also be used in the processing of any kind of material regardless of whether it is a fruit, vegetable, meat, dairy, and so forth. The imaging technique could be used for monitoring various quality characteristics, such as to measure weight or volume; to check for proper placement of food components (e.g., cream, jam); to monitor proper sealing of pouches, jars, and bottles; and to check barcodes, best-before dates, batch numbers, and labels.

11.2.1 Typical product flow in food processing industry

The flow diagram in Figure 11.1 shows a general product flow and processing operation in a food processing plant. Based on a specific product and specific process, a lot of different steps may be added or reduced from this flow diagram, but this gives a basic idea of the steps involved.

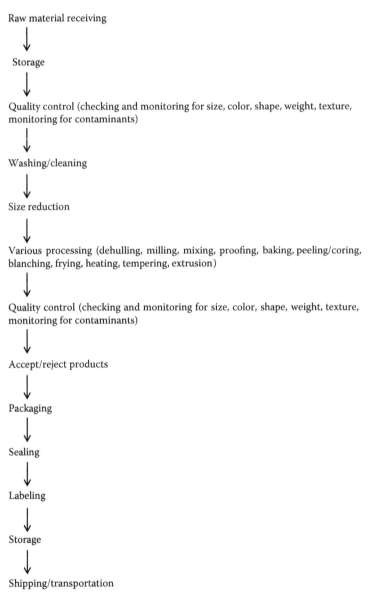

Figure 11.1 Line diagram of typical product flow in a processing plant.

There is a constant drive for automation in the food industry. Automation based on machine vision could be incorporated in many stages depending on, for example, the need of the industry and government requirements. A machine vision system could typically be located at the raw material receiving step to ensure that the products are not mixed with other unwanted materials and that the raw material meets the basic requirements. An imaging system could monitor the various processing operations and check the products for various specifications, maximum or minimum temperature achieved, proper filling, drying, and other quality attributes. Packaging, sealing, and labeling are also critical operations and require total monitoring for proper packaging and traceability requirements. The ability of machine vision to monitor sealing and packaging has become the most important capability of imaging systems.

11.3   Current uses of imaging-based automation in agriculture and food industries

11.3.1   Agriculture

11.3.1.1   Weeding

Weeding is an important task in crop production and it requires periodical monitoring and action, otherwise the yield of the crop is significantly reduced. Manual weeding is a laborious, time-consuming, and expensive process. The Farm Technology Group of Wageningen University along with Allied Vision Technologies developed a mobile imaging system that can be hauled by a tractor. This system has two digital cameras that perform two functions: localization of the plants against the ground and identification of plants as either weed or crop. The identified weeds are then treated with a herbicide microsprayer (Figure 11.2).

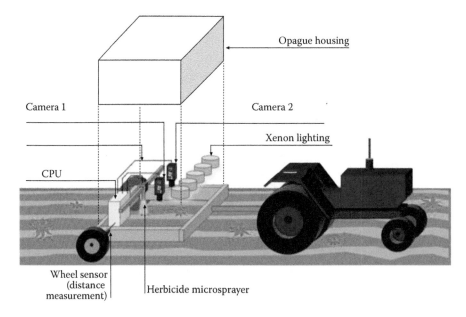

Figure 11.2 Weed treatment using machine vision. (From Allied Vision Technologies, 2010, Imaging makes agriculture greener, Allied Vision Technologies GmbH, Germany, http://www.alliedvisiontec .com/us/news/news-display/article/imaging-makes-agriculture-greener.html; accessed December 16, 2013. With permission.)

Tillett and Hague Technology Ltd. (2014) recently developed a vision-based robotic system for precision based-spot application of herbicides to individual weeds in the field. They developed more than 350 vision-guided implements for various inter-row operations for a wide variety of agricultural and horticultural applications. The system, named Robocrop, is designed to guide inter-row cultivations and spraying accurately at high speed. The system is equipped with a video camera to send images to the computer, which calculates the lateral position relative to the crop and minimizes misalignment by activating a side-shifting mechanism. To differentiate plant material from the background, Robocrop uses greenness in color images, which also reduces the effect of shadows and sunlight.

Hemming and Rath (2001) developed a computer-vision-based automated system for identification of weeds under field conditions. They achieved a high classification accuracy of plants and weeds using morphological and color features.

11.3.1.2   Identification of plants in field/harvesting

Three-dimensional mapping of plants could be performed for spraying, yield analysis, and to detect diseases or crop damage. Researchers at Danish Technical Institute (Odense, Denmark) developed a utility vehicle mounted with GPS, laser rangefinder, camera, and sensor for scanning. Using this system 3D reconstruction of an orchard was performed. After 3D reconstruction, supervised learning techniques were used to identify and classify the plants. Once the plants are identified, the imaging system could be used for harvesting such crops. At Shanghai Jiao Tong University (Shanghai, China), researchers developed a robot and a vision system for harvesting strawberries (Wilson, 2013). Wall-Ye is a vine-pruning robot with a vision system and consists of two arms, GPS system, and six cameras (Figure 11.3). The system has the ability to prune 600 vines per day. The system is capable of pruning, desuckering (i.e., removing unproductive shoots), and collecting valuable information on vigor of vine stock and soil conditions (such as temperature, moisture, and pH) (Ackerman, 2012).

Lettuce bot, an agricultural robot with video cameras and visual recognition software, has been used for thinning of lettuce in Salinas Valley, California. The vision system identifies the lettuce that needs to be eliminated and squirts fertilizer that kills the unwanted

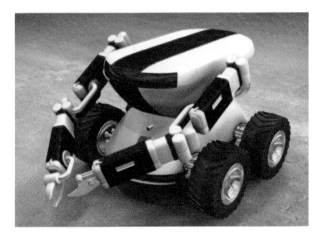

Figure 11.3 Wall-Ye vine pruning robot with vision system. (From Millot, C., Wall-ye.com, 2009. With permission.)

plants and enriches the soil. The Lettuce bot could replace at least two dozen workers and aid in the improved production of lettuce (Wozniacka and Chea, 2013).

New Holland North America (New Holland, Pennsylvania) and National Robotics Engineering Consortium (NREC) developed an automated harvester. The harvester consisted of vision cameras, frame grabbers, computers, and software. Three computers guided the harvester: a computer with vision processing software to collect image data, a second one to collect positional data to guide the path for the harvester, and a third computer for task management. The harvester was able to harvest 10 acres of alfalfa during a continuous 20 h. The speed of the harvester while cutting alfalfa was equal to the speed of a manual operator in the range of 5.6 to 7.2 km/h (3.5 to 4.5 mph) throughout the whole cutting time; however, manual harvesting speed fluctuates and gradually decreases in a short period of time. The harvester was ranked high for perfection of the cut and low failure rate, and has the critical advantage of reduced manpower required for the harvesting of vines (Wilson, 2001).

Remote controlled aircraft fitted with cameras fly over potato fields in the Hermiston, Oregon area to detect plants that do not get proper fertilizer and water. The system captures the reflected light in the wavelength region of 520 to 920 nm. Healthy plants strongly reflect NIR radiation, whereas stressed plants due to lack of water, nutrients, or insect infestation result in reduction in the level of reflected light. Thus, images could be used to determine healthy or stressed plants in the field. An imaging system (Tetracam) is used to sort grapes based on the quality of wine they may produce upon processing. Unmanned aerial vehicles (UAVs) are sent over vineyards to find the grapevines with the highest normalized difference vegetation index (NDVI) values, which indicate the fruits with high sugar content (Freebody, 2013).

At Michigan State University, a new vision-based harvesting cum sorting machine for apples has been developed and commercialized (Figure 11.4). The system could increase the efficiency of harvesting as well as sort the apples in the orchard into two or three grades (cull, processing, and fresh). Since the harvester also aids in sorting, inferior grade apples need not be sent to the packinghouse and hence prevents spoilage of good apples. At present, since sound and defective apples are harvested, combined, and shipped to

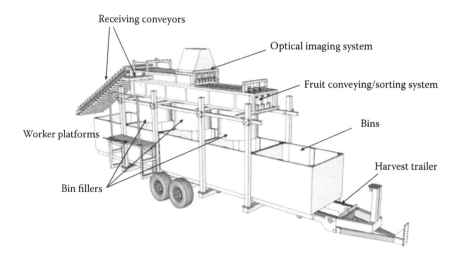

Figure 11.4 Vision-based system for harvesting and sorting apples. (From Renfu, L., Michigan State University, 2013. With permission.)

storage, it causes significant losses because defective ones are more prone to infestation by pests and diseases. The system could grade and sort apples at the rate of six to eight fruits per second (Renfu, 2013).

11.3.1.3 Grading/sorting

After harvesting, grading or sorting of fresh produce is a critical stage for quality monitoring. Manual grading and sorting is very time consuming and produces less accurate results. Imaging techniques for grading and sorting of vegetables and fruits could speed up and improve the efficiency of the process. National Frozen Foods (Burlington, Washington), which handles about 25 to 29 million kilograms (55 to 65 million pounds) of vegetables per year, initially used manual inspection for sorting vegetables. It installed a machine vision system for sorting and grading vegetables. Peas were sorted based on color features; the grading of beans requires more sophisticated algorithms involving feature and shape extraction to determine stem or skin defects. Manual and other color sorting systems remove three to four good peas for every defective pea, whereas the machine vision system removes 1.5 to 2 good peas for every defective pea reducing waste by half. The change of product just requires loading of particular software and hence the process line could be switched for different vegetables with ease. The complete process of cleaning, sorting, blanching, inspection, and freezing takes about 15 minutes for 680 kg (1500 pounds) of peas (Haystead, 1997).

It is estimated that in North America, more than 30% of fruits and vegetables are discarded even before they reach the grocery shelves due to the imperfection in the shape, size, or color, or external damage in the product. Those products that reach grocery stores can remain unsold and end up in landfills. A French multinational company, MAF Roda Agrobotic (http://maf-roda.com/en/), designs and manufactures equipment for grading, sorting, packing, washing, and palletization of fresh fruits and vegetables. An experimental machine vision system for sorting apples is shown in Figure 11.5. The vision system comprised of high-resolution CMOS (complementary metal-oxide silicon) cameras, acquisition board, and LED lighting has the ability to perform optical sizing, color sorting, and detection of any external damage. Grading and sorting of fruits and vegetables at the early

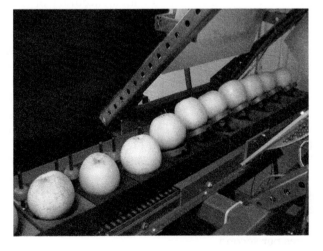

Figure 11.5 An experimental machine vision system for sorting apples. (From Bennedsen, B.S. et al., *Computers and Electronics in Agriculture*, 48, 92, 2005. With permission.)

stage could help in diverting the imperfect size of miscolored produce to be used for other applications (Overbury, 2010). The fruit sorters designed by MAF Roda have 1 to 10 parallel lanes, and the numbers of lanes determine the processing capacity of the machine. The system comes with 1 to 64 outlets that can handle various types of fruits ranging from melons to cherry tomatoes and are capable of sorting 10 to 15 fruits per second. One of the machine vision systems is called Globalscan. It acquires 20 color images and 20 infrared images for each fruit for 100% surface inspection.

A machine vision system for sorting wine grapes was developed by Fraunhofer Institute for Optronics, System Technologies and Image Exploitation (IOSB). The harvested grapes are passed along the conveyer belt at a speed of 3 m/s to the optical sorting system where the images of fruits are captured by a high-speed line scan camera. The images are evaluated in milliseconds, and foreign objects, such as stones, twigs, and insects, are blown out using compressed air, and the cleaned grapes are also sorted based on quality grades and passed on to the container. The machine vision system processes several tonnes of grapes in an hour, which saves the winemakers a significant amount of time and energy (Carroll, 2013).

Iris Vision (Stemmer Imaging) has developed a machine vision system to process carrots. Prewashed carrots between 150 and 300 mm long at any orientation are carried on a conveyer. By measuring how rapidly a carrot decreases in thickness, the system locates the point where the carrot should be cut (D. Wilson, 2012). Odenberg, a major food sorting system manufacturer (Dublin, Ireland), developed a vision-based system for sorting fruits and vegetables. The system can handle a variety of fresh produce, such as potatoes, carrot, cucumber, tomatoes, berries, peaches, pears, and dried fruits. with a capacity of 25,000 kg/h.

Sugar-end defects are a major quality deteriorating factor in grading of potatoes. Potatoes with these defect have a high concentration of reducing sugar (such as fructose, glucose, and starch concentration) on one end of the potatoes that when fried, the sugar caramalizes and results in a dark brown color at one end and a golden brown color at the other end. The sugar-end defects are not visible in the 380 to 780 nm spectrum but are visible at wavelengths around 1300 nm. Hence, a machine vision system with a near-infrared (NIR) camera was built to detect sugar-end defects. The system could classify and reject potatoes with more than 5% sugar-end defects with an accuracy of 91.7% and throughput of 16 t/h of potatoes (Burgstaller and Groinig, 2012).

Dates are a tricky fruit to handle because they are sticky and vary greatly in size. Com-N-Sense (Kfar Monash, Israel) and Lugo Engineering (Talme Yaffe, Israel) developed a machine vision system for sorting dates fed on V-shaped vibration feeders (Figure 11.6). The images are acquired from four cameras provided with uniform and white lighting. The dates are sorted at a rate of 1400 dates/min. In the future, the machine vision system will be modified to add a weight in the motion component to measure the weight of the dates. By measuring the width and height, an approximate volume could be determined, which along with the weight data could be used to determine the moisture content of dates and thereby sort the dates based on the juicy nature of the fruit (*Vision Systems Design*, 2012). Smart Vision Works (2011) developed two sorting systems using an infrared camera for dates: a color sorter for grading dates based on color and a quick sorter for grading dates based on size and amount of skin separation. The sorting machine could sort based on 12 grades of maturity and 8 quality grades. The processing speed of the system varied between 30 to 180 dates per second.

Color sorters using machine vision are also available for pulses, peanuts, coffee beans, melon, and pumpkin seeds. These systems come with CCD cameras and high-speed ejector

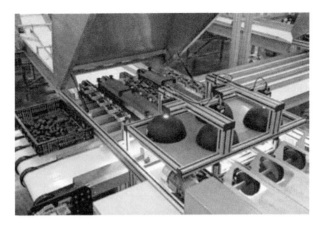

Figure 11.6 Machine vision system for sorting dates. (From Com-N-Sense, 2012. With permission.)

valves to sort different types of seeds. The advanced design aspect provides the ability to sort various seed sizes with different sorting modes (Hongshi Hitech, Anhui, China).

11.3.2 Food

Food production and processing is a complex process and requires continuous monitoring of products and processes. Maintaining the quality of final products by continuously supervising the incoming raw materials and rigorous control of production process are crucial for the success of the food processing industry. The most potential use of X-ray imaging in the food industry is the detection of contamination in the food products. Contamination could be of any object such as glass, stone, plastic, rubber, or other undesired materials present in the product. In many commercial food processing plants, including bottled mushrooms, fruit salad, salad leaves, baked products, pies, confectionary, dairy, meat, and poultry, X-ray imaging is used for detection of contaminants.

The imaging technique is widely used for monitoring of product defects such as oversize or undersize products. For instance, presence of a cavity inside a chocolate bar or block of butter; uneven boundary of crackers, chocolate bars, and cheese; and presence of split or cracks in sausages can be detected. The imaging technique is widely used for monitoring and inspection of packaging of various food materials and proper sealing of containers. Since many processed food materials are now packed in small containers made of different materials, proper sealing of the package is very critical; otherwise the product will be rejected. In commercial food processing and packaging units, imaging is used for monitoring of proper packaging and sealing of various food products.

11.3.2.1 Bakery inspection

Machine vision could be used for monitoring chocolate cakes and the proper placement of chocolate and jam in the middle of the cake (Davies, 2000). Inspection of cream biscuits is a challenge because a layer of cream should be sandwiched between the two wafer biscuits with the biscuits properly aligned and without the cream popping out of the biscuit. Machine vision has been used for monitoring of proper placement of cream and alignment of wafer biscuits in the manufacture of cream biscuits (Davies, 2001).

A machine vision technique has been used to develop a system to determine the size and weight of biscuits as they travel along the production line at the rate 3600 biscuits/min

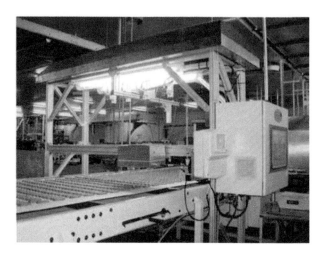

Figure 11.7 Machine vision system to determine the dimensions of the biscuit. (From Wilson, A., *Vision Systems Design*, 17, 2012. With permission.)

(Figure 11.7). Three cameras capture images that are used to determine the length and width of the biscuit, and by reconstructing a 3D image from the captured images, the height of the biscuit is determined (A. Wilson, 2012).

11.3.2.2   Pizza/tortilla

An imaging system with a 3D structured light inspection unit is used to measure the thickness profile. The system could monitor 7200 pizzas/h as they pass on a conveyer at a speed of 0.5 to 1 m/s (Figure 11.8). After processing the captured image data, 3D image data are used to measure the height of the product at various locations on the surface. Pizzas that do not meet the expecetd quality dimensions such as height, width, or shape

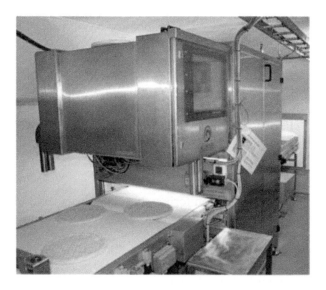

Figure 11.8 3D structured light system to measure diameter, thickness, and edge defects in pizza. (From Wilson, A., *Vision Systems Design*, 17, 2012. With permission.)

are diverted from the production line to a reject line. The same processing line could be used to monitor and inspect 40,000 tortillas/h (A. Wilson, 2012).

11.3.2.3 Cheese

A UK-based cheese maker developed an imaging system to detect improperly vacuum-sealed cheese bags. Proper sealing of a cheese bag is critical because even with one bag of improper sealing, mold growth could occur which may contaminate the entire batch resulting in huge losses. The surface of a cheese bag shows different reflective characteristics based on whether it was properly sealed. With proper sealing, the plastic bag is tightly wrapped on the uneven cheese blocks and light reflections occur from peaks of the wrap, whereas in an improperly sealed bag, a limited number of peaks appear and results in uniform reflection of light. As the vision system monitors and identifies improperly sealed packs, they are lifted from the main conveyer and transferred to a bypass conveyer (Flood and Bailey, 2013).

11.3.2.4 Monitoring fill levels

A machine vision system also aids in monitoring the fill level of fluid food products because a very narrow tolerance exists for under- or over-filling. Plastic containers are used in certain food applications, while glass bottles and jars are widely used because glass is strong and chemically inert. In the quality monitoring, checking for proper fill level is an important task because under- or over-filling of a bottle results in the rejection of the product. A machine vision system has the ability to check for proper filling and has been used in many commercial food industries such as sauce, ketchup, juice, and oil production facilities (Figure 11.9) (Omron Electronics, 2004b).

11.3.2.5 Label inspection and validation

In the processed food product, best before or use by date is a critical factor for consumers to let them know if the product is safe for them to consume. Also, label mix-ups may result in potential liability concerns if the product contains any allergens or expensive product recalls. Monitoring of labels by a manual process is tedious, cumbersome, and prone to errors. Important information regarding the date of manufacture or best-before date has become a mandatory requirement of food regulatory authorities. A machine vision system offers the best solution for monitoring best-before dates in food products. For instance, V-Viz Ltd. has an intelligent date inspection system that confirms date integrity

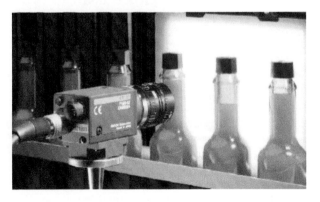

Figure 11.9 Machine vision system monitors under- or over-filled containers. (Omron Electronics, 2004b. Courtesy of Omron Automation and Safety.)

by verifying that every single product barcode matches the expected code. Any product that fails or has a misaligned date is tracked to a reject system and verified that the specific product does not reach the consumer (Figure 11.10). V-Viz Ltd. also provides a label inspection system based on machine vision to monitor the proper positioning of labels. If a system has successive reject items, the system automatically shuts down by preventing more containers from being improperly labeled, ultimately reducing waste (V-Viz Ltd., 2014a).

Machine Vision Consulting (MVC) has a machine-vision-based label inspection system for verification of the presence of label, position validation, presence of correct label, skewness and wrinkled label identification, bar code inspection, and optical character verification. The system operates at a speed of 900 parts per minute (PPM). MVC also has a commercial machine-vision-based 360-degree package inspection system that provides accurate 360-degree inspection of a package in a single image. The system provides noncontact, 100% inspection of product labels of jars, bottles, and vials at the rate of 750 PPM. The system is located on top of a conveyor and uses multiple digital cameras to acquire various images of the product that are then assembled into one image (Machine Vision Consulting Inc., 2013).

The Kraft Foods Canada processing facility produces 30 different sauces at the rate of 265 bottles per minute. It originally had a laser-based scanner to scan the labels, and the major problem was that it could only read codes in a small field of view. Hence, when a label design is changed, the code may be in a different position that requires the position of the laser scanner to be changed, which often times results in errors. When Kraft installed

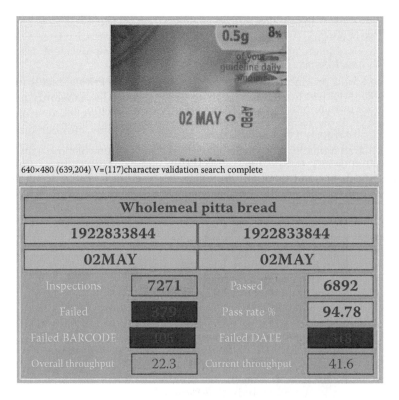

Figure 11.10 Intelligent date inspection system using machine vision. (From V-Viz Ltd., 2014a, Intelligent date inspection system, http://www.v-viz.com/Docs/iDiSDataSheet.pdf; accessed January 27, 2014. With permission.)

machine-vision-based technology, the algorithm searches the entire image and identifies the position of code, and reads it. The accuracy of labeling increased to 99.9% (Lewis, 2013).

The machine vision system performs optical character verification (OCV) or optical character recognition (OCR) to ensure that the date is printed clearly on packages. The OCV/OCR technology has seen great improvement in recent years and enhanced reliability. Also, the machine vision system located after labeling prevents imperfectly labeled bottles or cartons from entering the supply chain, which reflects poorly on the brand name (Figures 11.11 and 11.12) (Omron Electronics, 2004a). For OCR/OCV, the rule of thumb is that the stroke width should be at least 3 pixels wide for the smallest character and an area

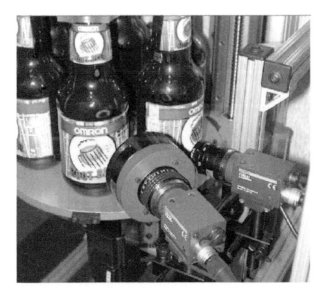

Figure 11.11 Machine vision system inspecting date or lot code. (Omron Electronics, 2004b. Courtesy of Omron Automation and Safety.)

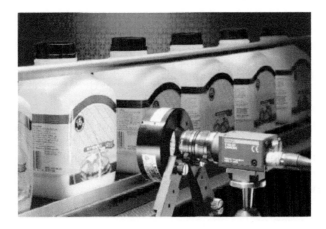

Figure 11.12 Machine vision system monitoring torn or perfect labels. (Omron Electronics, 2004b. Courtesy of Omron Automation and Safety.)

covered by a typical character should be about 20–25 pixels by 20–25 pixels. The best OCR system should have an accuracy of 99.9% (Zuech, 2000a). Vision systems can also grade bar codes to ensure that the product contains good contrast, and a clear and complete code that can be read throughout the flow chain of the product. A robust vision system not only grades but also rejects a product if it fails the inspection, also indicating if the device marking the barcode is running low on ink to prevent any further rejection of products. Most machine vision systems could identify and read a bar code placed at any orientation as long as the bar code lies within the camera's field of view. Of the different types of lighting, ring lighting is best suited for barcode inspection because poor lighting affects the ability of machine vision system to read the bar codes. Ring lights utilizing LEDs provide a lifetime of 100,000 h (Evanger, 2010).

11.3.2.6   Sealing inspection

Proper sealing of food containers is critical because a small flaw in sealing may result in product leakages ultimately leading to contamination and rejection of the whole lot. Manual inspection or other sealing inspections just look for evidence of gross leakage rather than monitoring subtle leakage, which may not be clearly visible but may create quality issues later in the supply chain. The machine vision system is used by many manufacturers to check for sealing integrity. Machine Vision Consulting (MVC) uses a machine vision system that ensures proper closure of seals in pouches. The system could detect major and minor seal defects and operates at a 0.5% false reject rate and 0.06% false accept rate. The MVC also employs a machine vision system for inspection of foil lids on various types of food containers that inspects lids at the rate of 10/s (Machine Vision Consulting Inc., 2013). Silgan Equipment developed a machine-vision-based bottle inspection system capable of inspecting 1200 bottles/min. The system ensures that bottles are filled, capped, and sealed, and an extra level of protection is provided by adding a form of tamper bands wrapped around the cap. Consumers are satisfied with the presence of tamper bands, which provide an extra level of security and conserve the freshness of the product. The machine vision system has three cameras that provide complete 360° inspection of sealing (*Vision Systems Design*, 2007).

The cap closure and sealing monitoring has become a crucial stage in packaging and sealing of food products. Eagle Vision Systems provides a closure inspection system based on machine vision for monitoring bottles, cans, and jars. The image of each closure passing the machine vision unit is compared to the ideal or standard image. The imperfect caps deviate from the actual standard images and hence are easily rejected from the product line. The system has a high speed of 60,000 units/h and random product orientation is possible. The system has an inspection accuracy of greater than 99% and false rejection rate of less than 0.1% (Eagle Vision Systems, 2013).

11.3.2.7   To determine weak chain link in conveyer

HJ Heinz is one of the most popular food brands and has the largest food processing complex in Europe. It is very critical for the plant to operate 24/7 to meet requirements. Even if a single link fails in the chain link system used to convey cans, significant damage could occur to the machine and the product. To avoid this damage, a machine vision system was installed to identify even very small cracks in the link that would appear before the chain fails. An LED backlight is positioned behind the chain and a camera is placed in front of the chain. The dimension on the chain link increased as it cracks and if the dimension exceeds a threshold, a red warning light activates which enables the operator to stop the line to check for failed links (V-Viz Ltd., 2014b).

11.3.2.8 Meat

A study conducted by David Caple & Associates reveals that over 50% of work-related injuries in meat processing facilities are due to repetitive manual operations. Machine vision could provide a safer and better solution by replacing hard manual labor. Jarvis (Middletown, Connecticut), one of the largest producers of meat processing equipment, developed a vision-based robot to cut beef carcasses. With the combination of a high-speed robot controller and 3D vision guidance, the system has performed accurate cutting operations since 2007 in major meat processing facilities (*Vision Systems Design*, 2008).

In a meat processing facility, meat is cut or diced to appropriate size and moved along the conveyer at a normal rate of 2722 kg/h (6000 pounds/h). A metal detector normally monitors the meat for the presence of any contamination, but plastics or lighter material often moves along the conveyer and may end up on consumers' plates. But a machine vision system provides color difference monitoring, which could identify plastic pieces or other lightweight materials in the meat processing line. Researchers at Georgia Institute of Technology (Atlanta, Georgia) along with its industrial partner Gainco Inc. (Gainesville, Georgia) developed a low cost machine vision system with a Sony CCD camera that scans the belt twice for detection of foreign objects (Hogan, 2005).

A machine vision system developed by Georgia Institute of Technology was tested at Gold Kist poultry processing plant (Carrollton, Georgia) for automating the visual-inspection-related tasks in the poultry industry. The technology, called a systemic screener, was installed at the beginning of poultry processing line and the cameras determine the defects on birds and defects caused by systemic diseases (septicemia or toxemia). The good ones pass on to the next stage for processing, while those with defects are removed from the processing line (The Meat Site, 2013). The machine vision application has potential in the processing facility because many operations are tough tasks for the human laborer, and incorporation of imaging technique in the processing facility will benefit the laborers and improve the efficiency of the process.

11.4 Advantages and limitations of machine vision technology

11.4.1 Advantages

The major advantages of automating the food industry are increased speed and efficiency of the operation, increased production throughput, and reduced human labor. Although the cost of initial investment for installation of automatic technologies may be expensive, the operating cost could be significantly reduced. For instance, Ellips, a Dutch company (Eindhoven, The Netherlands), installed a vision system for sorting cherries in which more than 2400 employees were hired for sorting cherries. By installing a vision system, the cost of labor could be significantly reduced. The cherries graded using the vision system were 80% to 90% accurate compared to 40% to 50% accuracy in the mechanical grading system (Hardin, 2012a).

Other advantages include improved quality control compared to manual labor because certain tasks in quality checking in the food industry are monotonous and create boredom for the human supervisors, which may affect accuracy and efficiency. Automated technologies, however, perform consistently throughout the day without any slowdown or decreased efficiency. In machine vision technology, once the criteria for grading are established, it will be applied consistently throughout the entire product line without even the slightest variation in checking for quality standards. More than identifying the defect in products, the machine vision system also has the ability to count the number of defective products, which could be used to set tolerance limits or the number of defects that could be allowed. It may also be possible to classify the defects, which could be used in the process of defect correction. A machine vision system could be used for on-line monitoring of the quality of the product rather than off-line monitoring. On-line monitoring provides a quick and easy quality check and does not delay the flow of the product.

In the food industry, the most commonly followed principle in defective product removal is to make an error based on caution by removing the product appearing to be defective rather than letting it go, which might result in more costly recalls. But false rejection on the other hand is a waste of resources and energy, which is a major cost factor and could account for reduction in profits or actually result in loss. Automation could result in improved workplace safety by avoiding human labor in some of the more difficult tasks. Recruiting and training skilled workers and supervisors for quality control of food products is becoming very difficult. The cost involved in recruiting, continuous training, and retaining of human laborers are becoming more expensive compared to the installation of a machine vision system.

Zuech and Miller (1989) stated the advantages of machine vision as increased productivity; reduced direct and indirect labor; increased utilization of equipment and space; reduction in inventory and waste; reduced lead times and setup times; reduced material handling costs; reduced error that could have occurred due to human inattentiveness, fatigue, or miscalculation; and on top of everything, increased customer satisfaction. Gümüş et al. (2011) stated that machine vision can provide accurate and fast identification and quality assessment of aquatic foods; perform classification based on size, shape, color, and other visual characteristics; and provide rapid inspection in a nondestructive, hygienic, and noncontact way.

Machine vision technique for the food processing industry could be viewed as a more hygienic option because fewer people come in contact with the food during processing and packaging. Also by using automation, the program can be switched from one task to another within a short time. The amount of damage caused by automation is much less compared to human counterparts. For instance, in packaging poppadum (a fried, thin, crisp Indian bread), the breakage was nil, which the human operators could never achieve (Mitsubishi Electric, 2013). Hence automated technologies could improve hygiene and reduce product waste.

Compared to manual quality control, a visual-based imaging system extracts and analyzes a large number of product features. Hence, acceptance or rejection of a product by an imaging system is more accurate than human inspectors; manual inspection is subjective and does not involve extensive analysis as does the machine vision system. Hence, on the quality aspects, imaging-based control is more acceptable and accurate than manual operation.

Many food and beverage packagers are installing vision systems at critical points in the packaging process to improve the quality and reduce product waste. Often, machine vision systems when installed in the early stage of processing remove defective products from the process at the early stage, thus saving the cost of further processing of defective products. Due to high labor costs and affordable vision system prices, even medium- and small-scale processors are able to install machine vision systems. Perfect products with no defects cannot be guaranteed with random sampling. Since machine vision could provide a 100% quality check on every product being produced, random sampling will soon become a thing of the past. Imaging could detect temperature abnormalities, and the actual temperatures of the product and processes, and hence could easily reject the product if it was under- or over-cooked, which may not be possible by manual operators.

Although the versatility of the human eye is far superior, weaknesses such as fatigue and distraction may cause significant losses for food processors. Compared to human vision, machine vision is far superior. Human beings use 10^{11} neurons to perform about 10^{15} operations per second, and human vision involves 2 billion years of evolutionary programming (Indiveri, 1985). In spite of these features, manual supervision is not on par with machine vision because of tiredness, fatigue, attention span distractions, inconsistency between individuals from day to day, overload of work, and other personal reasons. On the other hand, machine vision, even though not as superior as human vision, has high speed, repeatability, and accuracy.

The advancement in machine vision technology includes faster sensors that are capable of very high resolution and involve more complex image processing algorithms to perform more accurate quality monitoring tasks.

11.4.2   Concerns and limitations

Automated processes in the food or any industry are expensive and hence need to be flexible and configurable to adapt to changes in the near future. To reconfigure a production line successfully, it is essential to have a direct access to all the control elements such as switches, motors, and valves to the finest level of detail possible (Pinto, 2013).

Although machine vision could improve the quality monitoring of various food products, machine vision cannot duplicate human eyes' ability to send information to the brain or the brain's capacity to process the information and make final decisions based on the information. The capacity of the human eye and its judgment are better at times in evaluating subtle nuances. Decision making is very complex in a food quality evaluation, when the product does not lie exactly within the ideal range. Hence the performance of an imaging system decreases when the product lies outside the range of samples that were used for training purposes. Machine vision techniques are most successful in controlled environments, whereas in very noisy or uncontrolled backgrounds, performance of machine vision may not be satisfactory (Fabel, 1997). Machine vision systems just follow a set of instructions or rules, and do not have the intelligence to make decisions outside the set of instructions. However, manual inspectors sometimes make quick, intelligent decisions when required depending on special situations.

Quality monitoring by manual process is not significantly affected by lighting conditions or orientation of the product on the conveyer, whereas performance of a machine vision system is affected by poor lighting conditions and misalignment or disorientation of product flow. Hence, the limitations of machine vision include requirement of proper lighting and proper functioning of the parts associated with the imaging system. When product overlapping occurs, vision systems may not perform consistently. Another limitation with imaging application is when both sides of a product need to be examined for quality control purposes (Brosnan and Sun, 2004).

In machine vision monitoring, one of the main challenges is to optimize the elimination of unwanted product in the processing line. When product flow occurs in a discrete manner, elimination of defective or unwanted product is not a challenge, whereas when products are touching each other, there is a probability of good products being eliminated along with the defective ones, which increases the waste (Zuech, 2007).

Implementation of a machine vision system is still a daunting task that requires expert knowledge and experience. The application of machine vision requires development of advanced algorithms for every application, which requires skilled personnel.

11.4.3   Costs

In 2000, the average cost of a machine vision system was approximated at $35,000, which includes the hardware, software, and system integration. However, certain vision systems with limited applications are available for around $10,000. In a three-shift operation processing facility, the cost of a machine vision system could be recovered in less than a year. While all these numbers are rough estimations, actual estimation for cost savings requires a great deal of information and it varies significantly from one plant to another. To have an actual cost comparison for a manual process and an automated machine vision system, many questions need to be answered. Some typical parameters are number of processing lines, amount (or number) of materials being monitored (or graded or sorted) per hour, existing processing speeds, amount of labor required after installation of a machine vision system, accuracy of the existing and current system, value of waste or reject items, percentage of reject items being brought back into the actual processing line, number of shifts, total cost of production per piece or per unit quantity of existing and previous technique, total profit, and maintenance cost of the machine vision system. It is not possible to show a cost comparison statement between a manual processing line and machine vision system without every single detail. But it could be stated in a nutshell that with the savings in labor cost and the reduced cost of a machine vision system over the years, imaging systems in any food processing facility are economical and improve customer satisfaction (Zuech, 2000b).

The average cost of a thermal camera until a few years back was about $20,000, whereas the cost of a basic thermal imaging camera was $10,000 (PAEP, 2014). The cost of Wall-Ye, a robot-based vision system used for pruning grape vines, was around $32,000. It was predicted that Wall-Ye could save about $23 million per year for the wine industry through increased productivity and reduced yield losses (Ackerman, 2012).

Low cost machine vision systems, including the controller, camera, light source, keypad, lens, and cables, are available for as low as $4300 (Model: F 150, Omron Electronic Inc.). Better vision sensors that cost about $1500 can do what high-end sensors did a couple of years ago. Currently, cameras that can do pattern matching are available for $1000. Improvements in hardware and software have significantly reduced the price of the machine vision system (NASA Tech Briefs, 2008).

Machine vision systems have many applications in the engineering industry. A machine vision system for quality evaluation of casting surface inspection was developed by a few vendors. The basic cost of the equipment was quoted at $14,450, whereas the complete budget proposal ranged from $50,000 to $84,500. The cost included a two-phase design project in which phase one involved system design specification including hardware, software, and standards for grading defects. Phase two included the building of a complete machine vision inspection system and quality tests (Technikon, 2005). The cost of a machine vision system varies based on the requirement of the system specifications, which greatly depends on the actual type of automation to be performed. In general, the cost of hardware accounts for 60% of total system cost and the software 40% (CheckIn, 2012).

A snack food manufacturing company states that by installing a machine vision system to read the barcodes saved up to $250,000 per year. The original laser-based barcode reader was not effective in reading labels, which caused distortion and only resulted in 20% to 30% accuracy. To address the problem, an operator was assigned for all the three shifts to divert the boxes to correct locations when the barcode was not correctly identified. An operator for three shifts costs about $100,000 per year and the manual errors resulted in loss of $150,000 annually. Hence, the management of the company stated that installation of a machine vision system resulted in a savings of up to $250,000 annually (Lewis, 2013). Smart Vision Works (2011) developed a machine-vision-based date sorting system and stated that installation of the system resulted in reduction of labor costs around 45% without including the time and financial resources involved in hiring and training of labor.

Sperber (2012) states that fast, reliable, and safe inspection of products, packaging, and their labels is difficult through manual monitoring, whereas automated machine vision systems provide 100% safe and accurate monitoring that can meet compliance and quality standards. Also, the risk of false positive or true negatives varies from person to person while the risk is very minimal in machine vision systems. Manual inspectors are paid $50,000 to $60,000, whereas an automated machine vision system could cost $30,000 to $100,000. In a food or pharmaceutical company, a manual error of mislabeling a product and distributing it in the supply chain could cost anywhere in the range of $800,000 or more due to product recall. Hence, the cost of a machine vision system could be justified even by one occurrence of product quality deviation.

11.4.3.1 Maintenance of machine vision systems

All machine vision cameras are solid-state devices, that is, they experience minimal failure. The cameras are put under rigorous tests during manufacturing and hence if a product is not up to the mark, it fails at the initial stages of testing. Most machine vision cameras work more than 10 years without the need for any service or maintenance. Machine vision systems tend to last for longer time periods than the product they inspect. In other words, rather than the maintenance requirement, normal changes in the product design or process occur in a processing facility, which results in changes of the machine vision system (Hardin, 2012b).

Troubleshooting in machine vision systems can be categorized into three groups: optical, electrical, and mechanical. If the performance of the system is gradually affected, it is most probably associated with the amount of light received by the camera. When a machine vision system suddenly stops working, it is probably a mechanical problem due to vibration or impact, which knocked down the camera, lens, or lighting system. Electrical problems could occur due to poor connections or any problem arising due to poor cable connections. Machine vision systems require minimal preventive maintenance compared to other sophisticated equipment. If the environment of the processing facility is dusty or oily, it is better to keep the camera in an enclosure as it is easier to clean the enclosure than the lens. It is always better to have an adjustable lens rather than to move the camera. Most machine vision systems with LED lights perform consistently for years without any decrease in illumination, but fluorescent light may require occasional inspection (Sprovieri, 2010).

11.4.3.2 Myths about machine vision

The most common myth about machine vision is that it is too expensive to install and cannot be afforded by medium- and small-scale industries. The reason is that food processors always look at the initial cost of purchasing the machine vision system but ignore to account for the real cost in terms of waste, human labor, producing products with deviation, and reduced productivity. The cost of machine vision is very reasonable when all the benefits associated are calculated. Machine vision is also looked upon as a system with low flexibility in the production process. This is not true with modern sensors because they are easy to integrate in the production process and it is possible to reconfigure the system for product or process changes. With the current modern vision system, it is also possible to shift the unit from one production station to another and change the settings if a modification is required for a production line. Another myth about machine vision is that troubleshooting is difficult and disrupts the whole production process. But modern software packages are easy to learn and provide easy-to-follow information regarding troubleshooting. Also vision systems incorporate image logs that could be used to analyze and solve production problems. Another myth is that machine vision technology is not up to the expectations. But the development of machine vision technology is tremendous and is capable of performing 5000 inspections per minute and accuracy is down to hundredths of a millimeter. The fact that machine vision replaces human labor could be seen as the technology actually frees the labor from monotonous, boring jobs and provides an opportunity for them to be performing more challenging and beneficial work (Carter, 2014).

11.5   Future of machine vision in food and agriculture

11.5.1   Machine vision systems based on smart cameras versus PCs

In the machine vision industry, vision systems based on smart cameras are the latest innovation. A smart camera is a combination of a digital camera, processing, software, and communication in a single package. The major advantages of smart cameras are their simple and uncomplicated design, compact size, and fewer components, which results in lower cost of smart cameras compared to a PC-based system. Since smart cameras have a small number of moving parts, they require little maintenance. Also, the software components designed for smart cameras are relatively simple and hence does not require advanced computing skills for implementation of smart-camera-based machine vision systems.

On the other hand, the limitations of smart-camera-based machine vision systems are that due to their simple design, they have less processing ability than a PC-based system, and have limited range and a limited number of tasks that can be performed. The ability of smart cameras to upgrade is limited and hence expanding the functional range of these cameras to handle additional tasks is not possible. Due to higher processing power and higher speed, PC-based machine vision systems can handle complex machine vision tasks. PC-based machine vision systems are upgradeable and changing components is much easier (ThomasNet, 2014). Dawson (2011) states that smart cameras will take a huge market share and in the future will account for more than half the machine vision systems sold. Also, the machine vision market requires smarter algorithm to compensate for lighting.

11.5.2   Growth of machine vision

Machine vision technology is gradually replacing or complementing manual inspection in many industries including agriculture and food. Imaging technology is gradually automating the whole process starting from raw material procurement to various stages of processing, and finally into sealing and packaging. According to statistics from the Automated Imaging Association, in North America, the total sale of machine vision systems increased by 10% for the first quarter of 2013 and the increase in the sale of machine vision components is primarily due to the sale of cameras, which rose by 9% (Control Engineering, 2013).

According to a market research report, the market worth of machine vision systems and components is expected to reach $5 billion in 2018 at a compound annual growth rate of 8%. Among the machine vision market, PC-based machine vision systems held a majority of market share in 2012, while the fastest growing market segment is smart-camera-based machine vision systems. By 2018, the smart-camera-based systems are expected to hold more than 35% of the machine vision market share. Currently, the fastest growing market for machine vision is the Asia Pacific region followed by the European region, which contributed to 30% of overall market share in 2012 (Markets and Markets, 2013).

With government and food regulatory organizations' demand on traceability of food products, it is estimated that machine-vision smart cameras and bar code readers will have a market worth of $2 billion by 2018. Locating an error at an early stage is the key for cost reduction in the food industry. Whether it is a mislabeled product, unreadable barcode, or mismatched lid, it becomes a costly error if it gets into the supply chain. It becomes more complicated if it happens to contain any allergens or mislabeled allergen products (Spinner, 2013).

In the future, machine vision systems and robots will completely aid in the harvesting of fruits and crops. Already such system have been developed at Shanghai Jiao Tong University for harvesting of strawberries. Grading and sorting of crops using machine vision systems is no longer in the research phase; they are already in use for grading and sorting potatoes, dates, carrots, and oranges. In the upcoming years, complete grading and sorting of agricultural products could be performed based on robots and imaging systems. After sorting, the products need to be wrapped and packed for further transportation to retailers and consumers. For complete automation of sorting and packing of agricultural products, the European Union has started a project called PicknPack that aims at automating the entire process. The complete system will consist of a vision-based robotic handling unit and a sensing unit that assesses the quality of the product before sending it to packaging. The vision-based robotic hand then picks the product from the harvest bin and places it in the right position for packaging. After packaging, the products will be transported to their final destinations (Wilson, 2013). To automate food sorting and distribution, a French supermarket chain has designed and installed an industrial imaging system that can optimize the sorting and distribution of fresh agricultural produce and dairy products by handling at 3°C to 4°C, ideal for dairy products. The 7 foot long system with five CCD cameras operates at a speed of 4.8 m/s with OCR compatibility (*Vision Systems Design*, 2013).

Of the various imaging techniques available, the most commonly used imaging techniques in the food and agriculture industry are imaging in the visible spectrum, X-ray imaging, and thermal imaging. Other techniques are still in their infancy and may take a decade or so to be commercially available for food industry applications. With regard to X-ray imaging, in many commercial facilities, X-ray machines are placed toward the end of the process line to check for any contamination and final quality monitoring. But now, the trend is changing and many processing facilities are installing X-ray imaging at the beginning of the process line to also check the quality of incoming materials, so that defective materials could be rejected at an early stage, saving on cost and ensuring good quality, eventhough it requires additional investment.

The demand for machine vision systems is continuously growing with higher throughput requirements and strict quality standards, which have become mandatory for the food and agriculture industry. The future of machine vision in the food and agriculture industry seems very promising and has already moved far beyond the research phase. Many commercial applications of imaging systems have started to be implemented in the food and agriculture industries. In a couple of decades from now, machine vision will be part of every segment of the food and agriculture industry and imaging technology will dominate.

Until a decade ago, a malfunctioning machine vision system required a service engineer to visit the customer location to sort out the problem. But today, machine vision software utilize computational advantages and hence simple user interfaces are used rather than complicated features. With affordable prices and improved technology, the machine vision system market is rapidly growing and a more stable market growth is expected in the coming years. There is still unexplored potential for machine vision applications, such as criminology and forensics, entertainment and other areas, which has not been explored due to the higher price tag attached with machine vision system applications. With the availability of advanced, compact systems, machine vision systems are becoming more affordable and powerful, they will soon become a major contributor in more sectors.

The potential of machine vision in the food and agriculture industries is being extensively explored, and machine vision has replaced manual and other techniques in certain areas. But a large potential for machine vision still exists in the agri-food industry, and in the coming years, machine vision will become an irreplaceable technology and elevate efficiency, productivity, and quality.

References

Abdelhedi, S., K. Taouil, and B. Hadjkacem. 2012. Design of automatic vision based inspection system for monitoring in an olive oil bottling line. *International Journal of Computer Application* 51(21): 39–46.

Abdullah, A., N.K.N. Ismail, T.A.A. Kadir, J.M. Zain, N.A. Jusoh, and N.M. Ali. 2007. Agarwood grade determination system using image processing technique. In *Proceedings of International Conference on Electrical Engineering and Informatics*, 427–429.

Abdullah, M.Z., S.A. Aziz, and A.M.D. Mohamed. 2000. Quality inspection of bakery products using a color-based machine vision system. *Journal of Food Quality* 23: 39–50.

Abramowitx, M., and M.W. Davidson. 2010. Concepts in digital imaging technology. http://learn.hamamatsu.com/articles/scanningformats.html (accessed August 14, 2013).

Acciani, G., G. Brunetti, and G. Fornarelli. 2006. A multiple neural network system to classify solder joints on integrated circuits. *International Journal of Computational Intelligence Research* 2: 337–348.

Acevedo, C.A., O. Skurtys, M.E. Young, and J. Enrione. 2009. A non-destructive digital imaging method to predict immobilized yeast-biomass. *LWT—Food Science and Technology* 42: 1444–1449.

Ackerman, E. 2012. Wall-Ye robot is in your vineyard, pruning your vines. *IEEE Spectrum*, New York. http://spectrum.ieee.org/automaton/robotics/industrial-robots/wallye-robot- (accessed December 16, 2013).

Adedeji, A.A., and M.O. Ngadi. 2009. 3-D imaging of deep-fried chicken nuggets breading coating using X-ray micro-CT. *International Journal of Food Engineering* 5(4): 1–14.

Afek, U., J. Orenstein, and E. Nuriel. 1999. Steam treatment to prevent carrot decay during storage. *Crop Protection* 18: 639–642.

Akbari, H., Y. Kosugi, K. Kojima, and N. Tanaka. 2010. Detection and analysis of the intestinal Ischemia using visible and invisible hyperspectral imaging. *IEEE Transactions on Biomedical Engineering* 57(8): 2011–2017.

Akbari, H., L.V. Halig, D.M. Schuster, A. Osunkoya, V. Master, P.T. Nieh, G.Z. Chen, and B. Fei. 2012. Hyperspectral imaging and quantitative analysis for prostate cancer detection. *Journal of Biomedical Optics* 17(7): 1–10.

Alarousu, E., L. Krehut, T. Prykäri, and R. Myllylä. 2005. Study on the use of optical coherence tomography in measurements of paper properties. *Measurement Science and Technology* 16: 1131–1137.

Albregtsen, F., B. Nielsen, and H.E. Danielsen. 2000. Adaptive Gray level run length features from class distance matrices. *Proceedings of 15th International Conference on Pattern Recognition* 3: 738–741.

Al-Hiary, H., S. Bani-Ahmad, M. Reyalat, M. Braik, and Z. AlRahamneh. 2011. Fast and accurate detection and classification of plant diseases. *International Journal of Computer Applications* 17(1): 31–38.

Ali, M., and R. Parlapalli. 2010. Signal processing overview of optical coherence tomography systems for medical imaging. Texas Instruments Inc., Dallas, Texas. http://www.ti.com/lit/wp/sprabb9/sprabb9.pdf (accessed September 1, 2013).

Allied Vision Technologies. 2010. Imaging makes agriculture greener. Allied Vision Technologies GmbH, Germany. http://www.alliedvisiontec.com/us/news/news-display/article/imaging-makes-agriculture-greener.html (accessed December 16, 2013).

Alper, G. 2012. The future of machine vision. December 11. Adimec. http://info.adimec.com/blog posts/bid/93071/The-Future-of-Machine-Vision (accessed August 14, 2013).

Alramahi, B.A., and K.A. Alshibli. 2006. Applications of computed tomography to characterize the internal structure of geomaterials: Limitations and challenges. *Geotechnical special publication* 149: 88–95.

Altan, A., M.H. Oztop, K.L. McCarthy, and M.J. McCarthy. 2011. Monitoring changes in feta cheese during brining by magnetic resonance imaging and NMR relaxometry. *Journal of Food Engineering* 107: 200–207.

Aluze, D., F. Merienne, C. Dumont, and P. Gorria. 2002. Vision system for defect imaging, detection and characterization on a specular surface of a 3D object. *Image and Vision Computing* 20: 569–580.

American Cancer Society. 2012. Breast cancer overview. http://www.cancer.org/acs/groups/cid /documents/webcontent/003037-pdf.pdf.

Amin, M.H.G., K.P. Nott, and L.D. Hall. 2007. Quantitation by magnetic resonance imaging of heating of commercial baby foods in glass jars. *International Journal of Food Science and Technology* 42: 1408–1415.

Amodio, M.L., A.B. Cabezas-Serrano, G. Peri, and G. Colelli. 2011. Post-cutting quality changes of fresh-cut artichokes treated with different anti-browning agents as evaluated by image analysis. *Postharvest Biology and Technology* 61: 213–220.

Anami, B.S., and V.C. Burkpalli. 2009a. Color based identification and classification of boiled food grain images. *International Journal of Food Engineering* 5(5): 1–19.

Anami, B.S., and V.C. Burkpalli. 2009b. Texture based identification and classification of bulk sugary food objects. *International Journal on Graphics, Vision and Image Processing (GVIP)* 9(4): 9–14.

Andaur, J.E., A.R. Guesalaga, E.E. Agosin, M.W. Guarini, and P. Irarrazaval. 2004. Magnetic resonance imaging for non-destructive analysis of wine grapes. *Journal of Agricultural and Food Chemistry* 52: 165–170.

Andersen, K. 2003. X-ray technique for quality assessment. In *Quality of fish from catch to consumers: Labelling, monitoring and traceability*, ed. J.B. Luten, J. Oehlenschläger, and G. Ólafsdóttir, 283–286. The Netherlands: G. Wageningen Academic Publishers.

Ansari, A. 2009. *Radiation threats and your safety: A guide to preparation and response for professionals and community*. Chapman & Hall Publishers.

Antoun, B.R. and B. Song. 2012. "Thermal infrared imaging to study microstructural damage and failure in aluminum alloys." In Conference Proceedings of the Society for Experimental Mechanic Series 35, Bethel, CT, 115–117.

AOAC. 1995. *Official methods of analysis*, 16th ed. Washington, D.C.: AOAC International.

AOAC Official Method. 2008. Moisture and fat in meats by microwave and nuclear magnetic resonance analysis. June 2008.

Arabi, H., A.R. Kamali Asl, and S.M. Aghamiri. 2010. The effect of focal spot size on the spatial resolution of variable resolution X-ray CT scanner. *Iran Journal of Radiation Research* 8(1): 37–43.

Arevalo, J.K., D. Krivoy, and C.F. Fernandez. 2009. How does optical coherence tomography work? Basic principles. In *Retinal angiography and optical coherence tomography*, ed. J.F. Arevalo. New York: Springer.

Ariana, D.P., and R. Lu. 2008. Detection of internal defect in pickling cucumbers using hyperspectral transmittance imaging. *Transactions of the ASABE* 51: 705–713.

Ariana, D.P., R. Lu, and D.E. Guyer. 2006. Near-infrared hyperspectral imaging for detection of bruises on picking cucumbers. *Computers and Electronics in Agriculture* 53: 60–70.

Arifin, A.Z., and A. Asano. 2006. Image segmentation by histogram thresholding using hierarchical cluster analysis. *Pattern Recognition Letters* 27(13): 1515–1521.

Arivazhagan, S., R.N. Shebiah, S.S. Nidhyanandhan, and L. Ganesan. 2010. Fruit recognition using color and texture features. *Journal of Emerging Trends in Computing and Information Sciences* 1(2): 90–94.

Arivazhagan, S., R.N. Shebiah, S. Ananthi, and S.V. Varthini. 2013. Detection of unhealthy region of plant leaves and classification of plant leaf disease using texture features. *Agricultural Engineering International* 15(1): 211–217.

Arola, D.F., R.L. Powell, M.J. McCarthy, T. Li, and L. Ödberg. 1998. NMR imaging of pulp suspension flowing through an abrupt pipe expansion. *AIChe Journal* 44(12): 2597–2605.

Arora, N., D. Martins, D. Ruggerio, E. Tousimis, A.J. Swistel, M.P. Osborne, and R.M. Simmons. 2008. Effectiveness of a non-invasive digital infrared thermal imaging system in the detection of breast cancer. *The American Journal of Surgery* 196: 523–526.

Ascenti, G., C. Siragusa, S. Racchiusa, I. Lelo, G. Privitera, F. Midili, and S. Mazziotti. 2010. Stone-targeted dual-energy CT: A new diagnostic approach to urinary calculosis. *American Journal of Roentgenology* 195: 953–958.

Astley, M. 2012. Shielding curtain-less X-ray development offers hygienic option. Foodproduction daily.com, April 19. http://www.foodproductiondaily.com/Safety-Regulation/Shielding-curtain -less-x-ray-development-offers-hygienic-option-Thermo-Fisher (accessed October 25, 2012).

Attoh-Okine, N., I. Basheer, and D.H. Chen. 1999. Use of artificial neural networks in geomechanical and pavement systems. Transportation Research Board Circular E-C012. http://onlinepubs .trb.org/onlinepubs/circulars/ec012.pdf (accessed October 30, 2013).

Aursand, I.G., E. Veliyulin, and U. Erikson. 2006. Low field NMR studies of Atlantic Salmon (*Salmo salar*). In *Modern Magnetic Resonance*, ed. G.A. Webb, 905–913. The Netherlands: Springer.

Ayalew, G., N.M. Holden, P.M. Grace, and S.M. Ward. 2004. Detection of glass contamination in horticultural peat with dual-energy X-ray absorptiometry. *Computers and Electronics in Agriculture* 42(1): 1–17.

Babin, P., G. Della Valle, R. Dendievel, D. Lourdin, and L. Salvo. 2007. X-ray tomography for study of the cellular structure of extruded starches and its relations with expansion phenomenon and foam mechanical properties. *Carbohydrate Polymers* 68: 329–340.

Babu, K.N., S. Pothalaiah, and K.A. Babu. 2010. Image retrieval color, shape and texture features using content based. *International Journal of Engineering Science and Technology* 2(9): 4278–4287.

Bagavathiappan, S., B.B. Lahiri, T. Saravanan, J. Philip, and T. Jayakumar. 2013. Infrared thermography for condition monitoring—A review. *Infrared Physics and Technology* 60: 35–55.

Baiano, A., C. Terracone, G. Peri, and R. Romaniello. 2012. Application of hyperspectral imaging for prediction of physico-chemical and sensory characteristics of table grapes. *Computers and Electronics in Agriculture* 87: 142–151.

Ballerini, L., and I. Bocchi. 2006. Genetic programming for prediction of fat content in meat images. Workshop on Evolutionary Computation (GSICE2), Siena, Italy, September 15.

Ballerini, L., A. Högberg, G. Borgefors, A. Bylund, A. Lindard, K. Lundström, O. Rakotonirainy, and B. Soussi. 2002. A segmentation technique to determine fat content in NMR images of beef meat. *IEEE Transactions on Nuclear Science* 49(1): 195–199.

Balyasnikova, S., J. Löfgren, R. de Nijs, Y. Zamogilnaya, L. Højgaard, and B.M. Fischer. 2012. PET/MR in oncology: An introduction with focus on MR and future perspectives for hybrid imaging. *American Journal of Nuclear Medicine and Molecular Imaging* 2(4): 458–474.

Baranowski, P., J. Lipecki, W. Mazurek, and R.T. Walczak. 2008. Detection of watercore in Gloster apples using thermography. *Postharvest Biology and Technology* 47: 358–366.

Barbin, D.F., G. ElMasry, D. Sun, and P. Allen. 2012a. NIR hyperspectral imaging for fat quantification in minced pork. International Conference of Agricultural Engineering, July 8–12, Valencia, Spain.

Barbin, D.F., G. ElMasry, D. Sun, P. Allen, and N. Morsy. 2012b. Near-infrared hyperspectral imaging for grading and classification of pork. *Meat Science* 90: 259–268.

Barbin, D.F., G. ElMasry, D. Sun, P. Allen, and N. Morsy. 2013. Non-destructive assessment of microbial contamination in porcine meat using NIR hyperspectral imaging. *Innovative Food Science and Emerging Technologies* 17: 180–191.

Barcelon, E.G., S. Tojo, and K. Watanabe. 1999. X-ray CT imaging and quality detection of peach at different physiological maturity. *Transactions of ASAE* 42(2): 435–441.

Barcelon, E.G., S. Tojo, and K. Watanabe. 2000. Non-destructive ripening assessment of mango using and X-ray computed tomography. *Agricultural Engineering Journal* 9(2): 73–80.

Barker, D.A., T.A. Vouri, M.R. Hegedus, and D.G. Myers. 1992. The use of slice and aspect ratio parameters for the discrimination of Australian wheat varieties. *Plant Varieties and Seeds* 5(1): 47–52.

Barlis, P. 2009. Use of optical coherence tomography in interventional cardiology. *Interventional Cardiology* 1(1): 63–71.

Barnes, M., T. Duckett, G. Cielniak, G. Stroud, and G. Harper. 2010. Visual detection of blemishes in potatoes using minimalist boosted classifiers. *Journal of Food Engineering* 98: 339–346.

Barone, S., A. Paoli, and A.V. Razionale. 2006. A biomedical application combining visible and thermal 3D imaging. XVIII International Conference on Graphic Engineering, Barcelona, Spain, May 31–June 2.

Barreiro, P., J. Ruiz-Cabello, M.E. Fernandez-Valle, C. Oritz, and M. Ruiz-Altisent. 1999. Mealiness assessment in apples using MRI techniques. *Magnetic Resonance Imaging* 17: 275–281.

Barreiro, P., C. Ortiz, M. Ruiz-Altisent, J. Ruiz-Cabello, M.E. Fernández-Valle, I. Recasens, and M. Asensio. 2000. Mealiness assessment in apples and peaches using MRI techniques. *Magnetic Resonance Imaging* 18: 1175–1181.

Barton, J.F. 2012. Optical coherence tomography for the early detection of cancer. *Microscopy and Microanalysis* 18(2): 242–243.

Basheer, I.A., and M. Hajmeer. 2000. Artificial neural networks: Fundamental, computing, design and application. *Journal of Microbiological Methods* 43: 3–31.

Bashish, D.A., M. Braik, and S. Bani-Ahmad. 2011. Detection and classification of leaf disease using K-means based segmentation and neural-networks based classification. *Information Technology Journal* 10(2): 267–275.

Basset, O., B. Buquet, S. Abouelkaram, P. Delachartre, and J. Culioli. 2000. Application of texture image analysis for the classification of bovine meat. *Food Chemistry* 69: 437–445.

Bauer, W., F.T. Bessier, E. Zabier, and R.B. Bergmann. 2004. Computer tomography for nondestructive testing in the automotive industry. *Proceedings of the SPIE* 5535, 464–472. http://proceedings.spiedigitallibrary.org/proceeding.aspx?articleid=849686.

Baulain, U. 1997. Magnetic resonance imaging for the in vivo determination of body composition in animal science. *Computers and Electronics in Agriculture* 17: 189–203.

Beauvallet, C., and J. Renou. 1992. Applications of NMR spectroscopy in meat research. *Trends in Food Science and Technology* 3(8/9): 202–205.

Bechard, S.R., and G.R.B. Down. 1992. Infrared imaging of pharmaceutical materials undergoing compaction. *Pharmaceutical Research* 9(4): 521–528.

Beck, M., J. Goebbels, A. Burkert, B. Isecke, and R. Bäbler. 2010. Monitoring of corrosion processes in chloride contaminated mortar by electrochemical measurements and X-ray tomography. *Materials and Corrosion* 61(6): 475–479.

Beek, A.M., and A.C. Rossum. 2013. Cardiovascular magnetic resonance imaging in patients with acute myocardial infarction. *Heart* 96: 237–243.

Benady, M., and G.E. Miles. 1992. Locating melons for robotic harvesting using structured light. ASAE Paper No. 92-7021. St. Joseph, MI: ASAE.

Benediktsson, J.A., P.H. Swain, and O.K. Ersoy. 1990. Neural network approaches versus statistical methods in classification of multisource remote sensing data. *IEEE Transactions on Geoscience and Remote Sensing* 28(4): 540–552.

Bennedsen, B.S., D.L. Peterson, and A. Tabb. 2005. Identifying defects in images of rotating apples. *Computers and Electronics in Agriculture* 48: 92–102.

Bennett, C.W. 1969. Seed transmission of plant viruses. *Advances in Virus Research* 14: 221–261.

Bhatia, V., R. Bhatia, S. Dhindsa, and M. Dhindsa. 2003. Imaging of the vulnerable plaque: New modalities. *Southern Medical Journal* 96(11): 1142–1147.

Bhotmange, M. and P. Shastri. 2011. Application of artificial neural networks to food and fermentation technology. In *Artificial neural networks—Industrial and control engineering applications*. (Ed.) Kenji Suzuki, ISBN: 978-953-307-220-3.

BioOptics World Staff. 2011. Market and technology status update: Technology, applications and future directions: OCT in 2011 and beyond. *BioOptics World* 4(2).

Birgul, R. 2008. Monitoring macro voids in mortar by X-ray computed tomography. *Nuclear Instruments and Methods in Physics Research* 596(3): 459–466.

Bishop, C. 1995. *Neural networks for pattern recognition*. Oxford: Oxford University Press.

Blamire, A.M. 2008. The technology of MRI—The next ten years. *The British Journal of Radiology* 81: 601–617.

Blasco, J., N. Alexios, and E. Moltó. 2003. Machine vision system for automatic quality grading of fruit. *Biosystems Engineering* 85(4): 415–423.

Blasco, J., N. Aleixos, S. Cubero, J. Gómez-Sanchís, and E. Moltó. 2009. Automatic sorting of Satsuma (*Citrus unshiu*) segments using computer vision and morphological features. *Computers and Electronics in Agriculture* 66: 1–8.

Blink, E.J. 2004. The hardware. In *Basic MRI physics*, 6–9. http://www.mri-physics.net/bin/mri-physics-en-rev1.3.pdf (accessed April 20, 2013).

Boccara, M., W. Schwartz, E. Guiot, G. Vidal, R. Paepe, A. Dubois, and A. Boccara. 2007. Early chloroplastic alterations analysed by optical coherence tomography during harpin-induced hypersensitive response. *The Plant Journal* 50: 338–346.

Boesen, M., M. Østergaard, M.A. Cimmino, O. Kubassova, K.E. Jensen, and H. Bliddal. 2009. MRI quantification of rheumatoid arthritis: Current knowledge and future perspectives. *European Journal of Radiology* 71: 189–196.

Bolhouse, V. 1997. Fundamentals of machine vision, Robotic Industries Association. In *Proceedings of Coastal Sediments '87*, ed. American Society of Civil Engineers (ASCE), 468–483.

Boll, D.T., N.A. Patil, E.K. Paulson, E.M. Merkle, W.N. Simmons, S.A. Pierre, and G.M. Preminger. 2009. Renal stone assessment with dual-energy multi-detector CT and advanced post processing techniques: Improved characterization of renal stone composition-pilot study. *Radiology* 250(3): 813–820.

Bolo, F. 2007. A basic introduction to neural network. Department of Computer Science, University of Wisconsin-Madison. http://pages.cs.wisc.edu/~bolo/shipyard/neural/local.html (accessed October 31, 2013).

Boppart, S.A. 2003. Optical coherence tomography: Technology and applications for neuroimaging. *Psychophysiology* 40: 529–541.

Boppart, S.A., B.E. Bouma, C. Pitris, J.F. Southern, M.E. Brezinski, and J.G. Fujimoto. 1998a. In vivo cellular optical coherence tomography imaging. *Nature Medicine* 4: 861–864.

Boppart, S.A., M.E. Brezinski, C. Pitris, and J.G. Fujimoto. 1998b. Optical coherence tomography for neurosurgical imaging of intracortical melanoma. *Neurosurgery* 43: 834–841.

Bossi, R., and G. Georgeson. 1992. X-ray computed tomography analysis of castings. Proceedings of the 121st TMS Annual Meeting, San Diego, California, March 1–5.

Bossu, J., Ch. Gée, G. Jones, and F. Truchetet. 2009. Wavelet transform to discriminate between crop and weed in perspective agronomic images. *Computers and Electronics in Agriculture* 65: 133–143.

Bouma, B.E., G.J. Tearney, C.C. Compton, and N.S. Nishioka. 2000. High-resolution imaging of the human esophagus and stomach in vivo using optical coherence tomography. *Gastrointestinal Endoscopy* 51(4): 467–474.

Brant, F. 2000. The use of X-ray inspection techniques to improve quality and reduce costs. NDT.net, 5(5).

Braz, A.K.S., C.M. Aguiar, and S.L. Gomes. 2011. Evaluation of the integrity of dental sealants by optical coherence tomography. *Dental Materials* 27: e60–e64.

Brecht, J.K. 1991. Using X-ray computed tomography to non-destructively determine maturity of green tomatoes. *Horticultural Science* 26(1): 45–47.

Brennan, J. 2002. An introduction to digital radiography in dentistry. *Journal of Orthodontics* 29: 66–69.

Brenner, D.J., and M.A. Georgsson. 2005. Mass screening with CT colonography: Should the radiation exposure be of concern. *Gastroenterology* 129: 328–337.

Brezinski, M.E. 2006. Optical coherence tomography for identifying unstable coronary plaque. *International Journal of Cardiology* 107: 154–165.

Brezinski, M.E., G.J. Tearney, N.J. Weissman, S.A. Boppart, B.E. Bouma, M.R. Hee, A.E. Weyman, E.A. Swanson, J.F. Southern, and J.G. Fujimoto. 1997. Assessing atherosclerotic plaque morphology: Comparison of optical coherence tomography and high frequency intravascular ultrasound. *British Heart Journal* 77: 397–404.

Britton, D. 2003. The perfect buns: Digital imaging system on production line catches bad sandwich buns. Georgia Institute of Technology, Research News.

Brock, T.K. 2012. Infrared thermal cameras: Technology overview and buyers guide. Labcompare. http://www.labcompare.com/10-Featured-Articles/39062-Infrared-Thermal-Cameras-Technology-Overview-and-Buyers-Guide/ (accessed May 15, 2013).

Brosnan, T., and D. Sun. 2004. Improving quality inspection of food products by computer vision. *Journal of Food Engineering* 61: 3–16.

Brule, J.F. 1985. Fuzzy systems—A tutorial. University of Waterloo, Berkeley. https://www.cosc.brocku.ca/Offerings/4P79/fuzzytutorial.html (accessed October 30, 2013).

Budoff, M.J., M.L. Rasouli, D.M. Shavelle, A. Gopal, K.M. Gul, and S.S. Mao. 2007. Cardiac CT angiography (CTA) and nuclear myocardial perfusion imaging (MPI): A comparison in detecting significant coronary artery disease. *Academic Radiology* 14(3): 252–257.

Bulanon, D.M., T.F. Burks, and V. Alchanatis. 2008. Study on temporal variation in citrus canopy using thermal imaging for citrus fruit detection. *Biosystems Engineering* 101: 161–171.

Burgos-Artizzu, X.P., A. Ribeiro, A. Tellaeche, G. Pajares, and C. Fernández-Quintanilla. 2009. Improving weed pressure assessment using digital images from an experience-based reasoning approach. *Computers and Electronics in Agriculture* 65: 176–185.

Burgstaller, M., and M. Groinig. 2012. Spectral imaging sorts sugar end defects. *Vision Systems Design*, 17(2). http://www.vision-systems.com/articles/print/volume-17/issue-2/features/spectral-imaging-sorts-sugar-end-defects.html (accessed December 16, 2013).

Canadian Grain Commission (CGC). 2005. *Official grain grading guide.*

Canadian Nuclear Safety Commission. 2010. Radiation doses. http://www.cnsc-ccsn.gc.ca/eng/readingroom/radiation/radiation_doses.cfm (accessed January 10, 2013).

Canny, J. 1986. A computational approach to edge detection. *IEEE Transactions on Pattern Analysis and Machine Intelligence* 8(6): 679–698.

Cardenas-Weber, M., A. Hetzroni, and G.E. Miles. 1991. Machine vision to locate melons and guide robotic harvesting. ASAE Paper No. 91-7006. St. Joseph, MI: ASAE.

Carlson, B.S. 2002. Comparison of modern CCD and CMOS image sensor technologies and systems for low resolution imaging. Proceedings of IEEE Sensors, June 12–14, Orlando, Florida.

Carnier, P., L. Gallo, C. Romani, E. Sturaro, and V. Bondesan. 2004. Computer image analysis for measuring lean and fatty areas in cross sectioned dry-cured hams. *Journal of Animal Science* 82: 808–815.

Carroll, J. 2013. Vision system sorts wine grapes according to quality. *Vision Systems Design*. http://www.vision-systems.com/articles/2013/09/vision-system-sorts-wine-grapes-according-to-quality.html (accessed December 16, 2013).

Carter, S. 2014. Dispelling the myths about machine vision systems. SICK Sensor Intelligence, Melbourne, Australia. http://www.sick.com/au/en-us/home/pr/Whitepapers/Documents/SICK%20Avoiding%20quality%20control%20disasters%20with%20machine%20vision.pdf (accessed February 3, 2014).

CATSA. 2010. *X-ray safety awareness handbook.* Ottawa, Canada: Canadian Air Transport Security Association, Radiation Safety Institute of Canada.

Cauberg, E.C.C., D.M. de Bruin, D.J. Faber, T.G. van Leeuwen, J.M.C.H. de la Rosette, and T.M. de Reijke. 2009. A new generation of optical diagnostics for bladder cancer: Technology, diagnostic accuracy and future applications. *European Urology* 56: 287–297.

Caudill, M. 1987. Neural network primer: Part I. *AI Expert* 2(12): 46–52.

Cernadas, E., M.L. Durán, and T. Antequera. 2002. Recognizing marbling in dry-cured Iberian ham by multiscale analysis. *Pattern Recognition Letters* 23: 1311–1321.

Chacon, M.I., L. Aguilar, and A. Delgado. 2002. Definition and applications of fuzzy image processing scheme. In *Proceedings of the 10th IEEE Digital Signal Processing Workshop*, 102–107.

Chandarana, H., and V.S. Lee. 2009. Renal functional MRI: Are we ready for clinical application? *American Journal of Roentgenology* 192: 1550–1557.

Chanet, B., M. Fusellier, J. Baudet, S. Madec, and C. Guintard. 2009. No need to open the jar: A comparative study of magnetic resonance imaging results on fresh and alcohol preserved common carps (*Cyprinus carpio* [L. 1758], Cyprinidae, Teleostei). *Biodiversity* 332: 413–419.

Chang, T., Y. Hsia, and S. Liao. 2008. Application of digital infrared thermal imaging in determining inflammatory state and follow-up effect of methylprednisolone pulse therapy in patients with Graves' opthalmopathy. *Graefes Archive for Clinical and Experimental Ophthalmology*, 246(1): 45–49.

Chang, Y., and Y. Chen. 2006. An improved scheme of segmenting color food image by robust algorithm. In *23rd Workshop on Combinatorial Mathematics and Computation Theory*, 331–335.

Chanvrier, H., J.C. Gumy, and I. Blank. 2009. Food solid foams made from cereals: Assessment of the structure of extruded rice by X-ray tomography. Annual Micro-CT Meeting, Ghent, Belgium, April 22–24.

Chaunier, L., D.G. Valle, and D. Lourdin. 2007. Relationships between texture, mechanical properties and structure of cornflakes. *Food Research International* 40: 493–503.

Chavhan, G.B., P.S. Babyn, B. Thomas, M.M. Shroff, and E.M. Haacke. 2009. Principles, techniques and applications of T2-based MR imaging and its special applications. *RadioGraphics* 29(5): 1433–1499.

CheckIn. 2012. Inspection vision systems. Shumen, Bulgaria. http://www.checkin-bg.com/faq.html (accessed February 3, 2014).

Chelladurai, V., D.S. Jayas, and N.D.G. White. 2010. Thermal imaging for detecting fungal infection in stored wheat. *Journal of Stored Products Research* 46: 174–179.

Chen, K., and Ch. Qin. 2008. Segmentation of beef marbling based on vision threshold. *Computers and Electronics in Agriculture* 62: 223–230.

Chen, P., M.J. McCarthy, and R. Kauten. 1989. NMR for internal quality evaluation of fruits and vegetables. *Transactions of the ASAE* 32: 1747–1753.

Chen, P., J. McCarthy, R. Kauten, Y. Sarig, and S. Han. 1993. Maturity evaluation of avocados by NNMR methods. *Journal of Agricultural Engineering Research* 55: 177–187.

Chen, X. 2003. Detection of physical hazards in boneless poultry product using combined X-ray and laser range imaging technologies. PhD diss., University of Maryland.

Cheng, X., Y.R. Chen, Y. Tao, C.Y. Wang, M.S. Kim, and A.M. Lefcourt. 2004. A novel integrated PCA and FLD method on hyperspectral image feature extraction for cucumber chilling damage inspection. *Transcations of ASAE* 47(4): 1313–1320.

Chester, D.L. 1990. Why two hidden layers are better than one. In *Proceedings of the Joint International Conference on Neural Networks* 1: 265–268.

Chevallier, S., and A.L. Bail. 2012. X-ray microtomography to characterize the microstructure of bakery products. Annual Miro-CT Meeting, Brussels, Belgium, April 3–5.

Cho, B.K., W. Chayaprasert, and R.L. Stroshine. 2008. Effects of internal browning and watercore on low field (54 MHz) proton magnetic resonance measurements of T2 values of whole apples. *Postharvest Biology and Technology* 47: 81–89.

Choi, B., T.E. Milner, J. Kim, J.N. Goodman, G. Vargas, G. Aguilar, and J.S. Nelson. 2004. Use of optical coherence tomography to monitor biological tissue freezing during cryosurgery. *Journal of Biomedical Optics* 9(2): 282–286.

Choudhary, R., J. Paliwal, and D.S. Jayas. 2008. Classification of cereal grains using wavelet, morphological, colour, and textural features of non-touching kernel images. *Biosystems Engineering* 99: 330–337.

Chow, T.H., K.M. Tan, B.K. Ng, S.G. Razul, and C.M. Tay. 2009. Diagnosis of virus infection in orchid plants with high resolution optical coherence tomography. *Journal of Biomedical Optics* 14(1): 1–6.

Chtioui, Y., S. Panigrahi, and L.F. Backer. 1999. Rough sets theory as a pattern classification tool for quality assessment of edible beans. *Transactions of the ASAE* 42(4): 1145–1152.

Chu, A., C.M. Sehgal, and I.F. Greenleaf. 1990. Use of gray value distribution of run lengths for texture analysis. *Pattern Recognition Letters* 11: 415–420.

Chuang, C., C. Ouyang, T. Lin, M. Yang, E. Yang, T. Huang, C. Kuei, A. Luke, and J. Jiang. 2011. Automatic X-ray quarantine scanner and pest infestation detector for agricultural products. *Computers and Electronics in Agriculture* 77: 41–59.

Ciampa, A., M.T. Dell'Abate, O. Masetti, M. Valentini, and P. Sequi. 2010. Seasonal chemical-physical changes of PGI Pachino cherry tomatoes detected by magnetic resonance imaging (MRI). *Food Chemistry* 122: 1253–1260.

Ciupa, R., and A. Rogalski. 1997. Performance limitations of photon and thermal infrared detectors. *Opto-Electronics Review*, 5(4): 257–266.

Clare, S. 1997. Functional MRI: Methods and applications. PhD dissertation, University of Nottingham, England, United Kingdom.

Clark, A.T., J.S. Mangat, S.S. Tay, Y. King, C.J. Monk, P.A. White, and P.W. Ewan. 2007. Facial thermography is a sensitive and specific method for assessing food challenge outcome. *Allergy* 62: 744–749.

Clark, C.J., and D.M. Burmeister. 1999. Magnetic resonance imaging of browning development in "Braeburn" apple during controlled-atmosphere storage under high CO_2. *Horticultural Science* 34: 915–919.

Clark, C.J., P.D. Hockings, D.C. Joyce, and R.A. Mazucco. 1997. Application of magnetic resonance imaging to pre- and post–harvest studies of fruits and vegetables. *Postharvest Biology and Technology* 11: 1–21.

Clark, C.J., J.S. MacFall, and R.L. Bieleski. 1998. Loss of watercore from "Fuji" apple observed by magnetic resonance imaging. *Scentia Horticulturae* 71(4): 213–227.

Clements, J.C., A.V. Zvyagin, K.K.M.B.D. Silva, T. Wanner, D.D. Sampson, and W.A. Cowling. 2004. Optical coherence tomography as a novel tool for non-destructive measurement of the hull thickness of lupin seeds. *Plant Breeding* 123(3): 266–270.

Coherent. 2011. What is structured light. http://www.coherent.com/products/?1826/What-is -Structured-Light# (accessed October 1, 2013).

Collewet, G., P. Bogner, P. Allen, H. Busk, A. Dobrowolski, E. Olsen, and A. Davenel. 2005. Determination of the lean meat percentage of pig carcasses using magnetic resonance imaging. *Meat Science* 70: 563–572.

Conci, A., T.B. Borchartt, R. Resmini, L.S. Motta, M.J.A. Viana, L.C. Santos, R.C.F. Lima, E.M. Diniz, A.M. Santos, A.C. Paiva, and A.C. Silva. 2011. Biomedical use of infrared images. 18th International Conference on Systems, Signal and Image Processing, Sarajevo, Bosnia, and Herzegovina, June 16–18.

Connecting Industry. 2009. Machine meets meat inspection requirement. http://content.yudu .com/A1ghw0/FESept09/resources/20.htm (accessed December 20, 2012).

Conners, R.W., T. Cho, C.T. Ng, and T.H. Drayer. 1992. A machine vision system for automatically grading hardwood lumber. *Industrial Metrology* 2: 317–342.

Control Engineering. 2013. North America machine vision sales rising. http://www.controleng .com/search/search-single-display/north-america-machine-vision-sales-rising/bba 4f6495bb392f2de33acbdeaac271c.html (accessed February 3, 2014).

Cooke, T. 2002. Two variations on Fishers linear discriminant for pattern recognition. *IEEE Transactions on Pattern Analysis and Machine Intelligence* 24(2): 268–273.

Cornillon, P., and L.C. Salim. 2000. Characterization of water mobility and distribution in low and intermediate moisture food systems. *Magnetic Resonance Imaging* 18: 335–341.

Corvi, A., B. Innocenti, and R. Mencucci. 2006. Thermography used for analysis and comparison of different cataract surgery procedures based on phacoemulsification. *Physiological Measurement* 27: 371–384.

Costa, L.N., C. Stelletta, C. Cannizzo, M. Gianesella, D. Pietro Lo Fiego, and M. Morgante. 2007. The use of thermography on the slaughter-line for the assessment of pork and raw ham quality. *Italian Journal of Animal Science* 6(1): 704–706.

Couvreur, C., and P. Couvreur. 1997. Neural network and statistics: A naïve comparison. *Belgian Journal of Operations Research, Statistics, and Computer Sciences* 36(4).

Cowan, C.K. 1991. Automatic camera and light-source placement using CAD models. In *Workshop on Directions in Automated CAD-Based Vision*, 22–31.

Creber, S.A., J.S. Vrouwenvelder, M.C.M. van Loosdrecht, and M.L. Johns. 2010. Chemical cleaning of biofouling in reverse osmosis membranes evaluated using magnetic resonance imaging. *Journal of Membrane Science* 362: 202–210.

Curry, T.S., J.E. Dowdey, and R.C. Murry. 1990. *Christensen's physics of diagnostic radiology*, 4th ed. Philadelphia, PA: Lippincott Williams & Wilkins.

Czajkowski, J., T. Prykäri, E. Alarousu, J. Palosaari, and R. Myllylä. 2010. Optical Coherence tomography as a method of quality inspection for printed electronics products. *Optical Review* 17(3): 257–262.

Czajkowski, J., T. Fabritius, J. Ulański, T. Marszalek, M. Gazicki-Lipman, A. Nosal, R. Śliz, E. Alarousu, T. Prykäri, R. Myllylä, and G. Jabbour. 2011. Ultra-high resolution optical coherence tomography for encapsulation quality inspection. *Applied Physics B* 105: 649–657.

Dahmoush, H.M., A. Vossough, and T.P.L. Roberts. 2012. Pediatric high field magnetic resonance imaging. *Neuroimaging Clinics of North America* 22: 297–313.

Dalen, G.V., P. Nootenboom, L.J.V. Vliet, L. Voortman, and E. Esveld. 2007. 3D imaging, analysis and modelling of porous cereal products using X-ray microtomography. *Image Analysis and Stereology* 26: 169–177.

Dalen, G.V., S. Goh, A. Don, P. Nootenboom, and C. Gamonpilas. 2008. 3D imaging, analysis and modelling of bouillon cubes using X-ray microtomography. *Materials Engineering* 29(4): 396–402.

Danti, A., M. Madgi, and B.S. Anami. 2012. Mean and range color features based on identification of Indian leafy vegetables. *International Journal of Signal Processing, Image Processing and Pattern Recognition* 5(3): 151–160.

Das, A., M.V. Sivak, A. Chak, R.C. Wong, V. Westphal, A.M. Rollins, J. Willis, G. Isenberg, and J.A. Izatt. 2001. High-resolution endoscopic imaging of the GI tract: A comparative study of optical coherence tomography versus high-frequency catheter probe EUS. *Gastrointestinal Endoscopy* 54: 219–224.

Davenel, A., F. Seigneurin, G. Collewet, and H. Remignon. 2000. Estimation of poultry breast meat yield: Magnetic resonance imaging as a tool to improve the positioning of ultrasonic sensors. *Meat Science* 56(2): 153–158.

Davenel, A., S. Quellec, and S. Pouvreau. 2006. Non-invasive characterization of gonad maturation and determination of the sex of Pacific oysters by MRI. *Magnetic Resonance Imaging* 24: 1103–1110.

Davenel, A., R. Gonzalez, M. Suquet, S. Quellec, and R. Robert. 2010. Individual monitoring of gonad development in the European flat oyster *Ostrea edulis* by in vivo magnetic resonance imaging. *Aquaculture* 307(1 and 2): 165–169.

Davies, E.R. 2000. *Image processing for the food industry*. Singapore: World Scientific.

Davies, E.R. 2001. Some problems in food and cereal inspection and methods for their solution. *Proceedings of 5th International Conference on Quality Control by Artificial Vision (QCAV)*, 35–46.

Davies, P., and B.R. Silverstein. 1995. A comparison of neural nets to statistical classifiers for stubborn classification problems. In *International Conference on Acoustics, Speech and Signal Processing (ICASSP)* 5: 3467–3470.

Dawson, B. 2011. Machine vision: The future of machine vision. *Quality Magazine*, November 2011. http://www.qualitymag.com/articles/print/90617-machine-vision-the-future-of-machine-vision (accessed August 14, 2013).

Debska, B., and B. Suzowska-Świder. 2011. Application of artificial neural network in food classification. *Analytica Chimica*, 705: 283–291.

Deck, S.H., C.T. Morrow, P.H. Heinemann, and H.J. Sommer. 1995. Comparison of neural network and traditional classifier for machine vision inspection of potatoes. *Applied Engineering in Agriculture* 11(2): 319–326.

Defraeye, T., V. Lehmann, D. Gross, C. Holat, E. Herremans, P. Verboven, B.E. Verlinden, and B.M. Nicolai. 2013. Application of MRI tissue characterisation of "Braeburn" apple. *Postharvest Biology and Technology* 75: 96–105.

Del Fiore, A., M. Reverberi, A. Ricelli, F. Pinzari, S. Serranti, A.A. Fabbri, G. Bonifazi, and C. Fanelli. 2010. Early detection of toxigenic fungi on maize by hyperspectral imaging analysis. *International Journal of Food Microbiology* 144: 64–71.

Deng, L. 2011. An overview of deep structured learning for information processing. Proceedings of Asian-Pacific Signal and Information Processing Annual Summit and Conference (APSIPA-ASC), Xi'an, Shaanxi, China, October 19–21.

Deng, S., W.W. Cai, Q.Y. Xu, and B. Liang. 2010. Defect detection of bearing surfaces based on machine vision technique. In *International Conference on Computer Application and System Modeling*, 548–554.

Deshpande, A.S., M.P. Pillai, and A.N. Cheeran. 2010. X-ray imaging for non-destructive detection of spongy tissue in Alphonso mango. In *Computer vision and information technology: Advances and applications,* ed. K.V. Kale, S.C. Mehrotra, and R.R. Manza, 252–256. New Delhi, India: I.K. International Publishing House Pvt. Ltd.

De Silva, L.C., A. Pereira, and A. Punchihewa. 2005. Food classification using color imaging. In *Conference on Imaging and Vision Computing*, 1–6.

D'Esnon, G.A., G. Rabatel, R. Pellenc, R. Journeau, and M.J. Aldon. 1987. Magali: A self-propelled robot to pick apples. ASAE paper No. 87-1037. St. Joseph, MI: ASAE.

Dettori, L., and L. Semler. 2007. A comparison of wavelet, ridgelet, and curvelet-based texture classification algorithms in computed tomography. *Computers in Biology and Medicine* 37: 486–498.

Deych, R., and E. Dolazza. 2006. New trends in X-ray CT imaging. In *Radiation detectors for medical applications*, ed. S. Tavernier, A. Gektin, B. Grinyov, and W.W. Moses, 15–35. The Netherlands: Springer.

Dhawale, V.R., J.A. Tidke, and S.V. Dudul. 2013. Neural network based classification of pollen grains. In *International Conference on Advances in Computing, Communications and Informatics (ICACCI)*, 79–84.

Dirckx, C.J., S.A. Clark, L.D. Hall, B. Antalek, J. Tooma, J.M. Hewitt, and K. Kawaoka. 2000. Magnetic resonance imaging of the filtration process. *Fluid Mechanics and Transport Phenomena* 46(1): 6–14.

Dobranowski, J., A.H. Elzibak, A. Dobranowski, A. Farfus, C. Astill, A. Nair, A. Levinson, Y. Thakur, and M.D. Noseworthy. 2013. Medical imaging primer with a focus on X-ray usage and safety. Canadian Association of Radiologist. http://www.car.ca/uploads/standards%20guidelines /20130128_en_guide_radiation_primer.pdf.

Dobrusin, Y., and Y. Edan. 1992. Real-time image processing for robotic melon harvesting. ASAE Paper No. 92-3515.

Dogan, H. 2007. Non-destructive imaging of agricultural products using X-ray microtomography. *Microscopy Microanalysis* 13(2): 1316–1317.

Doster, T. 2011. Nonlinear dimensionality reduction for hyperspectral image classification. University of Maryland, Baltimore.

Douik, A., and M. Abdellaoui. 2010. Cereal grain classification by optimal features and intelligent classifiers. *International Journal of Computers, Communications and Control* 4: 506–516.

Dowlati, M., S.S. Mohtasebi, and M. Guardia. 2012. Application of machine vision techniques to fish quality assessment. *Trends in Analytical Chemistry* 40: 168–179.

Dowlati, M., S.S. Mohtasebi, M. Omid, S.H. Razavi, M. Jamzad, and M. Guardia. 2013. Freshness assessment of gilthead sea bream (*Sparus aurata*) by machine vision based on gill and eye color changes. *Journal of Food Engineering* 119: 277–287.

Du, C., and D. Sun. 2004a. Recent developments in the applications of image processing techniques for food quality evaluation. *Trends in Food Science and Technology* 15: 230–249.

Du, C., and D.W. Sun. 2004b. Shape extraction and classification of pizza base using computer vision. *Journal of Food Engineering* 64: 489–496.

Du, C., and D.W. Sun. 2006a. Automatic measurement of pores and porosity in pork ham and their correlations with processing time, water content and texture. *Meat Science* 72(2): 294–302.

Du, C., and D.W. Sun. 2006b. Estimating the surface area and volume of ellipsoidal ham using computer vision. *Journal of Food Engineering* 73(3): 260–268.

Duan, F., Y. Wang, and H. Liu, 2004. A real time machine vision system for bottle finish inspection. In *Control, Automatic, Robotics and Vision Conference* 2: 842–846.

Dubey, S.R., P. Dixit, N. Singh, and J.P. Gupta. 2013. Infected fruit part detection using k-means clustering segmentation technique. *International Journal of Artificial Intelligence and Interactive Multimedia* 2(2): 65–72.

Duce, S.L., T.A. Carpenter, and L.D. Hall. 1992. Nuclear magnetic resonance imaging of fresh and frozen courgettes. *Journal of Food Engineering* 16: 165–172.

Duncan, M.D., and M. Bashkansky. 1998. Subsurface defect detection in materials using optical coherence tomography. *Optics Express* 2(13): 540–545.

Duncker, P., and H. Spiecker. 2009. Detection and classification of Norway spruce compression wood in reflected light by means of hyperspectral image analysis. *International Association of Wood Anatomists Journal* 30(1): 59–70.

Eagle Vision Systems. 2013. Closure inspection. Naarden, The Netherlands. http://www.eaglevision .nl/index.php/basic-scout-reader-en-v2/items/10.html (accessed February 3, 2014).

Ebrahimi, E., K. Mollazade, and A. Arefi. 2011. Detection of greening in potatoes using image processing techniques. *Journal of American Science* 7(3): 243–247.

Ecker, R.D., S.J. Goerss, F.B. Meyer, A.A. Cohen-Gadol, J.W. Briton, and J.A. Levine. 2002. Vision of the future: Initial experience with intraoperative real-time high resolution dynamic infrared imaging. *Journal of Neurosurgery* 97: 1460–1471.

Edan, Y., H. Pasternak, I. Shmulevich, D. Rachmani, D. Guedalia, S. Grinberg, and E. Fallik. 1997. Color and firmness classification of fresh market tomatoes. *Journal of Food Science* 62(4): 793–796.

Edan, Y., D. Rogozin, T. Flash, and G.E. Miles. 2000. Robotic melon harvesting. *IEEE Transactions on Robotics and Automation* 16(6): 831–834.

Edinbarough, I., R. Balderas, and S. Bose. 2005. A vision and robot based on-line inspection monitoring system for electronic manufacturing. *Computers in Industry* 56: 986–996.

Edmund Optics Inc. 2013. Imaging Electronics 101: Camera types and interfaces for machine vision applications. http://www.edmundoptics.com/technical-resources-center/imaging/camera-types -and-interfaces-for-machine-vision-applications/?&viewall (accessed August 16, 2013).

Effendi, Z., R. Ramli, and J.A. Ghani. 2010. A back propagation neural networks for grading *Jatropha curcas* fruits maturity. *American Journal of Applied Sciences* 7(3): 390–394.

Egelberg, P., O. Månsson, and C. Peterson. 1995. Assessing cereal grain quality with a fully automated instrument using artificial neural network processing of digitized color video images. In *Proceedings of SPIE 2345*, 146–158.

Einen, O., B. Waagan, and M.S. Thomassen. 1998. Starvation prior to slaughter in Atlantic salmon (*Salmo salar*). I. Effects on weight loss, body shape, slaughter and fillet-yield, proximate and fatty acid composition. *Aquaculture* 166: 85–104.

ElMasry, G., and D. Sun. 2010. Principles of hyperspectral imaging technology. In *Hyperspectral imaging for Food Quality Analysis and Control*, ed. S. Sun. San Diego: Academic Press, 3–44.

ElMasry, G., N. Wang, A. ElSayed and M. Ngadi. 2007. Hyperspectral imaging for non-destructive determination of some quality attributes for strawberry. *Journal of Food Engineering* 81: 98–107.

ElMasry, G., D. Sun, and P. Allen. 2011a. Non-destructive determination of water holding capacity in fresh beef by using NIR hyperspectral imaging. *Food Research International* 44: 2624–2633.

ElMasry, G., D. Sun, P. Allen, and P. Ward. 2011b. Quality classification of cooked, sliced turkey hams using NIR hyperspectral imaging system. *Journal of Food Engineering* 103: 333–344.

ElMasry, G., D.F. Barbin, and D. Sun. 2012a. Meat quality evaluation by hyperspectral imaging technique: An overview. *Critical Reviews in Food Science and Nutrition* 52: 689–711.

ElMasry, G., M. Kamruzzaman, D. Sun, and P. Allen. 2012b. Principles and applications of hyperspectral imaging in quality evaluation of agro-food products: A review. *Critical Reviews in Food Science and Nutrition* 52: 999–1023.

Esser, F. 2013. An introduction to and brief history of digital imaging sensor technologies. *The Phoblographer*, July 31. http://www.thephoblographer.com/2013/07/31/an-introduction-to -and-brief-history-of-digital-imaging-sensor-technologies/ (accessed August 14, 2013).

Estrada, H., A.K. Sen, and M. Faruqi. 2004. Application of MRI tomography to characterization of the chloride ion permeability of regular and high performance concretes. In *Proceedings of International SAMPE Symposium and Exhibition*, 3011–3022.

Evanger, B. 2010. Technology update: Machine vision can ensure reliable, repeatable bar code inspection. *Control Engineering*, January. http://www.controleng.com/index.php?id=483&cHash =081010&tx_ttnews[tt_news]=38536 (accessed February 3, 2014).

Evans, S.D., A. Brambilla, D.M. Lane, D. Torreggiani, and L.D. Hall. 2002. Magnetic resonance imaging of strawberry (Fragaria vesca) slices during osmotic dehydration and air drying. *Lebensm.-Wiss.u-Technol.* 35: 177–184.

Fabel, G. 1997. Machine vision systems looking better all the time. *Quality Digest* 17(10): 62–64. http://www.qualitydigest.com/oct97/html/machvis.html (accessed February 6, 2014).

Falcone, P.M., A. Baiano, F. Zanini, L. Mancini, G. Tromba, D. Dreossi, F. Montanari, N. Scuor, and M.A. Del Nobile. 2005. Three-dimensional quantitative analysis of bread crumb by X-ray microtomography. *Journal of Food Science* 70(3): E265–E272.

Fan, C., and G. Yao. 2012. 3D imaging of tomato seeds using frequency domain optical coherence tomography. *Proceedings of SPIE*, vol. 8369.

FAO. 2011. Fisheries and aquaculture information and statistics services.

FAO. 2012. World review of fisheries and aquaculture. In *The state of world fisheries and aquaculture*, pt. 1.

FAO/OECD. 2012. Improving food systems for sustainable diets in a green economy, Working document. FAO/OECD Expert Meeting on Greening the Economy with Agriculture, Paris, France, September 5–7, 2011.

Faucitano, L., P. Huff, F. Teuscher, C. Gariepy, and J. Wegner. 2005. Application of computer image analysis to measure pork marbling characteristics. *Meat Science* 69: 537–543.

Feigin, D.S. 2010. Lateral chest radiograph: A systematic approach. *Academic Radiology* 17: 1560–1566.

Fellegari, R., and H. Navid. 2011. Determining the orange volume using image processing. In *International Conference on Food Engineering and Biotechnology (ICFEB)*, 180–184.

Feng, Y., D. Sun, G. ElMasry, and N. Morcy. 2012. Direct prediction of Enterobacteriaceae loads in chicken fillets using near infrared (NIR) hyperspectral imaging and support vector regression (SVR). International Conference of Agricultural Engineering, July 8–12, Valencia, Spain.

Fercher, A.F., C.K. Hitzenberger, W. Drexler, G. Kamp, and H. Sattmann. 1993. In vivo optical coherence tomography. *American Journal of Ophthalmology* 116: 113–114.

Fernández Pierna, J.A.F., P. Vermeulen, O. Amand, A. Tossens, P. Dardenne, and V. Baeten. 2012. NIR hypsersepctral imaging spectroscopy and chemoterics for the detection of undesirable substances in food and feed. *Chemometrics and Intelligent Laboratory Systems*, doi:10.1016/j .chemolab.2012.02.004.

Fiorino, G., C. Bonifacio, A. Malesci, L. Balzarini, and S. Danese. 2011. MRI in Crohn's disease—Current and future clinical applications. *Gastroenterology and Hepatology* 9: 23–31.

Firatligil-Durmus, E., E. Šárka, and Z. Bubník. 2008. Image vision technology for the characterisation of shape and geometrical properties of two varieties of lentil grown in Turkey. *Czech Journal of Food Science* 26(2): 109–116.

Fisheries and Aquaculture. 2009. The investigation of X-ray inspection for production of whole cooked whelk: Phase I and Phase II. Fisheries Technology and New Opportunities Program. Project Summary 0316-07-036/083. http://www.fishaq.gov.nl.ca/research_development/research /ftnop_summaries/0316_07_36_83_investigation_of_x_ray_inspection_for_whelk.pdf (accessed January 10, 2013).

Fito, P.J., M.D. Ortolá, R. De los Reyes, P. Fito, P., and E. De los Reyes. 2004. Control of citrus surface drying by image analysis of infrared thermography. *Journal of Food Engineering* 61: 287–290.

FLIR. 2011a. History of thermal imaging. *Security Sales and Integration*, July, A1–A8.

FLIR. 2011b. Thermal imaging guidebook for industrial applications. FLIR Systems AB. http://www .flirmedia.com/MMC/THG/Brochures/T820264/T820264_EN.pdf (accessed May 15, 2013).

FLIR. 2011c. Thermal imaging guideline for building and renewable energy applications. FLIR Systems AB, Täby, Sweden.

FLIR. 2012. FLIR application stories: Automation. http://www.flir.com/cs/emea/en/view /?id=42180 (accessed October 20, 2012).

FLIR. 2013a. Thermal imaging cameras in the food industry. FLIR Commercial Systems. http:// www.flir.com/cs/emea/en/view/?id=41781 (accessed May 15, 2013).

FLIR. 2013b. FLIR thermal imaging cameras help determine the functionality of anti-allergy medicine. http://www.flir.com/cs/emea/en/view/?id=41183 (accessed May 15, 2013).

Flood, N., and B. Bailey. 2013. Vision helps dairy spot slack cheese bags. *Vision Systems Design*, October 8, 18(9). http://www.vision-systems.com/articles/print/volume-18/issue-9/features/vision -helps-dairy-spot-slack-cheese-bags.html (accessed January 27, 2014).

Fojlaley, M., P.A. Moghadam, and S.A. Nia. 2012. Tomato classification and sorting machine vision using SVM, MLP, and LVQ. *International Journal of Agriculture and Crop Sciences* 4(15): 1083–1088.

Fokaides, P.A., and S.A. Kalogirou. 2011. Application of infrared thermography for the determination of the overall heat transfer coefficient (U-value) in building envelopes. *Applied Energy* 88: 4358–4365.

Folkestad, A., J.P. Wold, K. Rørvik, J. Tschudi, K.H. Haugholt, K. Kolstad, and T. Mørkøre. 2008. Rapid and non-invasive measurements of fat and pigment concentrations in live and slaughtered Atlantic salmon (*Salmo salar* L.). *Aquaculture* 280: 129–135.

Ford, H.D., R.P. Tatam, S. Landahl, and L.A. Terry. 2011. Investigation of disease in stored onions using optical coherence tomography. Proceedings of 4th International Conference on Postharvest Unlimited, Leavenworth, Washington, May 22–26.

Fornal, J., T. Jelinski, J. Sadowska, S. Grundas, J. Nawrot, A. Niewiada, J. Warchalewski, and W. Blaszczak. 2007. Detection of granary weevil *Sitophilus granaries* (L.) eggs and internal stages in wheat grain using soft X-ray and image analysis. *Journal of Stored Products Research* 43: 142–148.

Freebody, M. 2013. Farmers fuel growing market for imaging systems. *Photonics Spectra*, June. http:// www.photonics.com/Article.aspx?PID=5&VID=109&IID=692&Tag=Features&AID=54039 (accessed February 6, 2014).

Freeman, J., F. Downs, L. Marcucci, E.N. Lewis, B. Blume, and J. Rish. 1997. Multispectral and hyperspectral imaging: Applications for medical and surgical diagnostics. Proceedings of 19th International Conference IEEE/EMBS, Chicago, Illinois, October 30–November 2.

Freeman, J.E., S. Panasyuk, A.E. Rogers, S. Yang, and R. Lew. 2005. Advantage of intraoperative medical hyperspectral imaging for the evaluation of breast cancer resection bed for residual tumor. *Journal of Clinical Oncology* 23(16S): 709.

Freitas, A.Z., M. Zezell, N.D. Vieira, A.C. Ribeiro, and A.S.L. Gomes. 2006. Imaging carious human dental tissue with optical coherence tomography. *Journal of Applied Physics* 99: 024906.

Frisullo, P., J. Laverse, R. Marino, and M.A. Del Nobile. 2009. X-ray computed tomography to study processed meat microstructure. *Journal of Food Engineering* 94: 283–289.

Frisullo, P., A. Conte, and M.A. Del Nobile. 2010a. A novel approach to study biscuits and breadsticks using X-ray computed tomography. *Journal of Food Science* 75(6): E353–E358.

Frisullo, P., F. Licciardello, G. Muratore, and M.A. Del Nobile. 2010b. Microstructural characterization of multiphase chocolate using X-ray microtomography. *Institute of Food Technologists* 75(7): E469–E476.

Frize, M., C. Adèa, P. Payeur, G. Primio, J. Karsh, and A. Ogungbemile. 2011. Detection of rheumatoid arthritis using infrared imaging. *Proceedings of SPIE*, vol. 7962.

Fruit Logistica. 2012. The world of fresh produce. http://www.fruitlogistica.de/en/PressService /PressReleases/index.jsp?lang=en&id=177600 (accessed October 26, 2012).

Fujimoto, J.G. 2001. Optical coherence tomography. *Applied Physics* 2(4): 1099–1111.

Fujimoto, J.G., and M.E. Brezinski. 2003. Optical coherence tomography imaging. In *Biomedical photonics handbook*, ed. T. Vo-Dinh. Boca Raton, FL: Taylor & Francis.

Fujimoto, J.G., C. Pitris, S.A. Boppart, and M.E. Brezinski. 2000. Optical coherence tomography: An emerging technology for biomedical imaging and optical biopsy. *Neoplasia* 2: 9–25.

Gaber, K.A., C.R. McGavin, and I.P. Wells. 2005. Lateral chest X-ray for physicians. *Journal of the Royal Society of Medicine* 98: 310–312.

Gaemperli O, T. Schepis, I. Valenta, P. Koepfli, L. Husmann, H. Scheffel, S. Leschak, F.R. Eberli, T.F. Luscher, H. Alkadhi, and P.A. Kaufmann. 2008. Functionally relevant coronary artery disease: Comparison of 64-section CT angiography with myocardial perfusion SPECT. *Radiology* 248(2): 414–423.

Galloway, M.M. 1975. Texture analysis using gray level run lengths. *Computer Graphics and Image Processing* 4: 172–179.

Gan-Mor, S., R. Regev, A. Levi, and D. Eshel. 2011. Adapted thermal imaging for the development of postharvest precision steam-disinfection technology for carrots. *Postharvest Biology and Technology* 59: 265–71.

Garini, Y., I.T. Young, and G. McNamara. 2006. Spectral imaging: Principles and applications. *Cytometry* 69A: 735–747.

Garrido-Novell, C., D. Pèrez-Marin, J.M. Amigo, J. Fernández-Novales, J.E. Guerrero, and A. Garrido-Varo. 2012. Grading and color evolution of apples using RGB and hyperspectral imaging vision cameras. *Journal of Food Engineering* 113: 281–288.

Gat, N. 2000. Imaging spectroscopy using tunable filters: A review. In *Proceedings of SPIE* 4056, 50–64.

Gat, Y., G.N. Bachar, Z. Zukerman, A. Belenky, and M. Gorenish. 2004. Physical examination may miss the diagnosis of bilateral varicocele: A comparative study of 4 diagnostic modalities. *Journal of Urology* 172: 1239–1240.

GBI (Global Business Intelligence) Research. 2013. Global MRI systems market forecast to exceed $6 billion by 2018. http://www.giiresearch.com/press/7609.shtml (accessed April 20, 2013).

Gerbi, B.J. 2011. Radiation oncology. Health Physics Society. http://hps.org/publicinformation/ate /q1162.html (accessed June 6, 2013).

Gerrard, D.E., X. Gao, and J. Tan, 1996. Beef marbling and color score determination by image processing. *Journal of Food Science* 61: 145–148.

Geyer, S., and K. Gottschalk. 2008. Infrared thermography to monitor natural ventilation during storage of potatoes. *Agricultural Engineering International: CIGR Ejournal*, vol. 10.

Geyer, S., K. Gottschlalk, H.J. Hellebrand, and R. Schlauderer. 2004. Application of thermal imaging measuring system to optimise the climate control of potato stores, 1066–1067. AgEng Conference on Engineering the Future, Leuven, Belgium, September 12–16.

Ghazali, K.H., M.M. Mustafa, and A. Hussain. 2007. Color image processing of weed classification: A comparison of two feature extraction techniques. In *Proceedings of International Conference on Electrical Engineering and Informatics*, 607–610.

Ghazanfari, A., D. Wulfsohn, and J. Irudayaraj. 1998. Machine vision grading of pistachio nuts using gray-level histogram. *Canadian Agricultural Engineering* 40(1): 61–66.

Ghazanfari-Moghaddam, A. 1996. Machine vision classification of pistachio nuts using pattern recognition and neural networks. Ph.D. dissertation, University of Saskatchewan, Saskatchewan, Canada.

Giacinto, G., F. Roli, and L. Bruzzone. 1999. Combination of neural and statistical algorithms for supervised classification of remote sensing images. *Pattern Recognition Letters* 21: 385–397.

Giallorenzi, T.G. 2000. Optical technology in naval applications. *Optics and Photonic News* 11(4): 24–36.

Ginesu, G., D. Giusto, V. Märgner, and P. Meinlschmidt. 2004. Detection of foreign bodies in food by thermal image processing. *IEEE Transactions on Industrial Electronics* 51: 480–490.

Girolami, A., F. Napolitano, D. Faraone, and A. Braghieri. 2013. Measurement of meat color using a computer vision system. *Meat Science* 93: 111–118.

Gjerde, B. 1987. Predicting carcass composition of rainbow trout by computerized tomography. *Journal of Animal Breeding and Genetics* 104(1–5): 121–136.

Gladkova, N.D., E.V. Gubarkova, E.G. Sharabrin, V.I. Stelmashok, and A.E. Beimanov. 2012. The potential and limitations of intravascular optical coherence imaging. *Clinical and Translational Medicine* 4: 128–140.

Global Innovative Technology Co., Ltd. 2011. Lighting for machine vision. http://www.gitthailand .com/Lighting_for_Machine_Vision.htm (accessed October 2, 2013).

Goetz, A.F.H. 1995. Imaging spectrometry for remote sensing: Vision of reality in 15 years. In *Proceedings of SPIE* 2480, 2–13.

Gomez, R.B. 2002. Hyperspectral imaging, a useful technology for transportation analysis. *Optical Engineering*. 41(9): 2137–2143.

Gonzalez, J.J., R.C. Valle, S. Bobroff, W.V. Biasi, E.J. Mitcham, and M.J. McCarthy. 2001. Detection and monitoring of internal browning development in "Fuji" apples using MRI. *Postharvest Biology and Technology* 22: 179–188.

Gonzalez, R.C., and R.E. Woods. 2002. *Digital image processing*, 2nd edition. Delhi: Pearson Education Inc.

Goode, B.G. 2009. Optical coherence tomography: OCT aims for industrial application. *Laser Focus World*, September 1. http://www.laserfocusworld.com/articles/2009/09/optical-coherence -tomography-oct-aims-for-industrial-application.html (accessed September 5, 2013).

Gottschalk, K., and Cs. Mèszáros. 2012. IR thermometry for heat and mass transfer analysis of surface drying of fruit. 11th International Conference on Quantitative Infrared Thermography, Naples, Italy, June 11–14.

Gowen, A.A., C.P. O'Donnell, P.J. Cullen, G. Downey, and J.M. Frias. 2007. Hyperspectral imaging—An emerging process analytical tool for food quality and safety control. *Trends in Food Science and Technology* 18(2): 590–598.

Gowen, A.A., J. Burger, D.O. O'Callaghan, and C.P. O'Donnell. 2009a. Potential applications of hyperspectral imaging for quality control in dairy foods. Image Analysis for Agricultural Products and Processess, 1st International Workshop on Computer Image Analysis in Agriculture, Potsdam, Germany, August 27–28, 2009.

Gowen, A.A., M. Taghizadeh, and C.P. O'Donnell, C.P. 2009b. Identification of mushrooms subjected to freeze damage using hyperspectral imaging. *Journal of Food Engineering* 93: 7–12.

Gowen, A.A., B.K. Tiwari, P.J. Cullen, K. McDonnell, and C.P. O'Donnell. 2010. Applications in thermal imaging in food quality and safety assessment. *Trends in Food Science and Technology* 21: 190–200.

Granitto, P.M., H.D. Navone, P.F. Verdes, and H.A. Ceccatto. 2002. Weed seed identification by machine vision. *Computers and Electronics in Agriculture* 33: 91–103.

Grant, M., M. Bassett, M. Stewart, and J. Adès. 2011. Valuing food: The economic contribution of Canada's food sector. The Conference Board of Canada, Ottawa, Ontario, Canada.

Graser, A., C.R. Becker, M. Staehler, D.A. Clevert, M. Macari, N. Arndt, K. Nikolaou, W. Sommer, C. Stief, M.F. Reiser, and T.R. Johnson. 2010. Single phase dual-energy CT allows for characterization of renal masses as benign or malignant. *Investigative Radiology* 45(7): 399–405.

Graves, M. 2002. X-ray bone detection in further processed poultry production. In *Machine vision for the inspection of natural products*, ed. M. Graves and B. Batchelor. Heidelberg: Springer-Verlag.

Grift, T., Q. Zhang, N. Kondo, and K.C. Ting. 2008. A review of automation and robotics for the bioindustry. *Journal of Biomechatronics Engineering* 1(1): 37–54.

Grignon, B., L. Mainard, M. Delion, C. Hodez, and G. Oldrini. 2012. Recent advances in medical imaging: Anatomical and clinical applications. *Surgical and Radiologic Anatomy* 34: 675–686.

Groinig, M., M. Burgstaller, and M. Pail. 2011. Industrial application of a new camera system based on hyperspectral imaging for inline quality control of potatoes. 35th Annual Workshop of Austrian Association of Pattern Recognition (ÖAGM/AAPR), Graz, Styria, Austria, May 26–27.

Guevara-Hernandez, F., and J. Gomez-Gil. 2011. A machine vision system for classification of wheat and barley grain kernels. *Spanish Journal of Agricultural Research* 9(3): 672–680.

Guiheneuf, T.M., S.J. Gibbs, and L.D. Hall. 1997. Measurement of the inter-diffusion of sodium ions during pork brining by one-dimensional Na-23 magnetic resonance imaging (MRI). *Journal of Food Engineering* 31(4): 457–471.

Gujjar, H.S., and M. Siddappa. 2013. A method for identification of basmati rice grain of India and its quality using pattern recognition. *International Journal of Engineering Research and Applications* 3(1): 268–273.

Gümüş, B., M.Ö. Balaban, and M. Ünlüsayin. 2011. Machine vision applications to aquatic foods: A review. *Turkish Journal of Fisheries and Aquatic Sciences* 11: 171–181.

Gunasekaran, S. 1996. Computer vision technology for food quality assurance. *Trends in Food Science and Technology* 7: 245–256.

Gunasekaran, S. 2010. Computer vision systems. In *Nondestructive evaluation of food quality: Theory and practice*, ed. S.N. Jha. Berlin: Springer-Verlag.

Gupta, C., E.V. Casteele, and J.K. Chakravartty. 2009. Imaging of voids due to deformation in alloy steel using micro-focus X-ray beam. *Nuclear Instruments and Methods in Physics Research* B267: 3488–3490.

Gutierrez, J.A., A.P. Ruiz, S.R. Vaamonde, and I. Girbau. 2010. The application of hyperspectral image processing to the steel foundry process. International Surface Inspection Summit, Wuhan, China, March 4–5.

Gutierrez-Chico, J.L., E.E. Alegría-Barrero, R. Teijeiro-Mestre, P.H. Chan, H. Tsujioka, R. de Silva, N. Viceconte, A. Lindsay, T. Patterson, N. Foin, T. Akasaka, and C. di Mario. 2012. Optical coherence tomography: From research to practice. *European Heart Journal Cardiovascular Imaging* 13: 370–384.

Haff, R.P., and D.C. Slaughter. 2004. A real time X-ray assessment of wheat for infestation by the granary weevil, *Sitophilus granarius* (L.). *Transactions of ASAE* 47(2): 531–537.

Haff, R.P., and T.C. Pearson. 2007. An automatic algorithm for detection of infestations in X-ray images of agricultural products. *Sensors and Instrumentation for Food Quality* 1: 143–150.

Haff, R.P., and N. Toyofukku. 2008. X-ray detection of defects and contaminants in the food industry. *Sensors and Instrumentation for Food Quality* 2: 262–273.

Haff, R.P, D.C. Slaughter, Y. Sarig, and A. Kader. 2006. X-ray assessment of translucency in pineapple. *Journal of Food Processing and Preservation* 30: 527–533.

Hafsteinsson, H., and S. Rizvi. 1987. A review of sealworm problem. *Journal of Food Protection* 50(1): 70–84.

Hall, L.D., S.D. Evans, and K.P. Nott. 1998. Measurement of textural changes of food by MRI relaxometry. *Magnetic Resonance Imaging* 16(5/6): 485–492.

Hall, L.D., A.H.G. Amin, S. Evans, K. Nott, and L. Sun. 2001. Magnetic resonance imaging for industrial process tomography. *Journal of Electronic Imaging* 10(3): 601–607.

Hall-Beyer, M. 2007. The GLCM tutorial, version 2.10. http://www.fp.ucalgary.ca/mhallbey/tutorial.htm (accessed October 5, 2013).

Hamamatus. 2013. X-ray detectors. 198–218. http://www.hamamatsu.com/resources/pdf/ssd/e08_handbook_x-ray_detectors.pdf (accessed October 5, 2013).

Han, Y., and P. Shi. 2007. An efficient approach for fish bone detection based on image preprocessing and particle swarm clustering. *Communications in Computer and Information Science* 21: 940–948.

Han, Y.J., S.V. Bowers, and R.B. Dodd. 1992. Non-destructive detection of split-pit peaches. *Transactions of ASAE* 35(6): 2063–2067.

Hancz, C., R. Romvári, Z. Petrási, and P. Horn. 2003. Prediction of carcass quality traits of common carp by X-ray computerized tomography. *The Israeli Journal of Aquaculture* 55(1): 61–68.

Hanneschläger, G., A. Nemeth, C. Hofer, C. Goetzloff, J. Reussner, K. Wiesauer, and M. Leitner. 2011. Optical coherence tomography as a tool for non-destructive quality control of multi-layered foils. In *6th NDT in Progress, International Workshop of NDT Experts*, Prague, Czech Republic, October 10–12.

Haralick, R.M., K. Shanmugam, and I. Dinstein. 1988. Textural features for image classification. *IEEE Transaction Systems Manufacturing Cybernetics* 3(6): 610–621.

Hardin, W. 2012a. Machine vision helps food processors cut overhead costs. Automated Imaging Association. http://www.visiononline.org/vision-resources-details.cfm/vision-resources/Machine-Vision-Helps-Food-Processors-Cut-Overhead-Costs/content_id/3698 (accessed February 6, 2014).

Hardin, W. 2012b. The many faces of machine vision maintenance. Automated Imaging Association. http://www.visiononline.org/vision-resources-details.cfm/vision-resources/The-Many-Faces-of-Machine-Vision-Maintenance/content_id/3826/id/2/newsType_id/0 (accessed February 6, 2014).

Hartman, L.R. 2009. Really cool inspection of organic foods. *Packaging Digest*. http://www.packaging digest.com/article/355320-_Really_cool_inspection_of_organic_foods.php (accessed November 20, 2012).

Harvey, A.R., J. Lawlor, A.I. McNaught, and D.W. Fletcher-Holmes. 2002. Hyperspectral imaging for the detection of retinal disease. *Proceedings of SPIE* 4816, 325–335.

Hassan, G.M., and S.M. Al-Saqer. 2011. Pecan weevil recognition using support vector machine method. *American Journal of Agricultural and Biological Sciences* 6(4): 521–526.

Hassankhani, R., H. Navid, and H. Seyedarabi. 2012. Potato surface defect detection in machine vision system. *African Journal of Agricultural Research* 7(5): 844–850.

Hassoun, M.H. 1995. *Fundamentals of artificial neural networks*. Cambridge: MIT Press.

Hata, S. 1990. Vision systems for PCB manufacturing in Japan. In *IEEE Transaction, Production Engineering Research Laboratory Hitachi Ltd.*, 792–797.

Hatt, P.J., A. Davenel, P.A. Eliat, and S. Quellect. 2009. Magnetic resonance imaging as a means to assess the body growth and the gonad development of the oyster *Crassostrea gigas*. *Aquatic Living Resources* 22: 331–339.

Hatzakis, E., E. Archavlis, and P. Dais. 2007 Determination of glycerol in wines using 31P-NMR spectroscopy. *Journal of American Oil Chemists Soc*iety 84: 615–619.

Haystead, J. 1997. Machine vision speeds food processing and high speed sorting. *Vision Systems* 2(6). http://www.vision-systems.com/articles/print/volume-2/issue-6/features/feature-article/machine-vision-speeds-food-processing-and-high-speed-sorting.html (accessed January 27, 2014).

Haystead, J. 1999. Inspection system uses magnetic-resonance imaging to check food quality. *Vision Systems Design* 4(10). http://www.vision-systems.com/articles/print/volume-4/issue-10/features/feature-article/inspection-system-uses-magnetic-resonance-imaging-to-check-food-quality.html (accessed October 30, 2012).

Hecht-Nielsen, R. 1990. *Neurocomputing*. Reading, MA: Addison-Wesley.

Heidenreich, P. A., J.G. Trogdon, O.A. Khavjou, J. Butler, K. Dracup, M.D. Ezekowitz, E.A. Finkelstein, Y. Hong, S.C. Johnston, A. Khera, D.M. Lloyd-Jones, S.A. Nelson, G. Nicol, D. Orenstein, P.W.F. Wilson, and Y.J. Woo. 2011. Forecasting the future of cardiovascular disease in the United States: A policy statement from the American Heart Association. *Circulation* 123: 933–944.

Heindel, T.J., J.N. Gray, and T.C. Jensen. 2008. An X-ray system for visualizing fluid flows. *Flow Measurement and Instrumentation* 19: 67–78.

Heinemann, P.H., N.P. Pathare, and C.T. Morrow. 1996. An automated inspection station for machine-vision grading of potatoes. *Machine Vision and Applications* 9: 14–19.

Hellebrand, H.J., H. Beuche, M. Linke, B. Herold, and M. Geyer. 2001. Chances and shortcomings of thermal imaging in the evaluation of horticultural products. In *Physical Methods in Agricultural—Approach to Precision and Quality*, ed. J. Blahovec, and M. Libra, 112–117. Prague, Czech Republic.

Hemming, J., and T. Rath. 2001. Computer vision based weed identification under field conditions using controlled lighting. *Journal of Agricultural Engineering Research* 78(3): 233–243.

Henery, R.J. 1994. Classification. In *Machine learning, neural and statistical classification*, eds. D. Michie, D.J. Spiegelhalter, and C.C. Taylor, 6–16. Hertz, UK: Ellis Horwood.

Hermes, B., F. Spoler, A. Naami, J. Bornemann, M. Först, J. Grosse, G. Jakse, and R. Knüchel. 2008. Visualization of the basement membrane zone of the bladder by optical coherence tomography: Feasibility of non-invasive evaluation of tumor invasion. *Urology* 72: 677–681.

Hernández-Sánchez, N., B.P. Hills, P. Barreiro, and N. Marigheto. 2007. An NMR study on internal browning in pears. *Postharvest Biology and Technology* 44: 260–270.

Herremans, E., S. Chassagne-Berces, H. Chanvrier, A. Atoniuk, R. Kusztal, E. Bongaers, B.E. Verlinden, E. Jakubczyk, P. Estrade, P. Verboven, and B. Nicolai. 2011. Possibilities of X-ray nano-CT for internal quality assessment of food products. 11th International Congress on Engineering and Food, Athens, Greece, May 26.

Herremans, E., A. Melado, P. Barreiro, E. Bongaers, P. Estrade, P. Verboven, and B.M. Nicolai. 2012. InsideFood: X-ray CT and MRI study of watercore in apple. Micro CT User Meeting, Brussels, Belgium, April 3–5.

Heye, T., R.C. Nelson, L.M. Ho, D. Marin, and D.T. Boll. 2012. Dual-energy CT applications in the abdomen. *American Journal of Roentgenology* 199: S64–S70.

Hildebrandt, C., C. Raschner, and K. Ammer. 2010. An overview of recent application of medical infrared thermography in sports medicine in Austria. *Sensors* 10: 4700–4715.

Hills, B.P., and B. Remigereau. 1997. NMR studies of changes in subcellular water compartmentation in parenchyma apple tissue during drying and freezing. *International Journal of Food Science and Technology* 32: 51–61.

Hills, B.P., F. Babonneau, V.M. Quantin, F. Gaudet, and P.S. Belton. 1996. Radial NMR microimaging studies of the rehydration of extruded pasta. *Journal of Food Engineering* 27: 71–86.

Hobani, A.I., A.M. Thottam, and K.A.M. Ahmed. 2003. Development of a neural network classifier for date fruit varieties using some physical attributes. Research Bulletin, 126, Agriculture Research Center, King Saudi University, 5–18.

Hogan, H. 2005. Machine vision checks chicken and confirms cookies. *Photonics Spectra,* October. http://www.photonics.com/Article.aspx?AID=23156 (accessed January 27, 2014).

Holliman, F.M., D. Davis, A.E. Bogan, T.J. Kwak, W.G. Cope, and J.F. Levine. 2008. Magnetic resonance imaging of live freshwater mussels. *Invertebrate Biology* 127(4): 396–402.

Holmes, J. 2009. OCT technology development: Where are we now? A commercial perspective. *Journal of Biophotonics* 2(6–7): 347–352.

Horigane, A.K., H. Toyoshhima, H. Hemmi, W.M.H.G. Engelaar, A. Okubo, and T. Nagata. 1999. Internal hollows in cooked rice grains (*Oryza sativa* cv. Koshihikari) observed by NMR micro imaging. *Journal of Food Science* 64(1): 1–5.

Horigane, A.K., S. Naito, M. Kurimoto, K. Irie, M. Yamada, H. Motoi, and M. Yoshida. 2006. Moisture distribution and diffusion in cooked spaghetti studied by NMR imaging and diffusion model. *Cereal Chemistry* 83(3): 235–242.

Hrynchak, P., and T. Simpson. 2000. Optical coherence tomography: An introduction to the technique and its use. *Optometry and Vision Science* 77(7): 347–356.

Hua, C., S. Huili, Y. Xiangxi, and C. Xin. 2011. Artificial neural network in food processing. Proceedings of the 30th Chinese Control Conference, Yantai, China, July 22–24.

Huang, D., E.A. Swanson, C.P. Lin, J.S. Schuman, W.G. Stinson, W. Chang, M.R. Hee, T. Flotte, K. Gregory, C.A. Puliafito, and J.G. Fujimoto. 1991. Optical coherence tomography. *Science* 254: 1178–1181.

Huang, M. 2013. Design PC-based line scan imaging systems. Adlink Technology Inc. http://www .adlinktech.com/solution/tech_forum.php?file=measure/20050926.htm.

Huang, Y., L.J. Kangas, and B.A. Rasco. 2007. Applications of artificial neural networks (ANNs) in food science and nutrition. *Critical Reviews in Food Science and Nutrition* 47(2): 113–126.

Humbe, V.T., Y.S. Patil, and Y.B. Patil. 2011. Study of image restoration techniques for remote sensing images in agriculture field. *International Journal of Machine Intelligence* 3(3): 138–141.

Husband, J., and G. Dombrowe. 2005. X-ray computed tomography—A truly remarkable medical development. *The British Journal of Radiology* 78: 97–98.

Ibarra, J.G., Y. Tao, and H. Xin. 2000. Combined IR imaging-neural network method for the estimation of internal temperature in cooked chicken meat. *Optical Engineering* 39(11): 3032–3038.

Ibarra-Castanedo, C., M. Susa, M. Klein, M. Grenier, J.M., Piau, W.B. Larby, A. Bendada, and X. Maldague. 2008. Infrared thermography: Principle and applications to aircraft materials. *Non-Destructive Testing Journal.* Available at http://www.ndt.net/article/aero2008/aero08_maldague.pdf.

Iftimia, N., D.X. Hammer, M. Mujat, V. Desphande, S. Cizginer, and W. Brugge. 2009. Optical coherence tomography imaging for cancer diagnosis and therapy guidance. 31st Annual International Conference of the IEEE EMBS, Minneapolis, Minnesota, September 2–6.

Ikonomakis, N., K.N. Plataniotis, M. Zervakis, and A.N. Venetsanopoulos. 1997. Region growing and region merging segmentation. In *13th International Conference on Digital Signal Processing,* 299–302.

Inanc, F. 2001. Feasibility of suing X-rays for quantification of agricultural products and chemicals. In *American Institute of Physics Conference Proceedings* 557, 545–552. http://dx.doi.org/10.1063/1.1373806.

Indiveri, G. 1985. Computation in neuromorphic analog VLSI systems. *Human Neurobiology* 4(4): 219–227.

Ishak, A.J., A. Hussain, and M.M. Mustafa. 2009. Weed image classification using Gabor wavelet and gradient field distribution. *Computers and Electronics in Agriculture* 66: 53–61.

Ishida. 2008. X-ray inspection system ensure chicken fillet quality. http://www.ishidaeurope.com/pr_stories/default.asp?newsID=129. (accessed December 20, 2012).

Ishida. 2009. An IX-GA X-ray inspection system protects your business in three important ways. http://www.ishidaeurope.com/our_products/qualitycontrol_solutions/xray_inspection/protection/ (accessed December 10, 2012).

Ishida, N., T. Kobayashi, M. Koizumi, and H. Kano. 1989. H-NMR imaging of tomato fruits. *Agricultural and Biological Chemistry* 53(9): 2363–2367.

Ivanitsky, G.R., E.P. Khizhnyak, A.A. Deev, and L.N. Khizhnyak. 2006. Thermal imaging in medicine: A comparative study of infrared systems operating in wavelength ranges of 3-5 and 8-12 μm as applied to diagnosis. *Biochemistry, Biophysics and Molecular Biology* 407: 59–63.

Izumi, Y., O. Teranuma, T. Sato, K. Uehara, H. Okada, S. Tokuda, and T. Sato. 2001. Development of flat panel X-ray image sensors. *SharpTechnical Journal* 80: 25.

Jackman, P., D.W. Sun, and P. Allen. 2009. Automatic segmentation of beef *longissimus dorsi* muscle and marbling by an adaptable algorithm. *Meat Science* 83: 187–194.

Jackson, E.S., and R.P. Haff. 2006. X-ray detection and sorting of olives damaged by fruit fly. ASABE Annual Meeting, Paper No. 066062.

Jahns, G., H.M. Nielsen, and W. Paul. 2001. Measuring image analysis attributes and modelling fuzzy consumer aspects for tomato quality grading. *Computers and Electronics in Agriculture* 31(1): 17–29.

Jain, A.K., J. Mao, and K.M. Mohiuddin. 1996. Artificial neural networks: A tutorial. *IEEE Computer* 29(3): 31–44.

Jang, I.K., B.E. Bouma, D.H. Kang, S.J. Park, S.W. Park, K.B. Seung, K.B. Choi, M. Shishkov, K. Schlendorf, E. Pomerantsev, S.L. Houser, H.T. Aretz, and G.J. Tearney. 2002. Visualization of coronary atherosclerosis plaques in patients using optical coherence tomography: Comparison with intravascular ultrasound. *Journal of the American College of Cardiology* 39: 604–609.

Jayas, D.S. 2012. Storing grains for food security and sustainability. *Agricultural Research* 1(1): 21–24.

Jayas, D.S, J. Paliwal, and N.S. Visen. 2000. Multi-layer neural networks for image analysis of agricultural products. *Journal of Agricultural Engineering Research* 77(2): 119–128.

Jenneson, P.M., W.B. Gilboy, E.J. Morton, and P.J. Gregory. 2003. An X-ray micro-tomography system optimised for the low dose study of living organisms. *Applied Radiation and Isotopes* 58: 177–181.

Jerrolds, J., and S. Keene. 2009. MRI safety at 3T versus 1.5T. *The Internet Journal of World Health and Societal Politics* 6(1).

Jeyamkondan, S., N. Ray, G.A. Kranzler, and N. Biji. 2000. Beef quality grading using machine vision. In *Proceedings of the Conference on Biological Quality and Precision Agriculture II,* 91–101.

Jiang, J., H. Chang, K. Wu, C. Ouyang, M. Yang, E. Yang, T. Chen, and T. Lin. 2008. An adaptive image segmentation algorithm for X-ray quarantine inspection of selected fruits. *Computers and Electronics in Agriculture* 60: 190–200.

Jiang, L.J., E.Y.K. Ng, A.C.B. Yeo, S. Wu, F. Pan, W.Y. Yau, J.H. Chen, and Y. Yang. 2005. A perspective on medical infrared imaging. *Journal of Medical Engineering and Technology* 29(6): 257–267.

Jiang, L., B. Zhu, X. Rao, G. Berney, and Y. Tao. 2007. Discrimination of black walnut shell and pulp in hyperspectral imagery using Gaussian kernel function approach. *Journal of Food Engineering* 81: 108–117.

Jiang, T., Y. Zhang, F. Cai, J. Qian, and S. He. 2010. Optical coherence tomography for identifying the variety of rice grains. Advances in Optoelectronics and Micro/Nano Optics, Guangzhou, China, December 3–6.

Jimènez, A.R., A.K. Jain, R. Ceres, and J.L. Pons. 1999. Automatic fruit recognition: A survey and new results using range/attenuation images. *Pattern Recognition* 32: 1719–1736.

Jolesz, F.A. 2005. Future perspectives for intraoperative MRI. *Neurosurgery Clinics of North America* 16: 201–213.

Jones, A.Z. 2013. The visible light spectrum. http://physics.about.com/od/lightoptics/a/vislight spec.htm (accessed August 16, 2013).

Jong, P.A., F.R. Long, J.C. Wong, P.J. Merkus, H.A. Tiddens, J.C. Hogg, and H.O. Coxson. 2006. Computed tomographic estimation of lung dimensions throughout the growth period. *European Respiratory Journal* 27: 261–267.

Jonkers, J. 2012. Fish feed gets hospital treatment. Skretting, Norway. http://www.skretting.com/Internet/SkrettingGlobal/webInternet.nsf/wPrId/ECCED6C9193F95D6C1257A2F00476FE4!OpenDocument (accessed November 5, 2012).

Jørgensen, B.M., and K.N. Jensen. 2006. Water distribution and mobility in fish products in relation to quality. In *Modern magnetic resonance*, ed. G.A. Webb, 905–908. The Netherlands: Springer.

Joshi, A., S. Bapna, and S. Chunduri. 2013. Comparison study of different pattern classifiers. http://www.music.mcgill.ca/~ich/classes/mumt621_13/classifiers/ComparisonParzenStudy.pdf (accessed October 30, 2013).

Josling, T. 1999. Globalization of the food industry and its impact on agricultural trade policy. Conference on Agricultural Globalization, Trade and the Environment, University of California at Berkeley, March 7–9.

Jun, W., M.S. Kim, K. Lee, P. Millner, and K. Chao. 2009. Assessment of bacterial biofilm on stainless steel by hyperspectral fluorescence imaging. *Sensing and Instrumentation for Food Quality and Safety* 3: 41–48.

Jun, W., G.O. Jeffrey, G. Feng, and S.H. Jun. 2011. Fourier descriptor with different shape signatures: A comparative study for shape based retrieval of kinematic constraints. *Chinese Journal of Mechanical Engineering* 47(5): 1–10.

Kadir, A., L.E. Nugroho, A. Susanto, and P.I. Santosa. 2011. Neural network application on foliage plant identification. *International Journal of Computer Applications* 29(9): 15–22.

Kalender, W.A. 2006. X-ray computed tomography. *Physics in Medicine and Biology* 51: R29–R43.

Kaliramesh, S., V. Chelladurai, D.S. Jayas, K. Alagusundaram, N.D.G. White, and P.G. Fields. 2013. Detection of infestation by Callosobruchus maculates in mung bean using near-infrared hyperspectral imaging. *Journal of Stored Products Research* 52: 107–111.

Kampman, B., F. Brouwer, F., and B. Schepers. 2008. Agricultural land availability and demand in 2020. Part of the AEAT managed study for the renewable fuels agency, CE Delft, The Netherlands.

Kamruzzaman, M., D. Barbin, G. ElMasry, D. Sun, and P. Allen. 2012a. Potential of hyperspectral imaging and pattern recognition for categorization and authentication of red meat. *Innovative Food Science and Emerging Technologies* 16: 316–325.

Kamruzzaman, M., G. ElMasry, D. Sun, and P. Allen. 2012b. Prediction of some quality attributes of lamb meat using near-infrared hyperspectral imaging and multivariate analysis. *Analytica Chimica Acta* 714: 57–67.

Kang, S.P., and H.T. Sabarez. 2009. Simple colour image segmentation of bicolour food products for quality measurement. *Journal of Food Engineering* 94: 21–25.

Kanovsky, J., O. Bocek, P. Cervinka, T. Ondrus, and P. Kala. 2012. Optical coherence tomography in interventional cardiology-Research field or future daily routine? *Cor et Vasa, The Czech Society of Cardiology* 54: E167–E175.

Karamichou, E., B.G. Merrell, W.A. Murray, G. Simm, and S.C. Bishop. 2007. Selection for carcass quality in hill sheep measured by X-ray computed tomography. *Animal* 1: 3–11.

Karimi, M., M. Fathi, Z. Sheykholeslam, B. Sahraiyan, and F. Naghipoor. 2012. Effect of different processing parameters on quality factors and image texture features of bread. *Bioprocess and Biotechniques* 2(5): 127.

Karunakaran, C., D.S. Jayas, and N.D.G. White. 2003a. X-ray image analysis to detect infestation caused by insects in grain. *Cereal Chemistry* 80(5): 553–557.

Karunakaran, C., D.S. Jayas, and N.D.G. White. 2003b. Soft X-inspection of wheat kernels infested by Sitophilus Oryzae. *Transactions of ASAE* 46(3): 739–745.

Karunakaran, C., D.S. Jayas, and N.D.G. White. 2004a. Detection of infestations by *Cryptolestes ferrugineus* inside wheat kernels using a soft X-ray method. *Canadian Biosystems Engineering* 46: 7.1–7.9.

Karunakaran, C., D.S. Jayas, and N.D.G. White. 2004b. Identification of wheat kernels damaged by red flour beetle using X-ray images. *Biosystems Engineering* 87(3): 267–274.

Karunakaran, C., D.S. Jayas, and N.D.G. White. 2004c. Detection of internal wheat seed infestation by *Rhyzopertha dominica* using X-ray imaging. *Journal of Stored Products Research* 40(5): 507–516.

Karunakaran, C., J. Paliwal, D.S. Jayas, and N.D.G. White. 2005. Comparison of soft X-rays and NIR spectroscopy to detect insect infestations in grain. ASAE Paper Number: 053139, ASAE Annual International Meeting, Tampa, Florida, July 17–20.

Kato, Y., M. Ichinoseki, T. Kamada, A. Kumagai, K. Onuma, and R. Himeno. 2007. Influences of meat organization on intensity distribution in magnetic resonance images. Sixth International Special Topic Conference on Information Technology Applications in Biomedicine (ITAB), Tokyo, November 8–11.

Katrašnik, J., F. Pernuš, and B. Likar. 2011. Illumination system characterization for hyperspectral imaging. *Proceedings of SPIE* vol. 7891, February 10.

Katrašnik, J., F. Pernuš, and B. Likar. 2013. A method for characterizing illumination systems for hyperspectral imaging. *Optics Express* 21(4): 4841–4853.

Kaur, A., and V. Chopra. 2012. A comparative study and analysis of image restoration techniques using different image formats. *International Journal for Science and Emerging Technologies with Latest Trends* 2(1): 7–14.

Kaur, H., and B. Singh. 2013. Classification and grading rice suing multi-class SVM. *International Journal of Scientific and Research Publications* 3(4): 1–5.

Kavdir, I., and D.E. Guyer. 2003. Apple grading using fuzzy logic. *Turkish Journal of Agriculture and Forestry* 27: 375–382.

Keagy, P.M., and F. Schatzki. 1991. Effect of image resolution on insect detection in wheat radiographs. *Cereal Chemistry* 68(4): 339–343.

Keagy, P.M., B. Parvin, and T.F. Schatzki. 1996. Machine recognition of navel orange worm damage in X-ray images of pistachio nuts. *LWT—Food Science and Technology* 29: 140–145.

Keeton, J.T., Hafley, B.S., S.M. Eddy, C.R. Moser, B.J. McManus, and T.P. Leffler. 2003. Rapid determination of moisture and fat in meats by microwave and nuclear magnetic resonance analysis. *Journal of AOAC International* 86(6): 1193–1202.

Kellicut, D.C., J.M. Weiswasser, S. Arora, J.E. Freeman, R.A. Lew, C. Shuman, J.R. Mansfield, and A.N. Sidawy. 2004. Emerging technology: Hyperspectral imaging. *Perspectives in Vascular Surgery and Endovascular Therapy* 16(1): 53–57.

Ketcham, R.A. 2012. X-ray computed tomography. Science Education Research Centre at Carleton College, Northfield, Minnesota. http://serc.carleton.edu/research_education/geochemsheets/techniques/CT.html (accessed February 10, 2013).

Ketcham, R.A., and W.D. Carlson. 2001. Acquisition, optimization and interpretation of X-ray computed tomographic imagery: Applications to the geosciences. *Computers and Geosciences* 27: 381–400.

Keyserlingk, J.R., P.D. Ahlgren, E. Yu, and N. Belliveau. 1998. Infrared imaging of the breast: Initial reappraisal using high-resolution digital technology in 100 successive cases of stage I and II breast cancer. *The Breast Journal* 4: 245–251.

Khaodhiar, L., T. Dinh, K.T. Schomacker, S.V. Panasyuk, J.E. Freeman, R. Lew, T. Vo, A.A. Panasyuk, C. Lima, J.M. Giurini, T.E. Lyons, and A. Veves. 2007. The use of medical hyperspectral technology to evaluate microcirculatory changes in diabetic foot ulcers and to predict clinical outcomes. *Diabetes Care* 30(4): 903–910.

Khare, C., and K.K. Nagwanshi. 2011. Image restoration technique with non-linear filters. *International Journal of Engineering Trends and Technology*, May–June, 1–5.

Khoje, S.A., S.K. Bodhe, and A. Adsul. 2013. Automated skin defect identification system for fruit grading based on discrete curvelet transform. *International Journal of Engineering and Technology* 5(4): 3251–3256.

Kiliç, K., I.H. Boyac, H. Köksel, and I. Küsmenoğlu. 2007. A classification system for beans using computer vision system and artificial neural networks. *Journal of Food Engineering* 78: 897–904.

Kim, D. G., T.F. Burks, J. Qin, and D.M. Bulanon. 2009. Classification of grapefruit peel diseases using color texture feature analysis. *International Journal on Agriculture and Biological Engineering* 2(3): 41–50.

Kim, M.S., Y.R. Chen, and P.M. Mehl. 2001. Hyperspectral reflectance and fluorescence imaging system for food quality and safety. *Transactions of ASAE* 44(3): 721–729.

Kim, S., and T.F. Schatzki. 2000. Apple watercore sorting system using X-ray imagery: I. Algorithm development. *Transactions of ASAE* 43(6): 1695–1702.

Kim, S., and T.F. Schatzki. 2001. Detection of pinholes in almonds through X-ray imaging. *Transactions of ASAE* 44(4): 997–1003.

Kim, S., P. Chen, M.J. McCarthy, and B. Zion. 1999. Fruit internal quality evaluation using on-line nuclear magnetic resonance sensors. *Journal of Agricultural Engineering Research* 74: 293–301.

Kim, T.H., T.H. Cho, Y.S. Moon, and S.H. Park. 1999. Visual inspection system for the classification of solder joints. *Pattern Recognition* 32: 565–575.

Knobelsdorff-Brenkenhoff, F., and J. Schulz-Menger. 2012. Cardiovascular magnetic resonance imaging in ischemic heart disease. *Journal of Magnetic Resonance Imaging* 36: 20–38.

Ko, J.P., S. Brandman, J. Stember, and D.P. Naidich. 2012. Dual-energy computed tomography: Concepts, performance and thoracic applications. *Journal of Thoracic Imaging* 27(1): 7–22.

Kobori, H., N. Gorretta, G. Rabatel, V. Bellon-Maurel, G. Chaix, J. Roger, and S. Tsuchikawa. 2013. Applicability of vis-NIR hyperspectral imaging for monitoring wood moisture content. *Holzforschung* 76(3): 307–314.

Koc, A.B. 2007. Determination of watermelon volume using ellipsoid approximation and image processing. *Postharvest Biology and Technology* 45: 366–371.

Kohonen, T. 1989. *Self-organization and associative memory*, 3rd edition. New York: Springer.

Koizumi, M., S. Naito, N. Ishida, T. Haishi, and H. Kano. 2008. A dedicated MRI for food science and agriculture. *Food Science and Technology Research* 14(1): 74–82.

Koller, D.M., G. Hannesschläger, M. Leitner, and J.G. Khinast. 2011. Non-destructive analysis of tablet coatings with optical coherence tomography. *European Journal of Pharmaceutical Sciences* 44: 142–148.

Kolstad, K. 2001. Fat deposition and distribution measured by computer tomography in three genetic groups of pigs. *Livestock Production Science* 67: 281–292.

Kong, S.G., Y. Chen, I. Kim, and M.S. Kim. 2004. Analysis of hyperspectral fluorescence images for poultry skin tumor inspection. *Applied Optics* 43(4): 824–833.

Kong, S.G., Z. Du, M. Martin, and T. Vo-Dinh. 2005. Hyperspectral fluorescence image analysis for use in medical diagnostics. In *Proceedings of SPIE*, vol. 5692.

Kopinga, K., and L. Pel. 1994. One-dimensional scanning of moisture in porous materials with NMR. *Review of Scientific Instruments* 65(12): 3673–3681.

Kopparapu, S.K. 2006. Lighting design for machine vision application. *Image and Vision Computing* 24(7): 720–726.

Kornaat, P.R., R.Y. Ceulemans, H.M. Kroon, N. Riyazi, M. Kloppenburg, W.O. Carter, T.G. Woodworth, and J.L. Bloem. 2005. MRI assessment of knee osteoarthritis: Knee Osteoarthritis Scoring System (KOSS) inter observer and intra observer reproducibility of a compartment based scoring system. *Skeletal Radiology* 34: 95–102.

Kotwaliwale, N., J. Subbiah, P.W. Weckler, G.H. Brusewitz, and G.A. Kranzler. 2003. Digital radiography for quality determination of small agricultural products: Development and calibration of equipment. ASABE Meeting Presentation, Las Vegas, Nevada, July 27–30.

Kotwaliwale, N., P.R. Weckler, G.H. Brusewitz, G.A. Kranzler, and N.O. Maness. 2007. Non-destructive quality determination of pecans using soft X-rays. *Postharvest Biology and Technology* 45: 372–380.

Kotwaliwale, N., K. Singh, A. Kalne, S.N. Jha, N. Seth, and A. Kar. 2011. X-ray imaging methods for internal quality evaluation of agricultural produce. *Journal of Food Science and Technology.* http://dx.doi.org/10.1007/s13197-011-0485-y.

Koyama, H., Y. Ohno, S. Seki, M. Nishio, T. Yoshikawa, S. Matsumoto, and K. Sugimura. 2013. Magnetic resonance imaging for lung cancer. *Journal of Thoracic Imaging* 28(3): 138–150.

Krähenbühl, A., B. Kerautret, I. Debled-Ennesson, F. Longuetaud, and F. Mother. 2012. Knot detection in X-ray CT images of wood. *Lecture Notes in Computer Science* 7432: 209–218.

Kubo, T., Y. Ino, T. Tanimoto, H. Kitabata, A. Tanaka, and T. Akasaka. 2011. Optical coherence tomography imaging in acute coronary syndromes. *Cardiology Research and Practice*, Article ID312978.

Kumar, R., P. Kulashekar, B. Dhanasekar, and B. Ramamoorthy. 2005. Application of digital image magnification for surface roughness evaluation using machine vision. *International Journal of Machine Tools and Manufacture* 45(2): 228–234.

Kung, C., M. Lee, and C. Hsieh. 2012. Development of an ultraspectral imaging system by using a concave monochromator. *Journal of Chinese Institute of Engineers*, 35(3): 329–342.

Kutis, I.S., V.V. Sapozhnikova, R.V., Kuranov, and V.A. Kamenskii. 2005. Study of the morphological and functional state of higher plant tissues by optical coherence microscopy and optical coherence tomography. *Russian Journal of Plant Physiology* 52(4): 559–564.

Kwong, R.Y., and E.K. Yucel. 2003. Computed tomography scan and magnetic resonance imaging. *Journal of American Heart Association* 108: e104–e106.

Kyotoku, B.B.C., and A.S.L. Gomes. 2007. Dental fiber-reinforced composite analysis using optical coherence tomography. *Optics Communications* 279: 403–407.

La Heji, E.J.L., P.J.A.M. Kerkhof, K. Kopinga, and L. Pel. 1996. Determining porosity profiles during filtration and expression of sewage sludge by NMR imaging. *AIChe Journal* 42(4): 953–959.

Labs, W. 2012. Tech update: Metal detection and X-ray inspection. *Food Engineering*, January 10. http://www.foodengineeringmag.com/articles/tech-update-metal-detection-xray-inspection- (accessed November 2, 2012).

Laghi, L., M.A. Cremonini, G. Placucci, S. Sykora, K. Wright, and B. Hills. 2005. A proton NMR relaxation study of hen quality. *Magnetic Resonance Imaging* 23: 501–510.

Lak, M.B., S. Minaee, J. Amiriparian, and B. Beheshti. 2011. Machine vision recognition algorithm development as the first stage of apple robotic harvesting. 39th Symposium on Actual Tasks on Agricultural Engineering, February 22–25, Opatija, Croatia.

Lammertyn, J., B. Nicolaï, K. Ooms, V. De Smedt, and J. De Baerdemaeker. 1998. Non-destructive measurement of acidity, soluble solids, and firmness of Jonagold apples using NIR-spectroscopy. *Transactions of the ASAE* 41(4): 1089–1094.

Lammertyn, J., T. Dresselaers, P. Van Hecke, P. Jancsók, M. Wevers, and B.M. Nicolaï. 2003. Analysis of the time course of core breakdown in "Conference" pears by means of MRI and X-ray CT. *Postharvest Biology and Technology* 29: 19–28.

Landahl, S., L.A. Terry, and H.D. Ford. 2012. Investigation of diseased onion bulbs using data processing of optical coherence tomography images. Proceedings of 6th International Symposium on Edible *Alliaceae*. Fukuoka, Japan, December 10.

Landis, E.N., and D.T. Keane. 2010. X-ray micro tomography. *Material Characterization* 61: 1305–1316.

Langelaan, H.C., F. Pereira da Silva, U.T. Velzen, J. Broeze, A.M. Matser, M. Vollebregt, and K. Schroën. 2013. Technology options for feeding 10 billion people—Options for sustainable food processing. Science and Technology Options Assessment (STOA) report, Brussels, European Union.

Lape, A., S. Jensen, V.L.S. Jeor, and C.A. Lendon. 2008. Use of X-ray micro computed tomography in the evaluation of bread crumb structure. *Microscopy and Microanalysis* 14(S2): 700–701.

Larbig, M., B. Burtin, L. Martin, H. Stamm, B. Luettig, J.M. Hohlfeld, and N. Krug. 2006. Facial thermography is a sensitive tool to determine antihistaminic activity: Comparison of levocetirizine and fexofenadine. *British Journal of Clinical Pharmacology* 62: 158–164.

Larraín, R.E., D.M. Schaefer, and J.D. Reed. 2008. Use of digital images to estimate CIE color coordinates of beef. *Food Research International* 41: 380–385.

Larsson, P.T., E.L. Hult, K. Wickholm, E. Petterson, and T. Iversen. 1999. CP/MAS 13C-NMR spectroscopy applied to structure and interaction studies on cellulose. *Solid State Nuclear Magnetic Resonance* 15(1): 31–40.

Latkany, P. 2006. Retinal disease: Evolving treatment approaches. *Medscape Ophthalmology.* http://www.medscape.org/viewarticle/549001 (accessed September 1, 2013).

Laurent, W., J.M. Bonny, and J.P. Renou. 2000. Muscle characterisation by NMR imaging and spectroscopic techniques. *Food Chemistry* 69: 419–426.

Lechner, T., Y. Sandin, and R. Kliger. 2013. Assessment of density in timber using X-ray equipment. *International Journal of Architectural Heritage: Conservation, Analysis, and Restoration* 7(4): 416–433.

Lee, C., S. Lee, J. Kim, H. Jung, and J. Kim. 2011. Optical sensing method for screening disease in melon seeds by using optical coherence tomography. *Sensors* 11: 9467–9477.

Lee, C., S. Lee, J. Kim, H. Jung, and J. Kim. 2012. The application of optical coherence tomography in the diagnosis of Marssonina Blotch in apple leaves. *Journal of the Optical Society of Korea* 16(2): 133–140.

Lee, S., and Y. Kim. 2008. In vivo visualization of the water refilling process in xylem vessels using X-ray micro-imaging. *Annals of Botany* 101(4): 595–602.

Lee, W.S., D.C. Slaughter, and D.K. Giles. 1999. Robotic weed control system for tomatoes. *Precision Agriculture* 1: 95–113.

Lee, Z.S., and R.S. Lo. 2002. Application of vision image cooperated with multi-light sources to recognition of solder joints of PCB. TAAI Artificial Intelligence and Applications, pp. 425–430.

Leemans, V., H. Magein, and M.F. Destain. 1998. Defect segmentation on Golden Delicious apples by using colour machine vision. *Computers and Electronics in Agriculture* 20: 117–130.

Lefcourt, A.M., M.S. Wiederoder, N. Liu, M.S. Kim, and Y.M. Lo. 2013. Development of a portable hyperspectral imaging system for monitoring the efficacy of sanitation procedures in food processing facilities. *Journal of Food Engineering* 117: 59–66.

Leinonen, I., and H.G. Jones. 2004. Combining thermal and visible imagery for estimating canopy temperature and identifying plant stress. *Journal of Experimental Botany* 55(401): 1423–1231.

Leitgeb, R., C.K. Hitzenberger, and A.F. Fercher. 2003. Performance of Fourier domain vs. time domain optical coherence tomography. *Optics Express* 11(8): 889–894.

Leitner, M., G. Hannesschläger, A. Saghy, A. Nemeth, S. Chassagne-Berces, H. Chanvrier, E. Herremans, and B.E. Verlinden. 2011. Optical coherence tomography for quality control and microstructure analysis in food. 11th International Congress on Engineering and Food, Athens, Greece, May 22–26.

Lemström, G. 1995. Color line-scan technology in industrial applications. In *Proceedings of SPIE Vol. 2588, Intelligent Robots and Computer Vision XIV: Algorithms, Techniques, Active Vision, and Materials Handling*, 190–199.

Lenthe, J.H., E.C. Oerke, and H.W. Dehne. 2007. Digital infrared thermography for monitoring canopy health of wheat. *Precision Agriculture* 8: 15–26.

Leta, F.R., F.F. Feliciano, I.L. de Souza, and E. Cataldo. 2005. Discussing accuracy in an automatic measurement system using computer vision techniques. *ABCM Symposium Series in Mechatronics*, vol. 2, November 6–11, Ouro Preto, Brazil.

Létal, J., D. Jirák, L. Suderlová, and M. Hájek. 2003. MRI "texture" analysis of MR images of apples during ripening and storage. *LWT—Food Science and Technology* 36: 719–727.

Leung, M.K., and B.A. Standish. 2013. Optical coherence tomography for imaging biological tissue. In *Handbook of 3D machine vision: Optical metrology and imaging*, ed. S. Zhang, 316–334. Boca Raton, FL: Taylor & Francis.

Levi, P., R. Falla, and R. Pappalardo. 1988. Image controlled robotics applied to citrus fruit harvesting. Procedures, ROVISEC-VII, Zurich.

Lewis, J. 2013. Machine vision improves safety, productivity for food and beverage manufacturers. *Plant Engineering*, September, 47–50. http://bt.e-ditionsbyfry.com/publication/frame.php?i=176363&p=&pn=&ver=flex (accessed February 6, 2014).

Li, J., J. Tan, and P. Shatadal. 2001. Classification of tough and tender beef by image texture analysis. *Meat Science* 57: 341–346.

Li, Q. 2012. Hyperspectral imaging technology used in tongue diagnosis. In *Recent advances in theories and practice of Chinese Medicine*, ed. H. Kuang, 111–136. Shanghai, China.

Li, X.D., S.A. Boppart, J. Van Dam, H. Mashimo, M. Mutinga, W. Drexler, M. Klein, C. Pitris, M.L. Krinsky, M.E. Brezinski, and J.G. Fujimoto. 2001. Optical coherence tomography: Advanced technology for the endoscopic imaging of Barrett's esophagus. *Endoscopy* 32: 921–930.

Li, Z. 2006. Robotic food processing now with x-ray vision. Food processing.com, September 16. http://www.foodprocessing.com.au/articles/1133-Robotic-food-processing-now-with-x-ray-vision (accessed November 2, 2012).

Lim, K.S., and M. Barigou. 2004. X ray micro-computed tomography of cellular food products. *Food Research and international* 37(10): 1001–1012.

Liming, X., and Z. Yanchao. 2010. Automated strawberry grading system based on image processing. *Computers and Electronics in Agriculture* 71S: S32–S39.

Lin, S.C., C.H. Chou, and C.H. Su. 2007. A development of visual inspection system for surface mounted devices on printed circuit board. In *Proceedings of the 33rd Annual Conference of the IEEE industrial Electronics Society*, 2440–2445.

Lin, W.C., J.W. Hall, and A. Klieber, 1993. Video imaging for quantifying cucumber fruit color. *Horticulture Technology* 3(4): 436–439.

Lindegaard, H.M., J. Vallø, K. Hørslev-Petersen, P. Junker, and M. Østergaard. 2006. Low-cost, low field dedicated extremity magnetic resonance imaging in early rheumatoid arthritis: A 1 year follow-up study. *Annals of the Rheumatic Diseases* 65: 1208–1212.

Linden, V.V., R. Vereycken, C. Bravo, H. Ramon, and J.D. Baerdemaeker. 2003. Detection technique for tomato bruise damage by thermal imaging. *Acta Horticulturae* 599: 389–394.

Lippmann, R.P. 1987. An introduction to computing with neural nets. In *IEEE Acoustics, Speech and Signal Processing* 4: 4–22.

Litwiller, D. 2001. CCD vs CMOS: Facts and fiction. *Photonics Spectra* 154–157.

Liu, H., Y. Liu, T. Yu, and N. Ye. 2010. Usefulness of diffusion-weighted MR imaging in the evaluation of pulmonary lesions. *European Radiology* 20: 807–815.

Liu, J., J. Shen, Z. Shen, and R. Liu. 2012. Grading tobacco leaves based on image processing and generalized regression neural network. In *IEEE International Conference on Intelligent Control, Automatic Detection and High End Equipment*, 89–93.

Liu, P., R.M. Groves, and R. Benedictus. 2012. Quality assessment of aerospace materials with optical coherence tomography. *Proceedings of SPIE*, vol. 8430.

Liu, Y., and R. Dias. 2002. Evaluation of packaged defects by thermal imaging techniques. Proceedings from the 28th International Symposium for Testing and Failure Analysis, November 3–7, Phoenix, Arizona.

Liu, Z., H. Wang, and Q. Li. 2012. Tongue tumor detection in medical hyperspectral images. *Sensors* 12: 162–174.

Ljungberg, S., and O. Jönsson. 2002. Infrared thermography—A tool to map temperature anomalies of plants in a greenhouse heated by gas fired infrared heaters. In *Proceedings of SPIE*, vol. 4710, 399–405.

Loeb, G., and J.K. Barton. 2003. Imaging botanical subjects with optical coherence tomography: A feasibility study. *Transactions of ASAE* 46(6): 1751–1757.

Loma Systems. 2012. X-ray marks the spot for Central Food Services. http://www.loma.com/documents/2012_cfs.pdf (accessed November 30, 2012).

Loma Systems/Cintex. 2007. Loma serves up the perfect dessert. http://www.loma.co.uk/newsletters/november2007/index.html (accessed November 30, 2012).

Lou, H., Y. Hu, B. Wang, and H. Lu. 2012. Dried jujube classification using support vector machine based on fractal parameters and red green and blue intensity. *International Journal of Food Science and Technology* 47(9): 1951–1957.

Lu, G.M., Y.E. Zhao, L.J. Zhang, and U.J. Schoepf. 2012. Dual-energy CT of the lung. *American Journal of Roentgenology* 199: S43–S50.

Lu, J., J. Tan, P. Shatadal, and D.E. Gerrard. 2000. Evaluation of pork colour by using computer vision. *Meat Science* 56: 57–60.

Lü, Q., J. Cai, Y. Li, and F. Wang. 2010. Real time non-destructive inspection of chestnuts using X-ray imaging and dynamic threshold. In *World Automation Congress (WAC) 2010*, 365–368.

Lu, R. 2003. Detection of bruises on apples using near-infrared hyperspectral imaging. *Transactions of ASAE* 46(2): 523–530.

Lu, R., and Y. Peng. 2006. Hyperspectral scattering for assessing peach fruit firmness. *Biosystems Engineering* 93(2): 161–171.

Lu, R.S., Y.F. Li, and Q. Yu. 2001. On-line measurement of the straightness of seamless steel pipes using machine vision technique. *Sensors and Actuators* 94: 95–101.

Lukac, R., K.N. Plataniotis, D. Hatzinakos, and M. Aleksic. 2006. A new CFA interpolation framework. *Signal Processing*, 86(7), 1559–1579.

Luo, R., and R.L. Lytton. 2011. Determination of crack size distribution in asphalt mixtures. *Transportation Research Record* 2210: 113–121.

Luo, X., D.S. Jayas, and S.J. Symons. 1999a. Comparison of statistical and neural network methods for classifying cereal grains using machine vision. *Transactions of ASAE* 42(2): 413–419.

Luo, X.Y., D.S. Jayas, and S.J. Symons. 1999b. Identification of damaged kernels in wheat using a colour machine vision system. *Journal of Cereal Science* 30(1): 49–59.

Ma, R., C. Liu, K. Deng, S.J. Song, D.P. Wang, and L. Huang L. 2010. Cerebral artery evaluation of dual energy CT angiography with dual source CT. *Chinese Medical Journal* 123(9): 1139–1144.

Macedo, A., P.E. Cruvinel, R.Y. Inamasu, L.A.C. Jorge, J.M. Naime, A. Torreneto, C.M.P. Vaz, and S. Crestana. 1999. Micrometric X-ray CT scanner dedicated to soil investigation. IEEE International Multi-Conference on Circuit Systems Communications and Computers, Nigata, Japan, July 13–15.

Machine Vision Consulting Inc. 2013. Vision inspection for defect detection. http://www.machinevc.com/ (accessed February 6, 2014).

Mahesh, S. 2011. Long wavelength near-infrared hyperspectral imaging for classification and quality assessment of bulk samples of wheat from different growing locations and crop years. PhD dissertation, University of Manitoba, Winnipeg.

Mahesh, S., A. Manickavasagan, D.S. Jayas, J. Paliwal, and N.D.G. White. 2008. Feasibility of near-infrared hyperspectral imaging to differentiate Canadian wheat classes. *Biosystems Engineering* 101: 50–57.

Maini, R., and H. Agarwal. 2009. Study and comparison of various image edge detection techniques. *International Journal of Image Processing* 3(1): 1–12.

Majumdar, S. 1997. Classification of cereal grains using machine vision. Ph.D. dissertation, University of Manitoba, Winnipeg, Canada.

Majumdar, S., and D.S. Jayas. 2000a. Classification of cereal grains using machine vision. I. Morphology models. *Transactions of the ASAE* 43(6): 1669–1675.

Majumdar, S., and D.S. Jayas. 2000b. Classification of cereal grains using machine vision. II. Color models. *Transactions of the ASAE* 43(6): 1677–1680.

Majumdar, S., and D.S. Jayas. 2000c. Classification of cereal grains using machine vision. Texture models. *Transactions of the ASAE* 43(6): 1681–1687.

Majumdar, S., and D.S. Jayas. 2000d. Classification of cereal grains using machine vision. IV. Combined morphology, color, and texture models. *Transactions of the ASAE* 43(6): 1689–1694.

Malamas, E.N., E.G.M. Petrakis, M. Zervakis, L. Petit, and J. Legat. 2003. A survey on industrial vision systems, applications and tools. *Image and Vision Computing* 21: 171–188.

Mallick, P.K., and S. Rout. 2013. Identification and classification of similar looking food grains. *International Journal on Advanced Computer Theory and Engineering* 1(2): 139–144.

Manickavasagan, A., D.S. Jayas, and N.D.G. White. 2006. Non-uniformity of surface temperatures of grain after microwave treatment in an industrial microwave dryer. *Drying Technology* 24(12): 1559–1567.

Manickavasagan, A., D.S. Jayas, and N.D.G. White. 2008a. Thermal imaging to detect infestation by Cryptolestes *ferrugineus* inside wheat kernels. *Journal of Stored Products Research* 44: 186–192.

Manickavasagan, A., G. Sathya, D.S. Jayas, and N.D.G. White. 2008b. Wheat class identification using monochrome images. *Journal of Cereal Science* 47: 518–527.

Manickavasagan, A., D.S. Jayas, N.D.G. White, and F. Jian. 2008c. Thermal imaging of a stored grain silo to detect a hot spot. *Applied Engineering in Agriculture* 22(6): 891–897.

Manickavasagan, A., D.S. Jayas, N.D.G. White, and J. Paliwal. 2010. Wheat class identification using thermal imaging. *Food and Bioprocess Technology* 3: 450–460.

Manyak, M.J., N.D. Gladkova, J.H. Makari, A.M. Schwartz, E.V. Zagaynova, L. Zolfaghari, J.M. Zara, R. Iksanov, and F.I. Feldchtein. 2005. Evaluation of superficial bladder transitional cell carcinoma by optical coherence tomography. *Journal of Endourology* 19(5): 570–574.

Mar, N.S.S., P.K.D.V. Yarlagadda, and C. Fookes. 2011. Design and development of automatic visual inspection system for PCB manufacturing. *Robotics and Computer Integrated Manufacturing* 27: 949–962.

Marciani, L., M.S.J. Wickham, D. Bush, R. Faulks, J. Wright, and A.J. Fillery-Travis. 2006. Magnetic resonance imaging of the behavior of oil-in water emulsions in the gastric lumen of man. *British Journal of Nutrition* 95: 331–339.

Marel, 2013. X-ray bone detection. http://marel.com/Systems-And-Equipment/Poultry/Processes/Broilers/Deboning-and-skinning/1347/X-ray-Bone-Detection/1354/default.aspx (accessed November 30, 2012).

Marigheto, N., L. Venturi, and B. Hills. 2008. Two-dimensional NMR relaxation studies of apple quality. *Postharvest Biology and Technology* 48: 331–340.

Markets and Markets. 2013. Machine vision systems and components market. http://www.marketsandmarkets.com/PressReleases/machine-vision-systems.asp (accessed February 6, 2014).

Marofsky, N. 2012. A look back at the future. Technical Report: Machine Vision Developments.

Martens, H., A.K. Thybo, H.J. Andersen, A.H. Karlsson, S. Donstrup, H. Stodkilde-Jorgensen, and M. Martens. 2002. Sensory analysis for magnetic resonance image analysis: Using human perception and cognition to segment and assess the interior of potatoes. *LWT–Food Science and Technology* 35(1): 70–79.

Martin, D. 2007. A practical guide to machine vision lighting. Advanced illumination, Rochester, New York.

Martin, M.E., M.B. Wabuyele, K. Chen, P. Kasili, M. Panjehpour, M. Phan, B. Overholt, G. Cunningham, D. Wilson, R.C. Denove, and T. Vo-Dinh. 2006. Development of an advanced hyperspectral imaging system with applications for cancer detection. *Annals of Biomedical Engineering* 34(6): 1061–1068.

Martin, Y.L. 2001. Detection of added beet or cane sugar in maple syrup by the site-specific deuterium nuclear magnetic resonance (SNIF-NMR) method: Collaborative study. *Journal of AOAC International* 84(5): 1509–1152.

Marty-Mahe, P., P. Loisel, and D. Brossard. 2003. Colour image segmentation to detect defects on fresh ham. In *Proceedings of SPIE 5132*, 45–50.

Masters, T. 1994. *Practical neural network recipes in C++*. Boston: Academic Press.

Mateo, A., F. Soto, J.A. Villarejo, J. Roca-Dorda, F. De la Gandara, and A. García. 2006. Quality analysis of tuna meat using an automated color inspection system. *Aquacultural Engineering* 35: 1–13.

Mathworks. 1998. Fuzzy logic toolbox user's guide, version 2.1. Natick, MA: The Mathworks Inc.

Matsushima, U., W. Graf, S. Zabler, I. Manke, M. Dawson, G. Choinka, and W.B. Herppich. 2009. Synchrotron X-ray CT of rose peduncles-evaluation of tissue damage by radiation. *Image Analysis for Agricultural Products and Processes* 69: 128–131.

Maunu, S.L. 2002. NMR studies of wood and wood products. *Progress in Nuclear Magnetic Resonance Spectroscopy* 40(2): 151–174.

Mauritz, J.M.A., R.S. Morrisby, R.S. Hutton, C.H. Legge, and C.F. Kaminski. 2010. Imaging pharmaceutical tablets with optical coherence tomography. *Journal of Pharmaceutical Sciences* 99(1): 383–391.

McCarthy, M.J., E. Perez, and M. Ozilgen. 1991. Model for transient moisture profiles of a drying apple slab using the data obtained with magnetic resonance imaging. *Biotechnology Progress* 7: 540–543.

McCarthy, M.J., B. Zion, P. Chen, S. Ablett, A.H. Darke, and P.J. Lillford. 1995. Diamagnetic susceptibility changes in apple tissue after bruising. *Journal of the Science of Food and Agriculture* 67: 13–20.

McCarthy, M.J., J. Walton, and K. McCarthy. 2000. Magnetic resonance imaging: Analysis for confectionery products and processes. *The Manufacturing Confectioner* 80(6): 83–90.

McFarlane, N.J.B., R.D. Speller, C.R. Bull, and R.D. Tillett. 2003. Detection of bone fragments in chicken meat using X-ray backscatter. *Biosystems Engineering* 85(2): 185–199.

McCulloch, W.S. and W. Pitts. 1943. A logical calculus of the ideas immanent in nervous activity. *Bulletin of Mathematical Biophysics* 5: 115–133.

McGoverin, C.M., P. Engelbrecht, P. Geladi, and M. Manley. 2011. Characterisation of non-viable whole barley, wheat and sorghum grains using near-infrared hyperspectral data and chemometrics. *Analytical and Bioanalytical Chemistry* 401: 2283–2289.

McGovern, M., A. Senalik, G. Chen, F.C. Beall, and H. Reis. 2010. Detection and assessment of wood decay using X-ray computer tomography. In *Sensors and Smart Structures Technologies for Civil, Mechanical, and Aerospace Systems, Proceedings of SPIE*, vol. 7647. doi: 10.1117/12.843709.

McKellar, R.C., J. Odumeru, T. Zhou, A. Harrison, D.G. Mercer, J.C. Young, X. Lu, J. Boulter, P. Piyasena, and S. Karr. 2004. Influence of a commercial warm water/chlorine treatment on the shelf life of ready-to-use lettuce. *Food Research International* 37: 343–354.

McLaughlin, R.A., B.C. Quirk, A. Curatolo, R.W., Kirk, L. Scolaro, D. Lorenser, P.D. Robbins, B.A. Wood, C.M. Saunders, and D.D. Sampson. 2012. Imaging of breast cancer with optical coherence tomography needle probes: Feasibility and initial results. *IEEE Journal of Selected Topics in Quantum Electronics*, 18(3): 1184–1191.

Mcrory, N. 2010. Standing to the test. *Asia Food Journal*, September. http://www.asiafoodjournal.com/article/standing-to-the-test/7351 (accessed December 20, 2012).

Mebatsion, H.K., J. Paliwal, and D.S. Jayas. 2013. Automatic classification of non-touching cereal grains in digital images using limited morphological and color features. *Computers and Eelctronics in Agriculture* 90: 99–105.

Meglinski, I.V., C. Buranachai, and L.A. Terry. 2010. Plant photonics: Application of optical coherence tomography to monitor defects and rots in onion. *Laser Physics Letters* 7(4): 307–310.

Mehl, P.M., Y. Chen, M.S. Kim, and D.E. Chan. 2004. Development of hyperspectral imaging technique for the detection of apple surface defects and contaminations. *Journal of Food Engineering* 61: 67–81.

Mehrotra, K., C.K. Mohan, and S. Ranka. 1996. *Elements of artificial neural networks*. Cambridge: MIT Press.

Meigs, A.D., L.J. Otten, and T.Y. Cherezova. 2008. Ultraspectral imaging: A new contribution to global virtual presence. *IEEE A&E Systems Magazine*, 11–17.

Meinlschmidt, F., and V. Märgner. 2002. Detection of foreign substances in food using thermography. In *Proceedings of SPIE Thermosense XX1V*, vol. 4710, 565–571.

Melado, A., P. Barreiro, L. Rodriguez-Sinobas, M.E. Fernandez-Valle, J. Ruiz-Cabello, S. Chassagne-Berces, and H. Chanvrier. 2011. MRI texture analysis as means for addressing rehydration and milk diffusion in cereals. *Procedia Food Science* (11th International Congress on Engineering and Food) 1: 625–631.

Melles Griot. 2013. Machine vision lighting fundamentals. http://m.eet.com/media/1161576/4163-pg20_24.pdf (accessed October 2, 2013).

Melo, L.S.A., R.E. Araújo, A.Z. Freitas, D. Zezell, N.D. Vieira, J. Girkin, A. Hall, M.T. Carvalho, and A.S.L. Gomes. 2005. Evaluation of enamel dental restoration interface by optical coherence tomography. *Journal of Biomedical Optics* 10: 064027.

Memarian, N., and T. Chau. 2009. Infrared thermography as an access pathway for individuals with severe motor impairments. *Journal of NeuroEngineering and Rehabilitation* 6(11): 1–8.

Mendoza, F., P. Dejmek, and J.M. Aguilera. 2006. Calibrated color measurements of agricultural foods using image analysis. *Postharvest Biology and Technology* 41(3): 285–295.

Mendoza, F., P. Verboven, H.K. Mebatsion, G. Kerckhofs, M. Wevers, and B. Nicolaï. 2007. Three dimensional pore space quantification of apple tissue suing X-ray computed microtomography. *Planta* 226: 559–570.

Merla, A., and G.L. Romani. 2006. Functional infrared imaging in medicine: A quantitative diagnostic approach. Proceedings of 28th IEEE Annual International Conference, New York, August 30–September 3.

Merlot, S., A. Mustilli, B. Genty, H. North, V. Lefebvre, B. Sotta, A. Vavasseur, and J. Giraudat. 2002. Use of infrared thermal imaging to isolate Arabidopsis mutants defective in stomatal regulation. *The Plant Journal* 30(4): 601–609.

Mersch, S. 1987. Overview of machine vision lighting techniques. *Proceedings of SPIE 728*, 36–38.

Mery, D., and F. Pedreschi. 2005. Segmentation of colour food images using a robust algorithm. *Journal of Food Engineering* 66: 353–360.

Mery, D., I. Lillo, H. Loebel, V. Riffo, A. Soto, A. Cipriano, and J.M. Aguilera. 2011. Automated fish bone detection using X-ray imaging. *Journal of Food Engineering* 105: 485–492.

Mettler Toledo. 2009. *Safeline X-ray inspection guide.* Chapter 3: Choosing the right system, 17–18.

Michie, D., D.J. Spiegelhalter, and C.C. Taylor. 1994. Introduction. In *Machine learning, neural and statistical classification*, ed. D. Michie, D.J. Spiegelhalter, and C.C. Taylor, 1–5. Hertz, UK: Ellis Horwood.

Mikulska, D. 2006. Contemporary applications of infrared imaging in medical diagnostics. *Annales Academiae Medicae Stetinensis* 52(10): 35–39.

Milczarek, R.R., M.E. Saltveit, T.C. Garvey, and M.J. McCarthy. 2009. Assessment of tomato pericarp mechanical damage using multivariate analysis of magnetic resonance images. *Postharvest Biology and Technology* 52: 189–195.

Miri, T., and P. Fryer. 2008. Use of X-ray CT to characterize microstructure of bread and optimize the bread making process. Annual Skyscan User Meeting, Kontich, Belgium, June 15–17.

Miri, T., S. Bakalis, S.D. Bhima, and P.J. Fryer. 2006. Use of X-ray micro-CT to characterize structure phenomena during frying. International Union of Food Science and Technology, 13th World Congress of Food Science and Technology at Nantes, France, September 17–21.

Mitsubishi Electric. 2013. Food industry growing to new levels of automation. http://www.con nectingindustry.com/ProcessControl/food-industry-growing-to-new-levels-of-automation .aspx (accessed February 6, 2014).

Miyake, Y., K. Yokomizo, and N. Matsuzaki. 1998. Determination of unsaturated fatty acid composition by high-resolution nuclear magnetic resonance spectroscopy. *Journal of American Oil Chemists Society* 75(9): 1091–1094.

Mizoguchi, A., M. Sugawara, M. Nakamura, and K. Takeuchi. 2010. Application to non destructive physical method using X-ray CT imaging. Proceedings from the 36th International Symposium for Testing and Failure Analysis, Texas, November 14–18.

Mizushima, A., and R. Lu. 2013. An image segmentation method for apple sorting and grading using support vector machine and otsu's method. *Computers and Electronics in Agriculture* 94: 29–37.

Mladenov, M., S. Penchev, M. Dejanov, and M. Mustafa. 2011. Automatic classification of grain sample elements based on color and shape properties. *UPB Scientific Bulletin Series C* 73(4): 39–53.

Mohamed, A.K. 2003. Automation and computer integrated manufacturing in food processing industry: An appraisal. PhD dissertation, Dublin City University, Ireland.

Mohorič, A., F. Vergeldt, E. Gerkema, A. Jager, J. Duynhoven, G. Dalen, and H. Van As. 2004. Magnetic resonance imaging of single rice kernels during cooking. *Journal of Magnetic Resonance* 171: 157–162.

Mokhtar, A., M.A. Hussein, and T. Becker. 2011. Monitoring pasta production line using automated imaging technique. *Procedia Food Science* 1: 1173–1180.

Mokwa, R., and B. Nielsen. 2006. Non-destructive measurements of soil geotechnical properties using X-ray computed tomography. *GeoCongress* 2006: 1–6. http://dx.doi.org/10.1061/40803(187)47.

Monteiro, S.T., Y. Kosugi, K. Uto, and E. Watanabe. 2004. Towards applying hyperspectral imagery as an intraoperative visual aid tool. Proceedings of the Fourth IASTED International Conference, Marbella, Spain, September 6–8.

Monteiro, S.T., Y. Minekawa, Y. Kosugi, T. Akazawa, and K. Oda. 2007. Prediction of sweetness and amino acid content in soybean crops from hyperspectral imagery. *Journal of Photogrammetry and Remote Sensing* 62: 2–12.

Mora, C.R., L.R. Schimleck, S. Yoon, and C.N. Thai. 2011. Determination of basic density and moisture content of loblolly pine wood disks using a near infrared hyperspectral imaging system. *Journal of Near Infrared Spectroscopy* 19: 401–409.

Morales, R.A. 2002. Changes in identification and control of physical hazards since PR/HACCP. USDA/FSIS Technical Conference on Foreign Material Contaminants, Prerequisite Programs, and Validation, Omaha, NE.

Morita, K., J. Otani, T. Mukunoki, J. Hironaka, and K.D. Pham. 2007. Evaluation of vertical and lateral bearing capacity mechanism of pile foundations using X-ray CT. In *Proceedings of International Workshop on Recent Advances of Deep Foundation*, 217–223.

Morris, P., and A. Perkins. 2012. Diagnostic imaging. *The Lancet* 379(9825): 1525–1533.

Mosqueda, M.R P., E.W. Tollner, G.E. Boyhan, and R.W. McClendon. 2010. Predicting the economics of X-ray inspection technology in sweet onion packing houses using simulation modelling. *Biosystems Engineering* 105: 139–147.

Mousavi, R., T. Miri, P.W. Cox, and P.J. Fryer. 2007. Imaging food freezing using X-ray microtomography. *International Journal of Food Science and Technology* 42: 714–727.

Moya, R., and M. Tomazello-Filho. 2009. Wood density variation and tree ring demarcation in Gmelina arborea trees using X-ray densitometry. *Cerne* 15(1): 92–100.

Mühlenbruch, G., M. Das, G. Mommertz, M. Schaaf, S. Langer, A.H. Mahnken, J.E. Wildberger, A. Thron, R.W. Günther, and T. Krings. 2010. Comparison of dual-source CT angiography and MR angiography in preoperative evaluation of intra-and extracranial vessels: A pilot study. *European Radiology* 20: 469–476.

Mukane, S.M., and J.A. Kendule. 2013. Flower classification using neural network based image processing. *Journal of Electronics and Communications Engineering* 7(3): 80–85.

Mulaveesala, R., S.S.B. Panda, R.N. Mude, and M. Amarnath. 2012. Non-destructive evaluation of concrete structures by non-stationary thermal wave imaging. *Progress in Electromagnetics Research Letter*s 32: 39–48.

Munkevik, P., G. Hall, and T. Duckett. 2007. A computer vision system for appearance-based descriptive sensory evaluation of meals. *Journal of Food Engineering* 78: 246–256.

Mustafa, N.B.A., S.K. Ahmed, Z. Ali, W.B. Yit, A.A.Z. Abidin, and Z.A.M. Sharrif. 2009. Agricultural produce sorting and grading using support vector machines and fuzzy logic. In *IEEE International Conference on Signal and Image Processing Applications*, 391–396.

Nade, T., K. Fujita, M. Fujii, M. Yoshida, T. Haryu, S. Misumi, and T. Okumura. 2005. Development of X-ray computed tomography for live standing cattle. *Animal Science Journal* 76: 513–517.

Naes, T., T. Isaksson, T. Fearn, and T. Davies. 2002. *A user-friendly guide to multivariate calibration and classification*. Chichester, UK: NIR Publications.

Naganathan, G.K., L.M. Grimes, J. Subbiah, C.R. Calkins, A. Samal, and G.E. Meyer. 2008. Visible/near-infrared hyperspectral imaging for beef tenderness prediction. *Computers and Electronics in Agriculture* 64: 225–233.

Nakano, K. 1997. Application of neural networks to the color grading of apples. *Computers and Electronics in Agriculture* 18: 105–116.

Nandalur, K.R., B.A. Dwamena, A.F. Choudhri, M.R. Nandalur, and R.C. Carlos. 2007. Diagnostic performance of stress cardiac magnetic resonance imaging in the detection of coronary artery disease. *Journal of the American College of Cardiology* 50(14): 1343–1353.

Nanyam, Y., R. Choudhary, L. Gupta, and J. Paliwal. 2012. A decision-fusion strategy for fruit quality inspection using hyperspectral imaging. *Biosystems Engineering* 111: 118–125.

Narendra, V.G., and K.S. Hareesh. 2011. Cashew kernel classification using texture features. *International Journal of Machine Intelligence* 3(2): 45–51.

Narvankar, D.S., C.B. Singh, D.S. Jayas, and N.D.G. White. 2009. Assessment of soft X-ray imaging for detection of fungal infection in wheat. *Biosystems Engineering* 103: 49–56.

NASA Tech Briefs. 2008. Machine vision advances benefit motion applications. Vol. 32(8), August 1. http://www.techbriefs.com/component/content/article/23-ntb/features/feature-articles/9808 -15136-786 (accessed February 6, 2014).

Nashat, S., A. Abdullah, S. Aramvith, and M.Z. Abdullah. 2011. Support vector machine approach to real-time inspection of biscuits on moving conveyor belt. *Computers and Electronics in Agriculture* 75: 147–158.

Nasir, A.F.A, M.N.A. Rahman, and A.R. Mamat. 2012. A study of image processing in agriculture application under high performance computing environment. *International Journal of Computer Science and Telecommunications* 3(8): 16–24.

National Environmental Engineering Research Institute (NEERI). 1995. Investigation report on impacts of aquaculture farming and remedial measures in ecologically fragile coastal areas in the states of Andhra Pradesh and Tamil Nadu. National Environmental Engineering Research Institute, Nagpur, India.

National Heart, Lung and Blood Institute. 2007. Estimates for chronic obstructive pulmonary disease, asthma, pneumonia/influenza and other lung diseases. Bethesda, MD: National Heart, Lung and Blood Institute.

National Radiological Protection Board. 2010. Frequency of medical and dental x-ray examination in the UK 1997–1998. London: NRPB.

NATO (North Atlantic Treaty Organization) Research and Technology Organization. 1998. Advanced pattern recognition techniques, RTO Lecture Series 214, pp. 1–23.

Natterer, F., and E.L. Ritman. 2002. Past and future directions in X-ray computed tomography. *International Journal of Imaging Systems and Technology* 12: 175–187.

Nawrocka, A., E. Stepień, S. Grundas, and J. Nawrot. 2012. Mass loss determination of wheat kernels infested by granary weevil from X-ray images. *Journal of Stored Products Research* 48: 19–24.

Neethirajan, S., C. Karunakaran, D.S. Jayas, and N.D.G. White. 2006a. X-ray computed tomography image analysis to explain the airflow resistance differences in grain bulks. *Biosystems Engineering* 94(1): 545–555.

Neethirajan, S., C. Karunakaran, S. Symons, and D.S. Jayas. 2006b. Classification of vitreousness in durum wheat using soft X-rays and transmitted light images. *Computers and Electronics in Agriculture* 53(1): 71–78.

Neethirajan, S., D.S. Jayas, and C. Karunakaran. 2007a. Dual energy X-ray image analysis for classifying vitreousness in durum wheat. *Postharvest Biology and Technology* 45: 381–384.

Neethirajan, S., D.S. Jayas, and N.D.G. White. 2007b. Detection of sprouted wheat kernels using soft X-ray image analysis. *Journal of Food Engineering* 81: 509–513.

Nelson, M., and W.T. Illingworth. 1990. *A practical guide to neural nets*. Reading, MA: Addison-Wesley.

Nemeth, A., G. Hannesschläger, E. Leiss-Holzinger, K. Wiesauer, and M. Leitner. 2013. Optical coherence tomography—Applications in non-destructive testing and evaluation. In *Optical coherence tomography*, ed. M. Kawasaki, 163–185. Croatia: Intech Publishers.

Neuman, M., H.D. Sapirstein, E. Shwedyk, and W. Bushuk. 1989a. Wheat grain colour analysis by digital image processing I. Methodology. *Journal of Cereal Science* 10(3): 175–182.

Neuman, M., H.D. Sapirstein, E. Shwedyk, and W. Bushuk. 1989b. Wheat grain colour analysis by digital image processing II. Wheat class discrimination. *Journal of Cereal Science* 10(3): 182–183.

Newton Labs. 2013. Comparing line scan and area scan technologies. http://www.newtonlabs.com/line_systems.htm (accessed August 12, 2013).

Ng, E.Y.K. 2009. A review of thermography as promising non-invasive detection modality for breast cancer. *International Journal of Thermal Sciences* 48: 849–859.

Nguyen, T., T. Dresselaers, P. Verboven, G. D'hallewin, N. Culeddu, P. Van Hecke, and B. Nicolai. 2006. Finite element modelling and MRI validation of 3D transient water profiles in pears during postharvest storage. *Journal of the Science of Food and Agriculture* 86: 745–756.

Nicolaï, B.M., E. Lötze, A. Peirs, N. Scheerlinck, and K.I. Theron. 2006. Non-destructive measurement of bitter pit in apple fruit using NIR hyperspectral imaging. *Postharvest Biology and Technology* 40: 1–6.

Nikken, J.J., and G.P. Krestin. 2007. MRI of the kidney-state of the art. *European Radiology* 17: 2780–2793.

Nimesh, S., M.J. Delwiche, and R.S. Johnson. 1993. Image analysis methods for real time color grading of stone fruit. *Computers and Electronics in Agriculture* 9(1): 71–84.

Noh, H.K., and R. Lu. 2007. Hyperspectral laser-induced fluorescence imaging for assessing apple fruit quality. *Postharvest Biology and Technology* 43: 193–201.

Noordam, J.C., G.W. Otten, A.J.M. Timmermans, and B.V. Zwol. 2000. High speed potato grading and quality inspection based on a color vision system. *Proceedings of SPIE, Machine Vision Applications in Industrial Inspection VIII* 396: 206–220.

Norwegian Directorate of Health. 2009. World action on salt and health. Salt Action summary. http://www.worldactiononsalt.com/worldaction/europe/54014.html (accessed February 20, 2013).

Nott, K.P., S.D. Evans, and L.D. Hall. 1999a. Quantitative magnetic resonance imaging of fresh and frozen-thawed trout. *Magnetic Resonance Imaging* 17(3): 445–455.

Nott, K.P., S.D. Evans, and L.D. Hall. 1999b. The effect of freeze-thawing on the magnetic resonance imaging parameters of cod and mackerel. *LWT—Food Science and Technology* 32: 261–268.

OCS Checkweighers. 2013. X-ray scanners guarantee quality and product safety in dairies. http://www.dairyfoods.com/ext/resources/Case_Studies/AR-Mueller-Milch-en.pdf (accessed November 30, 2012).

Oerke, E.C., U. Steiner, H.W. Dehne, and M. Lindenthal. 2006. Thermal imaging of cucumber leaves affected by downy mildew and environmental conditions. *Journal of Experimental Botany* 57(9): 2121–2132.

Offermann, S., D. Bicanic, J.C. Krapez, D. Balageas, E. Gerkema, M. Chirtoc, M. Egee, K. Keijzer, and H. Jalink. 1998. Infrared transient thermography for noncontact, non-destructive inspection of whole and dissected apples and of cherry tomatoes at different maturity stages. *Instrumentation Science and Technology* 26(2–3): 145–155.

Ogawa, Y., N. Kondo, and S. Shibusawa. 2003. Inside quality evaluation of fruit by X-ray image. In *Proceedings of the IEEE/ASME International Conference on Advanced Intelligence Mechatronics*, 1360–1365, Kobe, Japan, July 20–24.

Ohali, Y.A. 2011. Computer vision based date fruit grading system: Design and implementation. *Journal of King Saud University—Computer and Information Sciences* 23: 29–36.

Ohno, Y., H. Koyama, M. Nogami, D. Takenaka, S. Matsumoto, M. Yoshimura, Y. Kotani, and K. Sugimura. 2007. Postoperative lung function in lung cancer patients: Comparative analysis of predictive capability of MRI, CT and SEPCT. *American Journal of Roentgenology* 189: 400–408.

Ohno, Y., H. Koyama, T. Yoshikawa, M. Nishio, S. Matsumoto, T. Iwasawa, and K. Sugimura. 2011. Pulmonary magnetic resonance imaging for airway diseases. *Journal of Thoracic Imaging* 26: 301–316.

Okada, Y., T. Kawamata, A. Kawashima, and T. Hori. 2007. Intraoperative application of thermography in extracranial-intracranial bypass surgery. *Operative Neurosurgery* 60(2): 362–365.

Okamoto, H., T. Murata, T. Kataoka, and S. Hata. 2007. Plant classification for weed detection using hyperspectral imaging with wavelet analysis. *Weed Biology and Management* 7(1): 31–37.

Okochi, T., Y. Hoshino, H. Fujii, and T. Mitsutani. 2007. Non-destructive tree ring measurements for Japanese oak and Japanese beech using micro-focus X-ray computed tomography. *Dendrochronologia* 24: 155–164.

Omid, M., M. Abbasgolipour, A. Keyhani, and S.S. Mohtasebi. 2010. Implementation of an efficient image processing algorithm for grading raisins. *International Journal of Signal and Image Processing* 1(1): 31–34.

Omron Electronics. 2004a. Automation trends. http://echannel.omron247.com:8085/marcom/pdf catal.nsf/PDFLookupByUniqueID/937455FFE865242986256E3800646772/$File/autotrens _FBpackagers_vision_2_04.pdf?OpenElement (accessed February 6, 2014).

Omron Electronics. 2004b. Packagers chose machine vision inspection to reduce waste and boost ROI. http://www.automation.com/library/articles-white-papers/vision-sensors-systems /packagers-choose-machine-vision-quality-inspection-to-reduce-waste-and-boost-roi (accessed January 16, 2014).

Osváth, S., and K. Szigeti. 2012. Novel X-ray imaging technology. *Port Technology International* 55: 126–127.

Otani, J., T. Mukunoki, Y. Obara, and K. Sugawara. 2000. Application of X-rays CT to soil and rock engineering. International Society of Rock Mechanics (ISRM) Symposium, Melbourne, Australia, November 19–24.

Otani, J., K. Pham, and J. Sano. 2006. Investigation of failure patterns in sand due to laterally loaded pile using X-ray CT. *Soils and Foundations* 46(4): 529–535.

Otani, J., Y. Watanabe, and B. Chevalier. 2010. Introduction of X-ray CT application in geotechnical engineering—Theory and practice. *IOP Conference Series: Material Science and Engineering* 10. http://dx.doi.org/10.1088/1757-899X/10/1/012089.

OuYang, A., R. Gao, Y. Liu, X. Sun, Y. Pan, and X. Dong. 2010. An automatic method for identifying different variety of rice seeds using machine vision technology. In *Sixth International Conference on Natural Computation*, 84–88.

Overbury, C. 2010. Application update: Machine vision saves fruit, by better sizing and sorting. *Control Engineering*, May. http://www.controleng.com/index.php?id=483&cHash=081010&tx _ttnews[tt_news]=38455 (accessed January 16, 2014).

Oztop, M.H., M. Rosenberg, Y. Rosenberg, K.L. McCarthy, and M.J. McCarthy. 2010. Magnetic resonance imaging (MRI) and relaxation spectrum analysis as methods to investigate swelling in
whey protein gels. *Journal of Food Science* 75(8): E508–E515.

Packaging Europe. 2009. Loma's advanced X4 X-ray inspection system guarantees the quality of
Germany's Brinkchen. http://www.packagingeurope.com/Packaging-Europe-News/32547
/Lomas-advanced-X4-Xray-inspection-system-guarantees-the-quality-of-Germanys
-Brinkchen.html (accessed November 20, 2012).

Paclík, P., R. Leitner, and R.P.W. Duin. 2006. A study on design of object sorting algorithms in the industrial applications using hyperspectral imaging. *Journal of Real-Time Image Processing* 1(1): 101–108.

PAEP (Pennsylvania Association of Environmental Professionals). 2014. Fluke thermography.
http://www.paep.org/p2e2/08/Fluke_Thermography_Presentation_Feb21.pdf   (accessed
February 6, 2014).

Paliwal, J., N.S. Shashidhar, and D.S. Jayas. 1999. Grain kernel identification using kernel signature.
Transactions of the ASAE 42(6): 1921–1924.

Paliwal. J., N.S. Visen, and D.S. Jayas. 2001. Evaluation of neural network architectures for cereal
grain classification using morphological features. *Journal of Agricultural Engineering Research*
79(4): 361–370.

Paliwal, J., N.S. Shashidhar, D.S. Jayas, and N.D.G. White. 2003. Comparison of a neural network and
a nonparametric classifier for grain kernel identification. *Biosystems Engineering* 85(4): 405–413.

Paliwal, J., D.S. Jayas, N.S. Visen, and N.D.G. White. 2005. Quantification of variations in machine
vision computed features of cereal grains. *Canadian Biosystems Engineering* 47: 7.1–7.6.

Palmieri, F., and U. Fiore. 2010. Network anomaly detection through nonlinear analysis. *Computers
and Security* 29: 737–755.

Panasyuk, S.V., S. Yang, D.V. Faller, D. Ngo, R.A. Lew, J.E. Freeman, and A.E. Rogers. 2007. Medical
hyperspectral imaging to facilitate residual tumor identification during surgery. *Cancer Biology
and Therapy* 6(3): 439–446.

Pandey, N., S. Krishna, and S. Sharma. 2013. Automatic seed classification by shape and color features using machine vision technology. *International Journal of Computer Applications Technology
and Research* 2(2): 208–213.

Pandharipande, S.L. 2004. *Artificial neural networks*. Nagpur: Central Techno Publications.

Parisky, Y.R., A. Sardi, R. Hamm, K. Hughes, L. Esserman, S. Rust, and K. Callahan. 2003. Efficacy
of computerized infrared imaging analysis to evaluate mammographically suspicious lesions.
American Journal of Roentgenology 180: 263–269.

Park, B., and Y. R. Chen. 2000. Real-time dual-wavelength image processing for poultry safety inspection. *Journal of Food Process Engineering* 23: 329–351.

Park, B., K.C. Lawrence, W.R. Windham, Y.R. Chen, and K. Chao. 2002. Discriminant analysis of
dual-wavelength spectral images for classifying poultry carcasses. *Computers and Electronics in
Agriculture* 33(3): 219–231.

Park, B., K.C. Lawrence, W.R. Windham, and D.P. Smith. 2006. Performance of hyperspectral imaging
system for poultry surface fecal contaminant detection. *Journal of Food Engineering* 75: 340–348.

Park, B., W.R. Windham, K.C. Lawrence, and D.P. Smith. 2007. Contaminant classification of poultry
hyperspectral imagery using a spectral angle mapper algorithm. *Biosystems Engineering* 96(3):
323–333.

Park, B., S. Yoo, W. Windham, K.C. Lawrence, G.W. Heitschmidt, M.S Kim, and K. Chao. 2010. Line-
scan hyperspectral imaging for real-time poultry fecal detection. *Proceeding of SPIE*, vol. 7676.

Parkin, D.M., F. Bray, J. Ferlay, and P. Pisani. 2005. Global cancer statistics, 2002. *CA: A Cancer Journal
for Clinicians* 55(2): 74–108.

Parrish, E., and A.K. Goksel. 1977. Pictorial pattern recognition applied to fruit harvesting. *Transactions
of ASAE* 20: 822–827.

Pascall, M.A., S. Ravishankar, K. Ghiron, B.T. Lee, and J.N. Johannessen. 2006. Evaluation of magnetic resonance for detection of bacterial contamination in low-acid, shelf stable packaged soy-
milk. *Journal of Food Protection* 69(7): 1668–1674.

Patel, V.C., R.W. McClendon, and J.W. Goodrum. 1998. Color computer vision and artificial neural
networks for the detection of defects in poultry eggs. *Artificial Intelligence Review* 12: 163–176.

Patil, N.K., V.S. Malemath, and R.M. Yadahalli. 2011. Color and texture based identification and classification of food grains using different color models and Haralick features. *International Journal on Computer Science and Engineering* 3(12): 3669–3680.

Pearce, K., G. Gardner, M. Ferguson, and D. Pethick. 2009. Dual X-ray absorptiometry accurately predicts carcass composition from live sheep and chemical composition of live and dead sheep. *Meat Science* 81(1): 285–293.

Pearce, R.S., and M. Fuller. 2001. Freezing of barley studied by infrared video thermography. *Plant Physiology*, 125: 227–240.

Peariso, D. 2008. X-ray examination of foods for foreign materials. In *Preventing foreign material contamination of foods*. Hoboken, NJ: Wiley-Blackwell.

Pernkopf, F., and P. O'Leary. 2003. Image acquisition techniques for automatic visual inspection of metallic surfaces. *NDT&E International* 36: 609–617.

Picón, A., O. Ghita, A. Bereciartua, J. Echazarra, P.F. Whelan, and P.M. Iriondo. 2012. Real-time hyperspectral processing for automatic non-ferrous material sorting. *Journal of Electronic Imaging* 21(1): 1–8.

Pinto, J. 2013. The future of industrial automation. Automation.com. http://www.automation.com /library/articles-white-papers/articles-by-jim-pinto/the-future-of-industrial-automation (accessed February 8, 2014).

Piotrowski, J., and A. Rogalski. 2004. Uncooled long wavelength infrared photon detectors. *Infrared Physics and Technology* 46: 115–131.

Pithadiya, K.J., C.K. Modi, and J.D. Chauhan. 2009. Comparison of optimal edge detection algorithms for liquid level inspection in bottles. In *Proceedings of Second International Conference on Emerging Trends in Engineering and Technology*, 447–452.

Plá, F., F. Juste, and F. Ferri. 1993. Feature extraction of spherical objects in image analysis: An application to robotic citrus harvesting. *Computers and Electronics in Agriculture* 8: 57–72.

Pla-Rucki, G.F., and M.O. Eberhard. 1995. Imaging of reinforced concrete: State of the art review. *Journal of Infrastructure Systems* 1: 134–141.

Plaza, A., P. Martínez, J. Plaza, and R. Pérez. 2005. Dimensionality reduction and classification of hyperspectral image data using sequences of extended morphological transformations. *IEEE Transactions on Geoscience and Remote Sensing*, 43(3): 466–479.

Podoleanu, A.G., J.A. Rogers, D.A. Jackson, and S. Dunne. 2000. Three dimensional OCT images from retina and skin. *Optics Express* 7: 292–298.

Poland, T.M., R.A. Haack, and T.R. Petrice. 1998. Chicago joins New York in battle with the Asian longhorned beetle. *Newsletter of the Michigan Entomological Society* 43(4): 15–17.

Posadas, D.A.N., A. Tannús, H. Panepucci, and S. Crestana. 1996. Magnetic resonance imaging as a non-invasive technique for investigating 3-D preferential flow occurring within stratified soil samples. *Computers and Electronics in Agriculture* 14: 255–267.

Postma, A.P., P.A. Hofman, A.A.R. Stadler, R.J. van Oostenbrugge, M.P.M. Tijssen, and J.E. Wildberger. 2012. Dual-energy CT of the brain and intracranial vessels. *American Journal of Roentgenology* 199: S26–S33.

Pouladzadeh, P., G. Villalobos, R. Almaghrabi, and S. Shirmohammadi. 2012. A novel SVM based food recognition method for calorie measurement applications. In *IEEE International Conference on Multimedia and Expo Workshops*, 495–498.

Pouvreau, S., M. Rambeau, J.C. Cochard, and R. Robert. 2006. Investigation of marine bivalve morphology by in vivo MR imaging: First anatomical results of a promising technique. *Aquaculture* 259: 415–423.

Prabuwono, A.S., R. Sulaiman, A.R. Hamdan, and A. Hasniaty. 2006. Development of intelligent visual inspection system (IVIS) for bottling machine. *Proceedings of IEEE TENCON*, November 14–17, Hongkong, China.

Pronost, N. 2013. Segmentation. In *Introduction to image processing*, Chap. 10. http://www.cs.uu.nl /docs/vakken/ibv/reader/chapter10.pdf (accessed October 10, 2013).

Prykäri, T., J. Czajkowski, E. Alarousu, and R. Myllylä. 2010. Optical coherence tomography as an accurate inspection and quality evaluation technique in paper industry. *Optical Review* 17(3): 218–222.

Pu, J., S. Gu, S. Liu, S. Zhu, D. Wilson, J.M. Siegfried, and D. Gur. 2012. CT based computerized identification and analysis of human airways: A review. *American Association of Physicists in Medicine,* 39(5): 2603–2616.

Puchalski, C., J. Gorzelany, G. Zagula, and G. Brusewitz. 2008. Image analysis for apple defect detection. *TEKA Komisji Motoryzacji Energetki Rolnictwa,* 8: 197–205.

Pydipati, R., T.F. Burks, and W.S. Lee. 2005. Statistical and neural network classifiers for citrus disease detection using machine vision. *Transactions of ASAE* 48(5): 2004–2014.

Qiao, J., M.O. Ngadi, N. Wang, C. Gariepy, and S.O. Prasher. 2007. Pork quality and marbling level assessment using a hyperspectral imaging system. *Journal of Food Engineering* 83: 10–16.

Qin, J. 2010. Hyperspectral imaging instruments. In *Hyperspectral imaging for food quality analysis and control,* ed. D.W. Sun, 129–172. San Diego: Academic Press.

Qin, J., and R. Lu. 2005. Detection of pits in tart cherries by hyperspectral transmission imaging. *Transactions of ASAE* 48(5): 1963–1970.

Qin, J., T.F. Burks, D.G. Kim, and D.M. Bulanon. 2008. Classification of citrus peel diseases using color texture feature analysis. Proceedings of Food Processing Automation Conference, Providence, Rhode Island, June 28–29, 2008.

Rabatel, G. 1988. A vision system for Magali, the fruit picking robot. International Conference on Agricultural Engineering, AGENG88 Paper 88293, March 2–6, Paris, France.

Radiological Society of North America. 2012. Computed Tomography (CT)-Body. http://www.radio logyinfo.org/en/info.cfm?pg=bodyct.

Rahkonen, J., and H. Jokela. 2003. Infrared radiometry for measuring plant leaf temperature during thermal weed control treatment. *Biosystems Engineering* 86(3): 257–266.

Ramos-Cabrer, P., J.P.M. Van Duynhoven, H. Timmer, and K. Nicolay. 2006. Monitoring of moisture redistribution in multicomponent food systems by use of magnetic resonance imaging. *Journal of Agricultural and Food Chemistry* 54: 672–677.

Randeberg, L.L., E.L. Larsen, and L.O. Svaasand. 2010. Characterization of vascular structures and skin bruises using hyperspectral imaging, image analysis and diffusion theory. *Journal of Biophotonics* 3(1–2): 53–65.

Rangamani, S., J. Varghese, L. Li, L. Harvey, J.M. Hammel, S.E. Fletcher, K.F. Duncan, D.A. Danford, and S. Kutty. 2012. Safety of cardiac magnetic resonance and contrast angiography for neonates and small infants: A 10-year single-institution experience. *Pediatric Radiology* 42: 1339–1346.

Rao, A.R. 1996. Future directions in industrial machine vision: A case study of semiconductor manufacturing applications. *Image and Vision Computing* 14: 3–19.

Rao, D.S.P. 2008. Infrared thermography and its applications in civil engineering. *The Indian Concrete Journal:* 41–50.

Rao, P.S., and S. Renganathan. 2002. New approaches for size determination of apple fruits for automatic sorting and grading. *Iranian Journal of Electrical and Computer Engineering* 1(2): 90–97.

Rashidi, M., M. Gholami, and S. Abbassi. 2009. Cantaloupe volume determination through image processing. *Journal of Agricultural Science and Technology* 11: 623–631.

Rashmi, S., and S. Mandar. 2011. Textural feature based image classification using neural network. In *International Conference on Advances in Computing, Communication, and Control Communications in Computer and Information Science,* eds. S. Unnikrishnan, S. Surve, and D. Bhoir, 125: 62–69.

Ravipati, G., W.S. Aronow, H. Lai, J. Shao, A.J. DeLuca, M.B. Weiss, A.L. Pucillo, K. Kalapatapu, C.E. Monsen, and R.N. Belkin. 2008. Comparison of sensitivity, specificity, positive predictive value, and negative predictive value of stress testing versus 64-multislice coronary computed tomography angiography in predicting obstructive coronary artery disease diagnosed by coronary angiography. *American Journal of Cardiology* 101(6): 774–775.

Reiss, S.M. 2011. Funding for OCT: Technologies, applications and businesses. *BioOptics World:* 4(2).

Rekha, P.N., R. Gangadharan, S.M. Pillai, G. Ramanathan, and A. Panigrahi. 2012. Hyperspectral image processing to detect the soil salinity in coastal watershed. IEEE—Fourth International Conference on Advanced Computing, Chennai, India, December 13–15.

Renfu, L. 2013. New apple harvesting system being developed. *Fruit Growers News,* June. http:// fruitgrowersnews.com/index.php/efgn/entry/new-apple-harvesting-system-being-devel oped-efgn-june-2013 (accessed January 16, 2014).

Renou, J.P., L. Foucat, and J.M. Bonny. 2003. Magnetic resonance imaging studies of water interactions in meat. *Food Chemistry* 82: 35–39.

Research Computing. 2005. Overview of geometric transformations. http://northstar-www.dartmouth.edu/doc/idl/html_6.2/Overview_of_Geometric_Transformations.html (accessed October 7, 2013).

Reynolds, P. 2011. Orval Kent assures food safety with X-ray inspection system. *Packaging World*. http://www.packworld.com/machinery/inspection/orval-kent-assures-food-safety-x-ray-inspection (accessed November 20, 2012).

Ring, E.F.J., and K. Ammer. 2012. Infrared thermal imaging in medicine. *Physiological Measurement* 33: 33–46.

Rios-Cabrera, R., I. Lopez-Juarez, and H. Sheng-Jen. 2008. ANN analysis in a vision approach for potato inspection. *Journal of Applied Research and Technology* 6(2): 106–119.

Ritman, E.L. 2011. Current status of developments and applications of micro-CT. *Annual Review of Biomedical Engineering* 13: 531–552.

Rocha, A., D.C. Hauagge, J. Wainer, and S. Goldenstein. 2010. Automatic fruit and vegetable classification from images. *Journal of Computer and Electronics in Agriculture* 70(1): 96–104.

Rodionova, O.Y., L.P. Houmøller, A.L. Pomerantsev, P. Geladi, J. Burger, V.L. Dorofeyev, and A.P. Arzamastsev. 2005. NIR spectrometry for counterfeit drug detection: A feasibility study. *Analytica Chimica Acta* 549: 151–158.

Rodríguez-Pulido, F.J., D.F. Barbin, D. Sun, B. Gordillo, M.L. González-Miret, and F.J. Heredia. 2013. Grape seed characterization by NIR hyperspectral imaging. *Postharvest Biology and Technology* 76: 74–82.

Rogalski, A. 2012. History of infrared detectors. *Opto-Electronics Review* 20(3): 279–308.

Rogasik, H., I. Onasch, J. Brunotte, D. Jegou, and O. Wendroth. 2003. Assessment of soil structure using X-ray computed tomography. In *Applications of X-ray computed tomography in geosciences*, ed. F. Mees, R. Swennen, M. Van Geet, and P. Jacobs, 151–166. London: The Geological Society.

Rogers, J.D. 2000. Measurement of dimensional changes and movements in engineering components using X-ray radiographic imaging. *Measurement Science and Technology* 11: 857–864.

Roig F.A., A. Calderón, N. Naves, A. Somoza, C.S. Lisi, and M.T. Fo. 2008. Poplar wood density assessed by X-ray densitometry: New insights for inferring wood quality. Proceedings of the 51st International Convention of Society of Wood Science and Technology, Concepción, Chile, November 10–12.

Roli, F., G. Giacinto, and G. Vernazza. 1997. Comparison and combination of statistical and artificial neural network. In *Neurocomputation in remote sensing data analysis*, ed. I. Kanellopoulos, G. Wilkinson, F. Roli, and J. Austin, 117–124. Berlin: Springer.

Romvári, R., C.S. Hancz, Z.S. Petrási, T. Molnár, and P. Horn. 2002. Non-invasive measurement of fillet composition of four freshwater fish species by computer tomography. *Aquaculture International* 10: 231–240.

Rosenblatt, R. 1962. *Principles of neurodynamics*. New York: Spartan Books.

Ruan, R., and J.B. Litchfield. 1992. Determination of water distribution and mobility inside maize kernels during steeping using magnetic resonance imaging. *Cereal Chemistry* 69(1): 13–17.

Ruan, R., S.J. Schmidt, A.R. Schmidt, and J.B. Litchfield. 1991. Nondestructuive measurement of moisture profiles and moisture diffusion coefficient in potato during drying and absorption by NMR imaging. *Journal of Food Process Engineering* 14: 297–313.

Rumelhart, D.E., G.E. Hinton, and R.J. Williams. 1986. Learning internal representation by error propagation. In *Parallel distributed processing: Exploration in the microstructure of cognition*, ed. D.E. Rumelhart and J.L. McClleland, vol. 1. Cambridge: MIT Press.

Russ, J.C. 1999. *The image processing handbook*, 3rd edition. Boca Raton, FL: CRC Press.

Rye, M. 1991. Prediction of carcass composition in Atlantic salmon by computerized tomography. *Aquaculture* 99: 35–48.

Sahoo, P.K., S. Soltani, and A.K.C. Wong. 1988. A survey of thresholding techniques. *Computer Vision, Graphics, and Image Processing* 41(2): 233–260.

Salas-Bringas, C., W.K. Jeksrud, O.I. Lekang, and R.B. Schüller. 2007. Noncontact temperature monitoring of a pelleting process using infrared thermography. *Journal of Food Process Engineering* 30(1): 24–37.

Saleh, S.A., and A.K. Aboulsoud. 2002. A general overview of solid states imaging sensor types. In *Proceedings of Third Workshop on Photonics and Its Application at Egyptian Engineering Faculties and Institutes*, 1–10.

Sánchez, A.J., W. Albarracin, R. Grau, C. Ricolfe, and J.M. Barat. 2008. Control of ham salting by using image segmentation. *Food Control* 19: 135–142.

Sander, T., H.H. Gerke, and H. Rogasik. 2008. Assessment of Chinese paddy-soil structure using X-ray computed tomography. *Geoderma* 145: 303–314.

Sandhu, D. 2013. Image segmentation based methodology for classification of various seed varieties. *International Journal of Research in Engineering and Advanced Technology* 1(2): 1–5.

Sankaran, S., J.M. Maja, S. Buchanon, and R. Ehsani. 2013. Huanglongbing (citrus greening) detection using visible, near infrared and thermal imaging techniques. *Sensors* 13: 2117–2130.

Sapirstein, H.D., and J.M. Kohler. 1995. Physical uniformity of graded railcar and vessel shipments of Canada Western Red Spring wheat determined by digital image analysis. *Canadian Journal of Plant Science* 75(2): 363–369.

Sapozhnikova, V.V., V.A. Kamenskii, and R.V. Kuranov. 2003. Visualization of plant tissues by optical coherence tomography. *Russian Journal of Plant Physiology* 50(2): 282–286.

Sapozhnikova, V.V., V.A. Kamenskii, R.V. Kuranov, I. Kutis, L.B. Snopova, and A.V. Myakov. 2004. In vivo visualization of *Tradescantia* leaf tissue and monitoring the physiological and morphological states under different water supply conditions using optical coherence tomography. *Planta* 219: 601–609.

Sasaki, K., H. Badarinarayan, T. Hori, and S. Oho. 2006. Study of micro-defects in aluminum casting using X-ray computed tomography. In *Simulation of aluminum shape casting processing: From alloy design to mechanical properties*, ed. W. Qigui, J.M.K. Matthew, and D.L. Peter. New Jersey: Wiley John & Sons.

Satti, V., A. Satya, and S. Sharma. 2013. An automatic leaf recognition system for plant identification using machine vision technology. *International Journal of Engineering Science and Technology* 5(4): 874–879.

Savakar, D. 2012. Identification and classification of bulk fruit images using artificial neural networks. *International Journal of Engineering an Innovative Technology* 1(3): 36–40.

Savakar, D.G., and B.S. Anami. 2009. Recognition and classification of food grains, fruits and flowers using machine vision. *International Journal of Food Engineering* 5(4), doi: 10.2202/1556-3758.1673.

Savnik, A., H. Malmskov, H.S. Thomsen, T. Bretlau. L.B. Graff, H. Nielsen, B. Danneskiold-Samsøe, J. Boesen, and H. Bliddal. 2001. MRI of the arthritic small joints: Comparison of extremity MRI (0.2 T) vs high-field MRI (1.5T). *European Radiology* 11: 1030–1038.

Saxena, A.K., and G.H. Willital. 2008. Infrared thermography: Experience from a decade of pediatric imaging. *European Journal of Pediatrics* 167: 757–764.

Sayinci, B., S. Ercisli, I. Ozturk, Z. Eryilmaz, and B. Demir. 2012. Determination of size and shape in the "Moro" blood orange and "Valencia" sweet orange cultivar and its mutants using image processing. *Notulae Botanicae Horti Agrobotanici* 40(1): 234–242.

Schaefer, A.L., S.D.M. Jones, A.C. Murray, A.P. Sather, and A.K.W. Tong. 1989. Infrared thermography of pigs with known genotypes for stress susceptibility in relation to pork quality. *Canadian Journal of Animal Science* 69: 491–495.

Schalkoff, R.J. 1997. *Artificial neural networks*. New York: McGraw-Hill.

Schatzki, T.F., and T.A. Fine. 1988. Analysis of radiograms of wheat kernels for quality control. *Cereal Chemistry* 65(3): 233–239.

Schatzki, T.F., R.P. Haff, R. Young, I. Can, L.C. Le, and N. Toyofuku. 1997. Defect detection in apples by means of X-ray imaging. *Transactions of ASAE* 40(5): 1407–1415.

Schenz, T.W., B. Dauber, C. Nicholls, C. Gardner, V.A. Scott, S.P. Roberts, and M.J. Hennesy. 1999. Online MR imaging for detection of spoilage in finished packages. *Food Science and Technology* 13(2): 92–96.

Schmermund, A., J. Rodermann, and R. Erbel. 2003. Intracoronary thermography. *Herz* 28(6): 505–512.

Schmoldt, D.L., P. Li, and A.L. Abbott. 1997. Machine vision using artificial neural networks with local 3D neighborhoods. *Computers and Electronics in Agriculture* 16: 255–271.

Schuman, J.S. 2012. Introduction to optical coherence tomography. FDA AGS Workshop, Pittsburgh, Pennsylvania, October 5.

Schumann, A. 1997. Neural networks versus statistics—A comparing study of their classification performance on well log data. In *Proceedings of 3rd Annual Conference on International Association for Mathematical Geology—IAMG'97*, 237–241.

Scott, R. 2013. Advantages of real time X-ray systems vs. automated in line X-ray systems. Total Quality Corporation, September 18. http://totalqualitycorp.com/advantages-of-real-time-x-ray-systems-vs-automated-in-line-x-ray-systems/ (accessed November 5, 2012).

Secca, M.F. 2006. Basic principles of MRI and F-MRI in neurosciences. Pan Arab NeuroRadiology Society, Beirut, Lebanon. http://www.panrs.org/doc/syllabus/ch1part1.pdf (accessed April 29, 2013).

Seetha, M., I.V. Muralikrishna, B.L. Deekshatulu, B.L. Malleswari, and N.P. Hegde. 2008. Artificial neural networks and other methods of image classification. *Journal of Theoretical and Applied Information Technology* 4(11): 1039–1053.

Segnini, S., P. Dejmek, and R. Öste. 1999. A low cost video technique for color measurement of potato chips. *LWT–Food Science and Technology* 32: 216–222.

Segtnan, V.H., M. Høy, O. Sørheim, A. Kohler, F. Lundby, J.P. Wold, and R. Ofstad. 2009. Non-contact salt and fat distributional analysis in salted and smoked salmon fillets using X-ray computed tomography and NIR interactance imaging. *Journal of Agricultural Food Chemistry* 57: 1705–1710.

Sela, E., Y. Cohen, V. Alchanatis, Y. Saranga, S. Cohen, M. Möller, M. Meron, A. Bosak, J. Tsipris, and V. Orolov. 2007. Thermal imaging for estimating and mapping crop water stress in cotton. In European Conference in Precision Agriculture, ed. J.V. Stafford, 365–371. The Netherlands: Wageningen Academic Publications.

Seng, W.C., and S.H. Mirisaee. 2009. A new method for fruits recognition system. International Conference on Electrical Engineering and Informatics (ICEEE), August 5–7, Selangor, Malaysia.

Serranti, S., A. Gargiulo, and G. Bonifazi. 2010. The utilization of hyperspectral imaging for impurities detection in secondary plastics. *The Open Waste Management Journal* 3: 56–70.

Serranti, S., D. Cesare, and G. Bonifazi. 2013. The development of a hyperspectral imaging method for the detection of *Fusarium*-damaged, yellow berry and vitreous Italian durum wheat kernels. *Biosystems Engineering* 115: 20–30.

Shahin, M.A., and E.W. Tollner. 1997. Apple classification based on watercore features using fuzzy logic. ASAE Paper No. 973077, St. Joseph, Michigan.

Shahin, M.A., and S.J. Symons. 2001. A machine vision system for grading lentils. *Canadian Biosystems Engineering* 43: 7.7–7.14.

Shahin, M.A., and S.J. Symons. 2012. Detection of fusarium damage in Canadian wheat using visible /near-infrared hyperspectral imaging. *Food Measurement* 6: 3–11.

Shahin, M.A., E.W. Tollner, R.D. Gitaitis, D.R. Sumner, and B.W. Maw. 2002. Classification of sweet onions based on internal defects using image processing and neural network techniques. *Transactions of ASABE* 45(5): 1613–1618.

Sharaf, M., D. Illman, and B. Kowalski. 1986. *Chemometrics*, 228. New York: Wiley.

Sharma, N., and L.M. Aggarwal. 2010. Automated medical image segmentation techniques. *Journal of Medical Physics* 35(1): 3–14.

Sharma, A., and A. Arbab-Zadeh. 2012. Assessment of coronary heart disease by CT angiography: Current and evolving applications. *Journal of Nuclear Cardiology* 19: 796–806.

Shedlock, D., T. Edwards, and C. Toh. 2011. X-ray backscatter imaging for aerospace applications. In *American Institute of Physics Conference Proceedings* 1335, 509–516. http://dx.doi.org/10.1063/1.3591894.

Shen, H., S. Li, D. Gu, and H. Chang. 2012. Bearing defect inspection based on machine vision. *Measurement* 45: 719–733.

Sherrod, P.H. 2003. Software for predictive modelling. http://www.dtreg.com/rbf.htm (accessed October 15, 2013).

Shinke, T., and J. Shite. 2010. Evaluation of stent placement and outcomes with optical coherence tomography. *Interventional Cardiology* 2(4): 535–543.

Shiranita, K., T. Miyajima, and R. Takiyama. 1998. Determination of meat quality by texture analysis. *Pattern Recognition Letters* 19: 1319–1324.

Shiranita, K., K. Hayashi, A. Otsubo, T. Miyajima, and R. Takiyama. 2000. Grading meat quality by image processing. *Pattern Recognition* 33: 97–104.

Shouche, S.P., R. Rastogi, S.G. Bhagwat, and J.K. Sainis. 2001. Shape analysis of grains of Indian wheat varieties. *Computers and Electronics in Agriculture* 33: 55–76.

Siciliano, D., K. Wasson, D. Potts, and R.C. Olsen. 2008. Evaluating hyperspectral imaging of wetland vegetation as a tool for detecting estuarine nutrient enrichment. *Remote Sensing of Environment* 112: 4020–4033.

Siddiqi, A.M., H. Li, F. Faruque, W. Williams, K. Lai, M. Hughson, S. Bigler, J. Beach, and W. Johnson. 2008. Use of hyperspectral imaging to distinguish normal, precancerous, and cancerous cells. *Cancer* 114: 13–21.

Siemens. 2011. Radiography: Plain X-rays. http://www.medicalradiation.com/types-of-medical -imaging/imaging-using-x-rays/radiography-plain-x-rays/ (accessed June 6, 2013).

Silva, C.S., and U. Sonnadara. 2013. Classification of rice grains using neural networks. In *Proceedings of Technical Sessions of Institute of Physics* 29: 9–14.

Silvén, O., and H. Kauppinen. 1994. Color vision based methodology for grading lumber. Proceedings of 12th International Conference on Pattern Recognition, vol. 1, October 9–13, Jerusalem, Israel.

Simonton, W., and D. Graham. 1996. Bayesian and fuzzy logic classification for plant structure analysis. *Applied Engineering in Agriculture* 12(1): 89–97.

Simpson, P.K. 1990. *Artificial neural systems: Foundations, paradigms, applications, and implementations.* New York: Pergamon Press.

Singh, C.B. 2009. Detection of insect and fungal damage and incidence of sprouting in stored wheat using near infrared hyperspectral and digital color imaging. Ph.D. dissertation, University of Manitoba, Winnipeg.

Singh, C.B., D.S. Jayas, J. Paliwal, and N.D.G. White. 2009a. Detection of sprouted and midge-damaged wheat kernels using near-infrared hyperspectral imaging. *Cereal Chemistry* 86(3): 256–260.

Singh, C.B., D.S. Jayas, J. Paliwal, and N.D.G. White. 2009b. Detection of insect-damaged wheat kernels using near-infrared hyperspectral imaging. *Journal of Stored Products Research* 45: 151–158.

Singh, C.B., D.S. Jayas, J. Paliwal, and N.D.G. White. 2012. Fungal damage detection in wheat using short wave near-infrared hyperspectral and digital color imaging. *International Journal of Food Properties* 15(1): 11–24.

Singh, J., and M. Kaur. 2012. Visual inspection of bakery products by texture analysis using image processing techniques. *IOSR Journal of Engineering* 2(4): 526–528.

Siripatrawan, U., Y. Makino, Y. Kawagoe, and S. Oshita. 2011. Rapid detection of *Escherichia coli* contamination in packaged fresh spinach using hyperspectral imaging. *Talanta* 85: 276–281.

Sites, P.W., and M.J. Dewilche. 1988. Computer vision to locate fruit on a tree. *Transactions of ASAE* 31(1): 257–263.

Sivanandam, S., M. Anburajan, R. Venkatraman, M. Menaka, and D. Sharath. 2012. Medical thermography: A diagnostic approach for type 2 diabetes based on non-contact infrared thermal imaging. *Endocrine* 42(2): 343–351.

Sivertsen, A.H., K. Heia, K. Hindberg, and F. Godtliebsen. 2012. Automatic nematode detection in cod fillets, *Gadus morhua* (L.) by hyperspectral imaging. *Journal of Food Engineering* 111: 675–681.

Skala, K., T. Lipić, I. Sović, L. Gjenero, and I. Grubišić. 2011. 4D thermal imaging system for medical applications. *Periodicum Biologorum* 13(4): 407–416.

Smart Vision Works. 2011. Automatic date sorting system. http://www.smartvisionworks.com/dates .php (accessed January 27, 2014).

Smith, D. 1999. Bones in boneless broiler breast meat is a legitimate concern. *World Poultry* 15(4): 35–36.

Smith, P.T., and N. Reddy. 2012. Application of magnetic resonance imaging (MRI) to study the anatomy and reproductive condition of live Sydney rock oyster, *Saccostrea glomerata* (Gould). *Aquaculture* 334–337: 191–198.

Sofradir EC Inc. 2013. Uncooled infrared detectors achieve high performance levels and cost targets. http://www.sofradir-ec.com/wp-uncooled-detectors-achieve.asp.

Sohaib, M., I. Haq, and Q. Mushtaq. 2012. Dimensionality reduction of hyperspectral image data using band clustering and selection through K-Means based on statistical characteristics of band images. *International Journal of Advanced Computer Science* 2(4): 146–151.

Somatilake, S., and A.N. Chalmers. 2007. An image based food classification system. In *Proceedings of Image and Vision Computing*, 260–265.

Sonego, L., R. Ben-Arie, J. Raynal, and J.C. Pech. 1995. Biochemical and physical evaluation of textural characteristics of nectarines exhibiting woolly breakdown: NMR imaging, X-ray computed tomography and pectin composition. *Postharvest Biology and Technology* 5: 187–198.

Song, H., and J.B. Litchfield. 1990. Nuclear magnetic resonance imaging of transient three-dimensional moisture distribution in an ear of corn during drying. *Cereal Chemistry* 67(6): 580–584.

Song, H.P., S.R. Delwiche, and M.J. Line. 1998. Moisture distribution in a mature soft wheat grain by three-dimensional magnetic resonance imaging. *Journal of Cereal Science* 27: 191–197.

Song, X., S. Jiang, S. Wang, J. Tang, and Q. Huang. 2013. Cross concept local Fisher discriminant analysis for image classification. In *Advances in Multimedia Modeling, 19th International Conference,* 407–416.

Space Computer Corporation. 2007. An introduction to hyperspectral imaging technology. http:// cant.ua.ac.be/sites/cant.ua.ac.be/files/courses/oe/Introduction_to_HSI_Technology.pdf.

Specht, D.F. 1990. Probabilistic neural networks. *Neural Networks* 3: 109–118.

Specht, D.F. 1991. A general regression neural network. *IEEE Transactions on Neural Networks* 2(6): 568–576.

Sperber, B. 2012. Justifying an automated vision inspection investment. Packaging World. http:// www.packworld.com/machinery/inspection/justifying-automated-vision-inspection-invest ment (accessed February 6, 2014).

Spinner, J. 2013. Traceability fuels $2 bn machine vision market. FoodProductiondaily.com. http:// www.foodproductiondaily.com/Packaging/Traceability-fuels-2bn-machine-vision-market (accessed February 6, 2014).

Sprawls, P. 1995. *Physical principle of medical imaging.* Madison, WI: Medical Physics Publishing.

Sprawls, P. 2000a. The imaging process. In *Magnetic resonance imaging: Principles, methods and techniques.* Madison, WI: Medical Physics Publishing.

Sprawls, P. 2000b. Magnetic resonance imaging system components. In *Magnetic resonance imaging: Principles, methods and techniques.* Madison, WI: Medical Physics Publishing.

Sprovieri, J. 2010. Machine vision: Trouble shooting vision systems. *Assembly Magazine.* http://www .assemblymag.com/articles/88697 (accessed February 6, 2014).

Stajnko, D., M. Lakota, M. Hočevar, and Z. Čmelik. 2003. Application of thermal imaging for estimating current yield in the apple orchard. *Die Bodenkultur,* 54(3): 171–180.

Stajnko, D., M. Lakota and M. Hocevar. 2004. Estimation of number and diameter of apple fruits in an orchard during the growing season by thermal imaging. *Computer and Electronics in Agriculture* 42(1): 31–42.

Stapley, A.G.F., T.M. Hyde, L.F. Gladden, and P.J. Fryer. 1997. NMR imaging of wheat grain cooking process. *International Journal of Food Science and Technology* 32: 355–375.

StatSoft, Inc., 2013. Electronic statistics textbook. http://www.statsoft.com/textbook/k-nearest -neighbors (accessed November 2, 2013).

Steckner, M.C. 2006. Advances in MRI equipment design, software, and imaging procedures. Hitachi Medical Systems America Inc., Orlando, Florida. http://www.aapm.org/meetings/amos2/pdf /26-5961-46702-744.pdf (accessed April 28, 2013).

Stemmer Imaging Ltd. 2013. Quality right down the line. http://www.stemmer-imaging.co.uk/en /technical+tips/1100-Line-scan-cameras (accessed August 10, 2012).

Stifter, D. 2007. Beyond biomedicine: A review of alternative applications and developments for optical coherence tomography. *Applied Physics* B88: 337–357.

Stoll, M., and H. Jones. 2007. Thermal imaging as a viable tool for monitoring plant stress. *International Journal of Vine and Wine Sciences* 41(2): 77–84.

Stoll, M., H.R. Schultz, and B. Berkelmann-Loehnertz. 2008. Exploring the sensitivity of thermal imaging for *Plasmopara viticola* pathogen detection in grapevines under different water status. *Functional Plant Biology* 35: 281–288.

Strachan, N.J.C. 1993. Length measurement of fish by computer vision. *Computers and Electronics in Agriculture* 8: 93–104.

Stuppy, W.H., J.A. Maisano, M.W. Colbert, P.J. Rudall, and T.B. Rowe. 2003. Three-dimensional analysis of plant structure using high-resolution X-ray computed tomography. *Trends in Plant Science* 8(1): 2–6.

Subash, H.M., and R.K. Wang. 2013. Optical coherence tomography: Technical aspect. In *Biomedical and optical imaging technologies*, ed. R. Linag. Boca Raton, FL: Taylor & Francis.

Subramanyam, H., S. Krishnamurthy, S. Subhadra, V.B. Dalal, G.S. Randhawa, and E.K. Chacko. 1971. Studies on internal breakdown, a physiological ripening disorder in Alphonso mangoes (*Mangifera indica* L.). *Tropical Science* 13: 203–210.

Sugiura, R., N. Noguchi, and K. Ishii. 2007. Correction of low-altitude thermal images applied to estimating soil water status. *Biosystems Engineering* 96(3): 301–313.

Sun, D., and C. Du. 2004. Segmentation of complex food images by stick growing and merging algorithm. *Journal of Food Engineering* 61: 17–26.

Sun, G., S.J. Hoff, B.C. Zelle, and M.A. Nelson. 2008. Development and comparison of back propagation and generalized regression neural network models to predict diurnal and seasonal gas and PM_{10} concentrations and emissions from swine buildings. *Transactions of ASAE* 51(2): 685–694.

Sun, T., C. Tseng, and M. Chen. 2010. Electric contacts inspection using machine vision. *Image and Vision Computing* 28: 890–901.

Suresha, M., N.A. Shilpa, and B. Sowmya. 2012. Apples grading based on SVM classifier. *International Journal of Computer Applications*, 27–30.

Suresh, A. and K.L. Shumnmuganathan. 2012. Feature fusion technique for colour texture classification system based on gray level co-occurrence matrix. *Journal of Computer Science* 8(12): 2106–2111.

Suzuki, Y., H. Okamoto, M. Takahashi, T. Kataoka, and Y. Shibata. 2012. Mapping the spatial distribution of botanical composition and herbage mass in pastures using hyperspectral imaging. *Japanese Society of Grassland Science* 58: 1–7.

Swanson, E.A., M.R. Hee, G.J. Tearney, and J.G. Fujimoto. 1996. Application of optical coherence tomography in non-destructive evaluation of material microstructure. *Summaries of Papers Presented at the Conference on Lasers and Electro-Optics, 1996*, 326–327.

Swennen, Q., G.P.J. Janssens, R. Geers, E. Decuypere, and J. Buyse. 2004. Validation of dual energy X-ray absorptiometry for determining in-vivo body composition of chickens. *Poultry Science* 83: 1348–1357.

Szabo, C.S., L. Babinsky, M.W.A. Verstegen, O. Vangen, A.J.M. Jansman, and E. Kanis. 1999. The application of digital imaging techniques in the in vivo estimation of the body composition of pigs: A review. *Livestock Production Science* 60 1–11.

Takeuchi, S., M. Fukuoka, Y. Gomi, M. Maeda, and H. Watanabe. 1997. An application of magnetic resonance imaging to the real time measurement of the change of moisture profile in a rice grain during boiling. *Journal of Food Engineering* 33: 181–192.

Tallada, J.G., D.T. Wicklow, T.C. Pearson, and P.R. Armstrong, 2011. Detection of fungus-infected corn kernels using near-infrared reflectance spectroscopy and color imaging. *Transactions of ASABE* 54(3): 1151–1158.

Tatzer, P., T. Panner, M. Wolf, and G. Traxler. 2005. Inline sorting with hyperspectral imaging in an industrial environment. In *Proceedings of SPIE* 5671.

Technikon LLC. 2005. Machine vision inspection system development cost study. Technikon report no. 1410-610. http://www.afsinc.org/files/1410-610%20machine%20vision%20inspection%20 public%20.pdf (accessed February 6, 2014).

Teledyne Dalsa Inc. 2014. Line scan imaging basics. Waterloo, Ontario, Canada.

The Meat Site. 2013. Machine vision technology to find defects. http://www.themeatsite.com/articles /1604/machine-vision-technology-to-find-defects (accessed February 6, 2014).

Thomas, A.D.H., M.G. Rodd, J.D. Holt, and C.J. Neill. 1995. Real-time industrial visual inspection: A review. *Real-Time Imaging* 1: 139–158.

Thomas, P., S.C. Saxena, R. Chandra, R. Rao, and C.R. Bhatia. 1993. X-ray imaging for detecting spongy tissue, an internal disorder in fruits of "Alphonso" mango. *Journal of Horticultural Science* 68: 803–806.

Thomas, P., A. Kannan, V.H. Degwekar, and M.S. Ramamurthy. 1995. Non-destructive detection of seed weevil-infested mango fruits by X-ray imaging. *Postharvest Biology and Technology* 5: 161–165.

Thomas, W.L. 2009. Thermal imaging cameras and their component parts. In *Thermal imaging cameras: Characteristics and performance*. Boca Raton, FL: Taylor & Francis.

ThomasNet. 2014. PC-based machine vision versus smart camera systems. http://www.thomasnet.com/articles/automation-electronics/smart-camera-versus-pc-based-machine (accessed February 6, 2014).

Thumm, A., M. Riddell, B. Nanayakkara, J. Harrington, and R. Meder. 2010. Near infrared hyperspectral imaging applied to mapping chemical composition in wood samples. *Journal of Near Infrared Spectroscopy* 18: 507–515.

Tian, Y., and L. Zhang. 2012. Study on the methods of detecting cucumber downy mildew using hyperspectral imaging technology. *Physics Procedia* 33: 743–750.

Tillett and Hague Technology Ltd. 2014. Some commercial applications—Robocrop vision guidance. Silsoe, England, UK.

Timmermans, A.J.M., and A.A. Hulzebosch. 1996. Computer vision system for on-line sorting of pot plants using an artificial neural network classifier. *Computers and Electronics in Agriculture* 15: 41–55.

Tingle, J.M., J.M. Pope, P.A. Baumgartner, and V. Sarafis. 1995. Magnetic resonance imaging of fat and muscle distribution in meat. *International Journal of Food Science and Technology* 30: 437–446.

Titova, T.P., V.G. Nachev, C.I. Damyanov, and P.I. Nikovski. 2013. Intelligent classifiers for nondestructive determination of food quality. *Automatic Control and Robotics* 12(1): 19–30.

Tizhoosh, H.R. 1997. *Fuzzy image processing: Introduction in theory and practice*. Berlin: Springer-Verlag.

Tizhoosh, H.R. 2012. Fuzzy image processing. University of Waterloo, Berkeley. http://tizhoosh.uwaterloo.ca/Fuzzy_Image_Processing/set.htm (accessed October 30, 2013).

Tjeerdsma, B.F., M. Boonstra, A. Pizzi, P. Tekley, and H. Militz. 1998. Characterization of thermal modified wood: Molecular reasons for wood performance improvement. *Holz als Roh- und Werkstoff* 56: 149–153.

Tollner, E.W., R.D. Gitaitis, K.W. Seebold, and B.W. Maw. 2005. Experiences with a food product X-ray inspection system for classifying onions. *Applied Engineering in Agriculture* 21(5): 907–912.

Tomazello, M., S. Brazolin, M.P. Chagas, J.T.S. Oliveira, A.W. Ballarin, and C.A. Benjamin. 2008. Application of X-ray technique in non-destructive evaluation of eucalypt wood. *Maderas. Ciencia y tecnología* 10(2): 139–149.

Tran, C.D. 2003. Infrared multispectral imaging: Principle and instrumentation. *Applied Spectroscopy Reviews* 38(2): 133–153.

Troum, O.M., O. Pimienta, and E. Olech. 2012. Magnetic resonance imaging applications in early rheumatoid arthritis diagnosis and management. *Rheumatic Disease Clinics of North America* 38: 277–297.

Troutman, M.Y., I.V. Mastikhin, B.J. Balcom, T.M. Eads, and G.R. Ziegler. 2001. Moisture migration in soft-panned confections during engrossing and aging as observed by magnetic resonance imaging. *Journal of Food Engineering* 48: 257–267.

TWI Ltd. 2012. Micro-focus X-ray. Cambridge, UK. http://www.twi.co.uk/technologies/ndt/advanced-ndt/micro-focus-x-ray/ (accessed February 18, 2012).

U.S. Food and Drug Administration (FDA). 2012a. Medical X-rays. http://www.fda.gov/Radiation-EmittingProducts/RadiationEmittingProductsandProcedures/MedicalImaging/MedicalX-Rays/default.htm# (accessed January 10, 2013).

U.S. Food and Drug Administration (FDA). 2012b. Radiation emitting products. http://www.fda.gov/Radiation-EmittingProducts/RadiationEmittingProductsandProcedures/MedicalImaging/ucm200086.htm (accessed March 30, 2013).

Unay, D., and B. Gosselin. 2006. Automatic defect segmentation of "Jonagold" apples on multispectral images: A comparative study. *Post-Harvest Biology and Technology* 42: 271–279.

Ureña, R., F. Rodríguez, and M. Berenguel. 2001. A machine vision system for seeds germination quality evaluation using fuzzy logic. *Computers and Electronics in Agriculture* 32: 1–20.

Vadivambal, R., V. Chelladurai, D.S. Jayas, and N.D.G. White. 2010a. Detection of sprout damaged wheat using thermal imaging. *Applied Engineering in Agriculture* 26(6): 999–1004.

Vadivambal, R., V. Chelldurai, D.S. Jayas, and N.D.G. White. 2010b. Determination of sprout damaged barley using thermal imaging. *Agricultural Engineering International CIGR Journal* 13(2): 1–6.

Valous, N.A., F. Mendoza, D. Sun, and P. Allen. 2009. Colour calibration of a laboratory computer vision system for quality evaluation of pre-sliced hams. *Meat Science* 81: 132–141.

Vapnik, V. 1995. *The nature of statistical learning theory.* New York: Springer-Verlag.

Vapnik, V.N. 1998. *Statistical learning theory.* Hoboken, NJ: John Wiley & Sons.

Vardasca, R., and R. Simoes. 2013. Current issues in medical thermography. *Topics in Medical Image Processing and Computational Vision* 8: 223–237.

Varith, J., G.M. Hyde, A.L. Baritelle, J.K. Fellman, and T. Sattabongkot. 2003. Non-contact bruise detection in apples by thermal imaging. *Innovative Food Science and Emerging Technologies* 4(2): 211–218.

Vasighi, M., and M. Kompany-Zareh. 2012. Classification ability of self-organizing maps in comparison with other classification methods. *Communications in Mathematical and Computer Chemistry* 70: 29–44.

Vassileva S., B. Tzvetkova, C. Katranoushkova, and L. Losseva. 2000. Neuro-fuzzy prediction of uricase production. *Bioprocess and Biosystems Engineering* 22(4): 363–367.

Vavrik, D., J. Dammer, J. Jakubek, I. Jeon, J. Jirousek, M. Kroupa, and P. Zlamal. 2011. Advanced X-ray radiography and tomography in several engineering applications. *Nuclear Instruments and Methods in Physics Research* A633: S152–S155.

Veliyulin, E., A. Borge, T. Singstad, I. Gribbestad, and U. Erikson. 2008. Post-mortem studies of fish using magnetic resonance imaging. In *Modern magnetic resonance*, ed. G.A. Webb, 959–966. The Netherlands: Springer.

Vengrinovich, V., S. Zolotarev, A. Kuntsevich, and G. Tillack. 2001. New technique for 2D and 3D X-ray image restoration of pipes in service given a limited access for observation. In *American Institute of Physics (AIP) Conference Proceedings* 557(1), 756–763. http://dx.doi.org/10.1063/1.1373833.

Verboven, P., A. Nemeth, M.K. Abera, E. Bongaers, D. Daelemans, P. Estrade, E. Herremans, M. Hertog, W. Saeys, E. Vanstreels, B. Verlinden, M. Leitner, and B. Nicolaï. 2013. Optical coherence tomography visualizes microstructure of apple peel. *Postharvest Biology and Technology* 78: 123–132.

Veraverbeke, E.A., P. Verboven, J. Lammertyn, P. Cronje, J. De Baerdemaeker and B.M. Nicolai. 2006. Thermographic surface quality evaluation of apple. *Journal of Food Engineering* 77(1): 162–168.

Vermaak, I., A. Viljoen, and S.W. Lindström. 2013. Hyperspectral imaging in the quality control of herbal medicines—The case of neurotoxic Japanese star anise. *Journal of Pharmaceutical and Biomedical Analysis* 75: 207–213.

Vernon, D. 1991. *Machine vision: Automated visual inspection and robot vision.* London: Prentice-Hall International.

Vestergaard, C., J. Risum, and J. Adler-Nissen. 2004. Quantification of salt concentrations in cured pork by computed tomography. *Meat Science* 68: 107–113.

Vidal, M., and J.M. Amigo. 2012. Pre-processing of hyperspectral images: Essential steps before image analysis. *Chemometrics and Intelligent Laboratory Systems* 17: 138–148.

Villiers, J., and E. Barnard. 1992. Back propagation neural nets with one and two hidden layers. *IEEE Transactions on Neural Networks* 4(1): 136–141.

Visen, N.S., J. Paliwal, D.S. Jayas, and N.D.J. White. 2004a. Image analysis of bulk grain samples using neural networks. *Canadian Biosystems Engineering* 46: 7.11–7.15.

Visen, N.S., D.S. Jayas, J. Paliwal, and N.D.G. White. 2004b. Comparison of two neural network architectures for classification of singulated cereal grains. *Canadian Biosystems Engineering* 46: 3.7–3.14.

Vision Doctor. 2009a. Line scan camera basics. http://www.vision-doctor.co.uk/line-scan-cameras.html (accessed August 10, 2012).

Vision Doctor. 2009b. Illumination techniques for line scan cameras. http://www.vision-doctor.co.uk/illumination-techniques/illumination-line-scan-camera.html (accessed August 12, 2013).

Vision Systems Design. 2007. Machine vision checks bottle cap seals. 12(12). http://www.vision-systems.com/articles/print/volume-12/issue-12/technology-trends/quality-control/machine-vision-checks-bottle-cap-seals.html (accessed February 6, 2014).

Vision Systems Design. 2008. Automated meat processing. 13(5). http://www.vision-systems.com/articles/print/volume-13/issue-5/features/industrial-automation-products/automated-meat-processing.html (accessed February 6, 2014).

Vision Systems Design. 2012. Food inspection: Automated system inspects dates at high speed. December 5, 17(6). http://www.vision-systems.com/articles/print/volume-17/issue-6/depart ments/technology-trends/food-inspection-automated-system-inspects-dates-at-high-speed .html (accessed February 6, 2014).

Vision Systems Design. 2013. Imaging system automates food sorting. 18(11). http://www.vision -systems.com/articles/print/volume-18/issue-11/departments/snapshots/imaging-system -automates-food-sorting.html (accessed February 6, 2014).

V-Viz Ltd. 2014a. Intelligent date inspection system. http://www.v-viz.com/Docs/iDiSDataSheet .pdf (accessed January 27, 2014).

V-Viz Ltd. 2014b. Heinz uses machine vision system to identify weakest link. http://www.v-viz .com/Docs/V-VizHeinzChainLink.pdf (accessed February 8, 2014).

Wagner, M.J., M. Loubat, A. Sommier, D. LeRay, G. Collewet, B. Broyart, H. Quintard, A. Davenel, G. Trystram, and T. Lucas. 2008. MRI study of bread baking: Experimental device and MRI signal analysis. *International Journal of Food Science & Technology* 43(6): 1129–1139.

Wang, G., and H. Yu. 2008. An outlook on X-ray CT research and development. *Medical Physics* 35(3): 1051–1064.

Wang, H., B. Dinwiddie, L. Jiang, P.K. Liaw, C.R. Brooks, and D.L. Klarstrom. 2000. Application of high speed-infrared imaging during mechanical fatigue tests. In *Proceedings of SPIE*, vol. 4020.

Wang, H., Y. Zong, S. Deng, E. Sun, and Y. Wang. 2011. Bearing characters recognition system based on LabVIEW. In *International Conference on Consumer Electronics, Communications and Networks*, 118–122.

Wang, J., and T.J. Blackburn. 2000. X-ray image intensifiers for fluoroscopy. *RadioGraphics* 20(5): 1471–1477.

Wang, J., K. Chang, C. Chen, K. Chien, Y. Tsai, Y. Wu, Y. Teng, and T.T. Shih. 2010. Evaluation of the diagnostic performance of infrared imaging of the breast: A preliminary study. *Biomedical Engineering Online* 9: 3–14.

Wang, N., F.E. Dowell, and N. Zhang. 2003. Determining wheat vitreousness using image processing and a neural network. *Transactions of ASAE* 46(4): 1143–1150.

Wang, S.Y., P.C. Wang, and M. Faust. 1988. Non-destructive detection of watercore in apple with nuclear magnetic resonance imaging. *Scientia Horticulturae* 25: 227–334.

Wang, S., W. Albabish, S. Nie, and M.F. Marcone. 2011. Comparison of NMR/MRI technique with other analytical methodologies in the field of food science and technology. International Union of Food Science and Technology and Institute of Food Technologist. http://worldfoodscience .com/cms/index.html@pid=1006201.html (accessed November 6, 2012).

Wang, Y.N., H.J. Liu, and F. Duan. 2005. A bottle finish inspect method based on fuzzy support vector machines and wavelet transform. In *International Conference on Machine Learning and Cybernetics* 8: 4588–4592.

Ward Systems Group, Inc. 1998. Frederick, Maryland.

Warmann, C., and V. Märgner. 2005. Quality control of hazel nuts using thermographic image processing. IAPR Conference on Machine Vision Applications, Tsukuba Science City, Japan, May 16–18.

Warriss, P.D., S.J. Pope, S.N. Brown, L.J. Wilkins, and T.G. Knowles. 2013. Estimating the body temperature of groups of pigs by thermal imaging. *Veterinary Records* 158: 331–334.

Washer, G., N. Bolleni, and R. Fenwick. 2010. Thermographic imaging of subsurface deterioration in concrete bridges. *Journal of Transportation Research Board* 2201: 27–33.

Weglarz, W.P., M. Hemelaar, K. van der Linden, N. Franciosi, G. van Dalen, C. Windt, H. Blonk, J. van Duynhoven, H. Van As. 2008. Real-time mapping of moisture migration in cereal based food systems with Aw contrast by means of MRI. *Food Chemistry* 106: 1366–1374.

Werbos, P.J. 1974. Beyond regression: New tools for prediction and analysis in the behavioral sciences. PhD dissertation, Harvard University, Cambridge, Massachusetts.

Werz, K., H. Braun, P. Martirosian, and F. Schick. 2010. Non-destructive characterization of the pulp of different kinds of apples and pears by magnetic resonance imaging. *Erwerbs-Obstbau* 52: 11–16.

Wielpütz, M., and H. Kauczor. 2012. MRI of the lung: State of the art. *Diagnostic and Intervention Radiology* 18: 344–353.

Wielpütz, M.O., M. Eichinger, and M. Puderbach. 2013. Magnetic Resonance Imaging of cystic fibrosis lung disease. *Journal of Thoracic Imaging* 28(3): 151–159.

Wiesauer, K., M. Pircher, E. Götzinger, S. Bauer, R. Engelke, G. Ahrens, G. Grützner, C.K. Hitzenberger, and D. Stifter. 2005. En-face scanning optical coherence tomography with ultra-high resolution for material investigation. *Optics Express* 13(3): 1015–1024.

Wiesauer, K., M. Pircher, E. Götzinger, C.K. Hitzenberger, R. Oster, and D. Stifter, 2007. Investigation of glass-fibre reinforced polymers by polarisation-sensitive, ultra high resolution optical coherence tomography: Internal structures, defects and stress. *Composition Science and Technology* 67: 3051–3058.

Wikibooks. 2012. Basic physics of nuclear medicine/MRI. http://en.wikibooks.org/wiki/Basic_Physics_of_Nuclear_Medicine/MRI_%26_Nuclear_Medicine (accessed October 7, 2013).

Wikibooks. 2013. Basic physics of nuclear medicine/X-ray CT in nuclear medicine. http://en.wikibooks.org/wiki/Basic_Physics_of_Nuclear_Medicine/X-Ray_CT_in_Nuclear_Medicine (accessed March 18, 2014).

Wildenschild, D., J.W. Hopmans, C.M.P. Vaz, M.L. Rivers, D. Rikard, and B.S.B. Christensen. 2002. Using X-ray computed tomography in hydrology: Systems, resolutions, and limitations. *Journal of Hydrology* 267: 285–297.

Williams, P., P. Geladi, G. Fox, and M. Manley. 2009. Maize kernel hardness classification by near infrared (NIR) hyperspectral imaging and multivariate data analysis. *Analytica Chimica Acta* 653: 121–130.

Wilson, A. 2001. Machine imaging system manages harvester. *Vision Systems Design* 6(2). http://www.vision-systems.com/articles/print/volume-6/issue-2/features/spotlight/machine-imaging-system-manages-harvester.html (accessed December 16, 2013).

Wilson, A. 2012. Vision software blends into food processing. *Vision Systems Design*, June 1, 17(6). http://www.vision-systems.com/articles/print/volume-17/issue-6/features/vision-software-blends-into-food-processing.html (accessed December 16, 2013).

Wilson, A. 2013. Machine vision: A look into the future. *Vision Systems Design*, December 5, 18(11). http://www.vision-systems.com/articles/print/volume-18/issue-11/features/machine-vision-a-look-into-the-future.html (accessed February 8, 2014).

Wilson, D. 2012. Vision systems help sort carrots. *Vision Systems Design*, February 8. http://www.vision-systems.com/articles/2012/02/vision-system-helps-sort-carrots.html (accessed January 27, 2014).

Wolberg, G. 1988. Geometric transformation techniques for digital images: A survey. Technical report CUCS-390-88. Department of Computer Science, Columbia University, New York.

Wölfel, M., and H.K. Ekenel. 2005. Feature weighted Mahalanobis distance: Improved robustness for Gaussian classifiers. 13th European Signal Processing Conference, EUSIPCO, Antalya, Turkey, September 4–8.

Woolford, T. 2011a. The future of X-ray inspection systems in the food industry. Manufacturing.Net, August 5. http://www.manufacturing.net/articles/2011/08/the-future-of-x-ray-inspection-systems-in-the-food-industry (accessed November 2, 2012).

Woolford, T. 2011b. The evolution of X-ray inspection system. http://www.foodprocessing.com.au/articles/49672-The-evolution-of-X-ray-inspection-systems?topic_id=1452 (accessed December 20, 2012).

Worldwatch Institute. 2011. Global meat production and consumption continue to rise. Washington, D.C, October 11. http://www.worldwatch.org/global-meat-production-and-consumption-continue-rise-1 (accessed November 4, 2012).

Worldwatch Institute. 2012. Global rain production at record high despite extreme climatic events. September 25. http://www.worldwatch.org/global-grain-production-record-high-despite-extreme-climatic-events-0 and http://www.worldwatch.org/node/5539 (accessed November 4, 2012).

Wozniacka, G., and T. Chea. 2013. Robots are designed to harvest delicate crops, replace workers. *The Commercial Appeal.* http://www.commercialappeal.com/news/2013/jul/16/robots-are-designed-to-harvest-delicate-crops/?print=1 (accessed December 16, 2013).

Wu, D., and D. Sun. 2013a. Colour measurements by computer vision for food quality control—A review. *Trends in Food Science and Technology* 29: 5–20.

Wu, D., and D. Sun. 2013b. Potential of time series hyperspectral imaging (TS-HIS) for non-invasive determination of microbial spoilage of salmon fish. *Talanta* 111: 39–46.

Wu, D., H. He, and D. Sun. 2012a. Non-destructive texture analysis of farmed Salmon using hyperspectral imaging technique. 7th International CIGR Technical Symposium, Stellenbosch, Africa.

Wu, Q., D. Zhu, C. Wang, Z. Ma, and J. Wang. 2012b. Recognition of wheat pre-harvest sprouting based on hyperspectral imaging. *Optical Engineering* 51(11): 1–7.

Wu, Q., X. Lou, Z. Zeng, and T. He. 2010. Defects inspecting system for tapered roller bearings based on machine vision. In *International Conference on Electrical and Control Engineering*, 667–670.

Xiao-bo, Z., Z. Jie-wen, L. Yanxiao, and M. Holmes. 2010. In-line detection of apple defects using three color cameras system. *Computers and Electronics in Agriculture* 70: 129–134.

Xing, J., S. Symons, M. Shahin, and D. Hatcher. 2010. Detection of sprout damage in Canada Western Red Spring wheat with multiple wavebands using visible/near-infrared hyperspectral imaging. *Biosystems Engineering* 106: 188–194.

Xradia. 2010. X-ray detectors. http://www.xradia.com/technology/basic-technology/detectors .php (accessed December 20, 2012).

Xu, D., A.S. Kurani, J.D. Furst, and D.S. Raicu. 2004. Run-length encoding for volumetric texture. In *Fourth IASTED International Conference on Visualization, Imaging and Image Processing (VIIP)*, 452–458.

Xu, H., S.F. Othman, and R.L. Magin. 2008. Monitoring tissue engineering using magnetic resonance imaging. *Journal of Bioscience and Bioengineering* 106(6): 515–527.

Yacob, Y., H. Ahmad, P. Saad, R.A.A. Raof, and S. Ismail. 2005. A comparison between X-ray and MRI in postharvest non-destructive detection method. Proceedings of the 3rd International Conference on Information Technology and Multimedia (ICIMU), Universiti Tenaga Nasional Selangor, Malaysia, November 22–24.

Yacob, Y.M., H. Ahmad, P. Saad, R.A.A. Raof, and S. Ismail. 2005. A comparison between X-ray and MRI in postharvest non-destructive detection method. Proceedings of International Conference on Information Technology and Multimedia at UNITEN (ICIMU'05), Malaysia. 22–24 Nov, 2005.

Yaffe, M.J., and J.A. Rowlands. 1997. X-ray detectors for digital radiography. *Physics in Medicine and Biology* 42: 1–39.

Yam, K.L., and S.E. Papadakis. 2004. A simple digital imaging method for measuring and analyzing color of food surfaces. *Journal of Food Engineering* 61: 137–142.

Yan, Z., M.J. McCarthy, L. Klemann, M.S. Otterburn, and J. Finley. 1996. NMR applications in complex food systems. *Magnetic Resonance Imaging* 14(7/8): 979–981.

Yang, F., L. Yang, Q. Yang, and L. Kang. 2009. Nondestructive detection of internal quality of apple using X-ray and machine vision. *IFIP Advances in Information and Communication Technology*. 295: 1699–1706.

Yang, C.C., S.O. Prasher, J.A. Landry, H.S. Ramaswamy, and A. Ditommaso. 2000a. Application of artificial neural networks in image recognition and classification of crop and weeds. *Canadian Agricultural Engineering* 42(3): 147–152.

Yang, C.C., S.O. Prasher, J.A. Landry, J. Perret, and H.S. Ramaswamy. 2000b. Recognition of weeds with image processing and their use with fuzzy logic for precision farming. *Canadian Agricultural Engineering* 42(4): 195–200.

Yang, C., S.O. Prasher, J. Landry, and H.S. Ramaswamy. 2003a. Development of an image processing system and fuzzy algorithm for site specific herbicide applications. *Precision Agriculture* 4: 5–18.

Yang, C., J.H. Everitt, M.R. Davis, and C. Mao. 2003b. A CCD camera based hyperspectral imaging system for stationary and airborne applications. *Geocarto International* 18(2): 71–80.

Yang, C., W. Jun, M.S. Kim, K. Chao, S. Kang, D.E. Chan, and A. Lefcourt. 2010. Classification of fecal contamination on leafy greens by hyperspectral imaging. In *Proceedings of SPIE*, vol. 7676.

Yang, E., M. Yang, L. Liao, and W. Wu. 2006. Non-destructive quarantine technique-potential application of using X-ray images to detect early infestations caused by Oriental Fruit Fly (*Bactrocera dorsalis*) in fruit. *Formosan Entomology* 26: 171–186.

Yang, Q. 1993. Classification of apple surface features using machine vision and neural networks. *Computers and Electronics in Agriculture* 9: 1–12.

Yazdi, L., A.S. Prabuwono, and E. Golkar. 2011. Feature extraction algorithm for fill level and cap inspection in bottling machine. In *International Conference on Pattern Analysis and Intelligent Robotics (ICPAIR)*, 47–52.

Ye, X., R.R. Ruan, C.K. Mok, L. Chen, F. Yu, P.L. Chen, C.J. Doona, and T.C.S. Yang. 2004. Monitoring yogurt fermentation process using magnetic resonance imaging and relaxometry. IFT Annual Meeting, Las Vegas, Nevada, July 12–16.

Yi, S., R.M. Haralick, and L.G. Shapiro. 1995. Optimal sensor and light source positioning for machine vision. *Computer vision and Image Understanding* 61(1): 122–137.

Yin, P. 2002. Maximum entropy-based optimal threshold selection using deterministic reinforcement learning with controlled randomization. *Signal Processing* 82: 993–1006.

York, T. 2011. Fundamentals of image sensor performance. http://www.cse.wustl.edu/~jain/cse567 -11/ftp/imgsens.pdf.

Yoshida, S., H. Masuda, C. Ishii, H. Tanaka, Y. Fujii, S. Kawakami, and K. Kihara. 2011. Usefulness of diffusion-weighted MRI in diagnosis of upper urinary tract cancer. *American Journal of Roentgenology* 196: 110–116.

Zagaynova, E. V., O.S. Streltsova, N.D. Gladkova, L.B. Snopova, G.V. Gelikonov, F.I. Feldchtein, and A.N. Morozov. 2001. In vivo optical coherence tomography feasibility for bladder disease. *Journal of Urology* 167: 1492–1496.

Zhang, D., and G. Lu. 2002. A comparative study of Fourier descriptors for shape representation and retrieval. In *5th Asian Conference on Computer Vision*, 202.

Zhang, D., and G. Lu. 2004. Review of shape representation and description techniques. *Pattern Recognition* 37: 1–19.

Zhang, J., Z. Chen, and G. Isenberg. 2009. Gastrointestinal optical coherence tomography: Clinical applications, limitations, and research priorities. *Gastrointestinal Endoscopy Clinics of North America* 19(2): 243–259.

Zhang, J.L., H. Rusinek, H. Chandarana, and V.S. Lee. 2013. Functional MRI of the kidneys. *Journal of Magnetic Resonance Imaging* 37: 282–293.

Zhang, L., and M.J. McCarthy. 2012a. Measurement and evaluation of tomato maturity using magnetic resonance imaging. *Postharvest Biology and Technology* 67: 37–43.

Zhang, L., and M.J. McCarthy. 2012b. Black heart characterization and detection in pomegranate using NMR relaxometry and MR imaging. *Postharvest Biology and Technology* 67: 37–43.

Zhang, L., Y. Jin, L. Lin, J. Li, and Y. Du. 2008. The comparison of CCD and CMOS sensors. Proceedings of SPIE, vol. 7157, International Conference on Optical Instruments and Technology: Advanced Sensor Technologies and Applications, November 18, Beijing, China.

Zhang, S., T. Takahashi, and H. Fukuchi. 1997. Apple detection using infrared thermal imaging. Part 1: Thermal distribution on apple tree and acquisition of apple binary image. *Journal of the Japanese Society of Agricultural Machinery* 59: 57–64.

Zhang, S., T. Takahashi, and H. Fukuchi. 1998. Apple detection using infrared thermal imaging. Part 3. Real time temperature measurement of apple tree. *Journal of the Japanese Society of Agricultural Machinery* 60: 89–95.

Zhao, J., J. Tow, and J. Katupitiya. 2005. On-tree fruit recognition using texture properties and color data. IEEE International Conference on Intelligent Robots and Systems, August 2–6, Alberta, Canada.

Zheng, C., and D. Sun. 2008. Image segmentation techniques. In *Computer vision technology for food quality evaluation*, ed. D. Sun, 37–56. Burlington, MA: Academic Press.

Zheng, C., D. Sun, and C. Du. 2006. Estimating shrinkage of large cooked joints during air-blast cooling by computer vision. *Journal of Food Engineering* 72: 56–62.

Zhong, S., Y. Shen, I. Ho, R.K. May, J.A. Zeitler, M. Evans, P.F. Taday, M. Pepper, T. Rades, K.C. Gordon, R. Müller, and P. Kleinebudde. 2011. Non-destructive quantification of pharmaceutical tablet coatings using terahertz pulsed imaging and optical coherence tomography. *Optics and Lasers in Engineering* 49: 361–365.

Zhou, L., V. Chalana, and Y. Kim. 1998. PC-based machine vision for real-time computer-aided potato inspection. *International Journal of Imaging Systems and Technology* 9: 423–433.

Zhou, T., A.D. Harrison, R. McKellar, J.C. Young, J. Odumeru, P. Piyasena, X. Lu, D.G. Mercer, and S. Karr. 2004. Determination of acceptability and shelf life of ready-to-use lettuce by digital image analysis. *Food Research International* 37: 875–881.

Zhu, H. 2009. New algorithm of liquid level of infusion bottle based on image processing. Proceedings of International Conference on Information Engineering and Computer Science, December 19–20, Wuhan, China.

Zink, F.E. 1997. X-ray tubes. *RadioGraphics* 17: 1259–1268.

Zion, B., P. Chen, and M.J. McCarthy. 1995. Detection of bruises in magnetic resonance images of apples. *Computers and Electronics in Agriculture* 13: 289–299.

Zschech, E., W. Yun, and G. Schneider. 2008. High-resolution X-ray imaging—A powerful non-destructive technique for applications in semiconductor industry. *Applied Physics:* A92: 423–429.

Zsom, T., W.B. Herppich, Cs. Balla, A. Fekete, J. Felföldi, and M. Linke. 2005. Study of water transpiration features of sweet pepper using a thermal imaging system and non-destructive quality monitoring during post-harvest storage. *Journal of Thermal Analysis and Calorimetry* 82: 239–243.

Zuech, N. 2000a. Evaluating machine vision applications. In *Understanding and applying machine vision*, 2nd ed., 303–308. New York: Marcel Dekker Inc.

Zuech, N. 2000b. Cost justification strategies for machine vision. Automated Imaging Association (AIA) Vision Online. http://www.visiononline.org/vision-resources-details.cfm/vision-resources /Cost-Justification-Strategies-for-Machine-Vision/content_id/1330 (accessed February 6, 2014).

Zuech, N. 2007. Current machine vision activities in the food industry. Automated Imaging Association (AIA) Vision Online. http://www.visiononline.org/vision-resources-details.cfm /vision-resources/Current-Machine-Vision-Activities-in-the-Food-Industry/content_id/1157 (accessed December 16, 2013).

Zuech, N., and R.K. Miller. 1989. Machine vision—A data acquisition system. In *Machine vision*, 1–18. New York: Van Nostrand Reinhold.

Zuzak, K.J., M.D. Schaeberle, M.T. Gladwin, R.O. Cannon, and I.W. Levin. 2001. Noninvasive determination of spatially resolved and time-resolved tissue perfusion in humans during nitric oxide inhibition and inhalation by use of a visible-reflectance hyperspectral imaging technique. *Circulation* 104: 2905–2910.

Index

Page numbers followed by f and t indicate figures and tables, respectively.

Printed and bound by CPI Group (UK) Ltd, Croydon, CR0 4YY

22/10/2024

01777614-0011